60 HIKES WITHIN 60 MILES

2ND Edition

HARRISBURG

Including Cumberland, Dauphin, Lancaster, Lebanon, Perry, and York Counties in Central Pennsylvania

Matt Willen

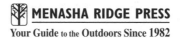

MENASHA RIDGE PRESS
Your Guide to the Outdoors Since 1982

60 Hikes Within 60 Miles: Harrisburg

Copyright © 2016 by Matt Willen
All rights reserved
Printed in the United States of America
Published by Menasha Ridge Press
Distributed by Publishers Group West
Second edition, fourth printing 2024

Project editor: Ritchey Halphen
Cover design: Scott McGrew
Text design: Annie Long; typesetting and layout: Leslie Shaw
Cartography: Scott McGrew, Tony Hertzel, and Matt Willen
Cover and interior photographs © Matt Willen, except where noted
Copyeditor: Susan Roberts McWilliams
Proofreaders: Laura Franck, Rebecca Henderson, Vanessa Lynn Rusch
Indexer: Ann Weik Cassar / Cassar Technical Services

Library of Congress Cataloging-in-Publication Data

Names: Willen, Matthew, author.
Title: 60 hikes within 60 miles, Harrisburg : including Cumberland, Dauphin, Lebanon,
    Lancaster, Perry, and York Counties / Matt Willen.
Other titles: Sixty hikes within sixty miles, Harrisburg
Description: Second Edition. | Birmingham : Menasha Ridge Press, [2016] | "Distributed by
    Publishers Group West"—T.p. verso. | Includes index.
Identifiers: LCCN 2016007370 | ISBN 978-1-63404-014-3 | ISBN 978-1-63404-015-0 (e-book)
Subjects: LCSH: Hiking—Pennsylvania—Harrisburg Region—Guidebooks. | Trails—
    Harrisburg Region—Guidebooks. | Harrisburg Region (Pa.)—Guidebooks.
Classification: LCC GV199.42.P42 W55 2016 | DDC 796.5109748/1—dc23
LC record available at lccn.loc.gov/2016007370

 MENASHA RIDGE PRESS

An imprint of AdventureKEEN
2204 First Ave. S., Suite 102
Birmingham, AL 35233
800-678-7006, fax 888-374-9016

Visit menasharidge.com for a complete listing of our books and for ordering information. Contact us at our website, at facebook.com/menasharidge, or at twitter.com/menasharidge with questions or comments. To find out more about who we are and what we're doing, visit blog.menasharidge.com.

DISCLAIMER This book is meant only as a guide to select trails in and around Harrisburg, Pennsylvania, and does not guarantee hiker safety in any way—you hike at your own risk. Neither Menasha Ridge Press nor Matt Willen is liable for property loss or damage, personal injury, or death that may result from accessing or hiking the trails described in this guide. Be especially cautious when walking in potentially hazardous terrains with, for example, steep inclines or drop-offs. Do not attempt to explore terrain that may be beyond your abilities. Please read carefully the introduction to this book, as well as safety information from other sources. Familiarize yourself with current weather reports and maps of the area you plan to visit (in addition to the maps provided in this guidebook). Be cognizant of park regulations, and always follow them. While every effort has been made to ensure the accuracy of the information in this guidebook, land and road conditions, phone numbers and websites, and other information are subject to change.

FOR JOE NOLD AND HERB KINCEY—
LONGTIME FRIENDS AND INSPIRATIONS

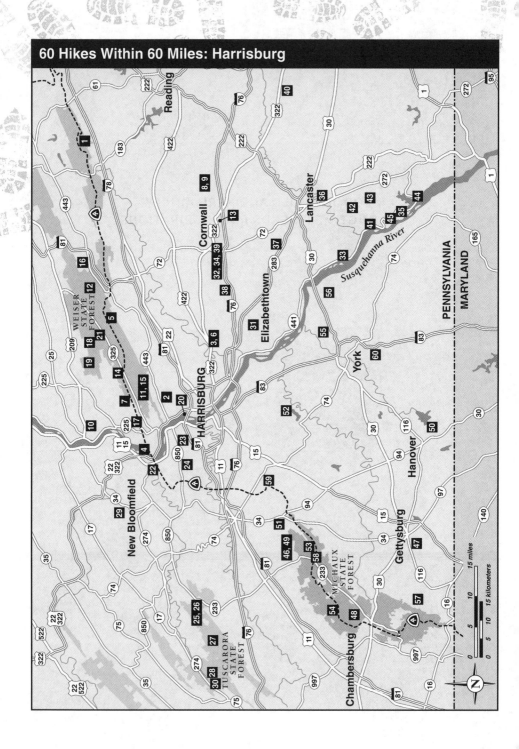

60 Hikes Within 60 Miles: Harrisburg

Table of Contents

Featured trail	Alternate trail	Appalachian Trail
Freeway	Highway with bridge	Minor road
Boardwalk	Unpaved road	
Railroad	Power line	Boundary line
Park/forest	Water body	River/creek/ intermittent stream

🔊 Amphitheater	● General point of interest	♻ Recycling area
🧍 Baseball field	⑦ Information kiosk	🚻 Restrooms
⌐ Bench	🗼 Lookout tower	👁 Scenic view
🚤 Boat launch	Marsh	⊏ Shelter
△ Campground	⊥ Monument	⟍ Sledding hill
🚣 Canoe access	🏠 Park office	⊙ Soccer field
⊺ Cemetery	P Parking area	🏊 Swimming access
⚘ Church	▲ Peak/hill	🎾 Tennis courts
／ Dam	🎏 Picnic area	🚶 Trailhead
∐ Drinking water	📷 Picnic shelter	🗑 Trash receptacle
🔥 Fire pit	🚽 Pit toilets	⌂ Tunnel (pedestrian)
🎣 Fishing access	🛝 Playground	🔭 Viewing platform
✕ Footbridge	📡 Radio tower	♿ Wheelchair access
●— Gate		

Acknowledgments

ANYONE WHO DOES ANY OF THESE HIKES owes a great debt of gratitude to all of the volunteers and employees of the state, county, local, public, and private organizations and foundations who have worked to construct and maintain the numerous trails in this area. Without their efforts, this book and the wonderful experiences I had while writing it would not have been possible.

So many people assisted me in many ways as I wrote this book. I am indebted to their kindness and wisdom. I would like to thank all of the folks who work for the Pennsylvania Bureau of Forestry, the Pennsylvania Department of Conservation and Natural Resources, and the Pennsylvania Game Commission for answering my endless questions with kindness and courtesy, and for pointing me in the right direction (figuratively and literally). In particular, I would like to thank the Susquehanna Appalachian Trail Club for providing me with the opportunity to share what I have learned with their members and for their encouragement. I also owe many thanks to the volunteers for the Lancaster County Conservancy that I ran into along the trails and who provided me with considerable information.

I am indebted to the folks at Menasha Ridge Press/AdventureKEEN for allowing me to write a new edition of this book. Tim Jackson was extremely helpful in working with me on developing a schedule and completing the project. Many thanks also go out to Molly Merkle, Allison Brown, Tanya Sylvan, Scott McGrew, Ritchey Halphen, Susan McWilliams, Laura Franck, Rebecca Henderson, Vanessa Rusch, and Ann Cassar for all of their assistance with various parts of this project. Thank you all for this opportunity.

Finally, this book would have been impossible without the assistance and support of all the friends that I have made over the past year; you all know who you are. And finally, I owe so many thanks to my sons, Jackson and Ian, who joined me, and encouraged me, and laughed with me through all of these hikes. They are my inspiration.

—*Matt Willen*

Foreword

WELCOME TO MENASHA RIDGE PRESS'S *60 Hikes Within 60 Miles,* a series designed to provide hikers with the information they need to find and hike the very best trails surrounding metropolitan areas.

Our strategy is simple: First, find a hiker who knows the area and loves to hike. Second, ask that person to spend a year researching the most popular and very best trails around. And third, have that person describe each trail in terms of difficulty, scenery, condition, elevation change, and other categories of information that are important to hikers. "Pretend you've just completed a hike and met up with other hikers at the trailhead," we told each author. "Imagine their questions, and be clear in your answers."

An experienced hiker and writer, Matt Willen has selected 60 of the best hikes in and around the Harrisburg metropolitan area. From Rocky Knob to the Gold Mine Trail, Matt provides hikers (and walkers) with a great variety of outings—and all within roughly 60 miles of Harrisburg.

You'll get more out of this book if you take a moment to read the Introduction explaining how to read the trail listings. The "Topographic Maps" section will help you understand how useful topos are on a hike, and will also tell you where to get them. And though this is a "where-to," not a "how-to" guide, readers who have not hiked extensively will find the Introduction of particular value.

As much for the opportunity to free the spirit as well as to free the body, let these hikes elevate you above the urban hurry.

All the best,
The Editors at Menasha Ridge Press

About the Author

MATT WILLEN is a writer, explorer, and photographer. He spends much of his time exploring little-known and remote places around the globe, most recently in areas above 50 degrees north latitude and below 50 degrees south. Matt is also the author of *The Best in Tent Camping: Pennsylvania* (Menasha Ridge Press). When he isn't on the road, he can be found messing around with his two sons, Jackson and Ian, or playing music. He lives just outside of Hershey, Pennsylvania.

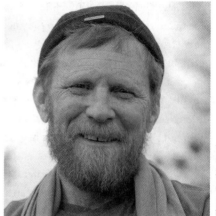

Photo: Cynthia Kasales

Preface

AS WITH THE FIRST EDITION, my objective in selecting hikes was to aim for variety. I wanted to provide hikes of various lengths and difficulties that provided access to different types of terrain and wildlife, and that would be accessible to all sorts of travelers, from seasoned hikers to families to people with special needs. With this edition I also strived to provide a more balanced distribution of hikes in the four principal quadrants of the region around Harrisburg. Admittedly, the distribution is weighted somewhat toward the Valley and Ridge Province region in the northeast; this is primarily because that area offers the greatest number of opportunities for diverse hikes, but it is also my favorite area to hike around here. I have tried to provide hikes that help people get outdoors and into nature. I think going out for walks is the best therapy for and antidote to the crazy lives that we live these days. We are so plagued by information, by multitasking, by cell phones, e-mail, and the like, that we tend to live more like extensions of machines rather than as human beings. People need to put that stuff aside for a while. A good hike can help us to slow down and notice what we have around us. Doing so makes us feel better. It helps keep people sensible and it helps to keep people from getting mean (in every sense of the word).

The area covered in this guidebook is all part of the lower Susquehanna River basin. All streams that you'll pass on these hikes eventually flow to the Susquehanna and then south to the Chesapeake Bay. The region can be divided into four major physiographic provinces, each of which offers a different kind of hiking experience.

If you draw a circle around Harrisburg, with a perimeter extending 60 miles from the center of the city, most of the northern half of that circle is home to the **Valley and Ridge Province,** which extends from the Maryland state line north and east toward Scranton and Wilkes-Barre. Characterized by long, level, rocky ridgetops separated by valleys of fertile farmland, the origins of these mountains date back 200–300 million years, from the major Allegheny mountain-building period. Because the rocks on the ridgetops are so hard, they are quite resistant to erosion. The exceptions to this rule, however, are the numerous water gaps that bisect the ridges at several points. The most prominent of these gaps are those along the Susquehanna River north of Harrisburg, where the river cuts directly through five different ridges as it makes its way south. Other smaller gaps are located throughout the region. The gaps are something of a geological anomaly: Water should theoretically follow the path of least resistance and make its way around a ridge rather than directly through it. Their origins are still contested by geologists, though current thought suggests that changes in the direction of flow of the Susquehanna River caused by periods of uplift of bedrock allowed river currents to capitalize on weaknesses in the upper strata.

The Valley and Ridge Province is home to several major hiking trails that pass through the region. The **Appalachian Trail (AT)** cuts through a long segment of the province, entering from the south just west of Harrisburg and then angling east and passing just north of Harrisburg parallel to Interstate 81. The **Tuscarora Trail** in Perry County is part of a 248-mile trail that extends from the AT in Shenandoah National Park to Pennsylvania. It was constructed as an alternate route to the busy AT corridor. Many people say that it offers more wilderness and solitude than the AT, and I would agree with that assessment. The trail extends 110 miles from the Maryland state line through the Valley and Ridge Province to Deans Gap on Blue Mountain, where it joins the AT west of Harrisburg. You'll also find the **Darlington Trail,** the **Horse-Shoe Trail,** and many side trails in these mountains, making for nearly limitless hiking opportunities. Large tracts of public land can be found in these mountains, administered by the Pennsylvania Bureau of Forestry, the Pennsylvania Department of Conservation and Natural Resources, or the Pennsylvania Game Commission.

The hiking in this region is characteristically rugged and remote. Many trails follow the paths of old haul roads built for moving coal and timber during the 19th century. They tend to be rather rocky, and almost inevitably entail a steep climb from a valley to the top of a ridge. A good pair of sturdy hiking boots is a wise investment for exploring this terrain. The area is home to black bear, white-tailed deer, bobcats, foxes, coyotes, and other woodland mammals. The abundance of birdlife, as throughout the entire region, is remarkable. The forest is typically hardwood and you'll find an enormous diversity of tree and plant life in the area.

To the south of the Valley and Ridge Province runs the **Great Valley Province.** The Great Valley (also referred to as the Cumberland Valley west of the Susquehanna and Lebanon Valley to the east) extends from New Jersey west and south along the east side of the Appalachian Mountains all the way to Georgia. The geology of this province is characterized by large areas of limestone, the origins of which date back to when the region was once underwater millions of years ago.

Much of the development in the central Pennsylvania region has taken place in the Great Valley. Harrisburg, Carlisle, Lancaster, and York are all located in it or on its edge. The area is home to many farms and is traversed by small tributaries of the Susquehanna River. The hikes in the Great Valley tend to be comparatively gentle, often following the paths of old railroad grades converted to rail-trails. The AT cuts directly north through it just east of Carlisle. This region is home to an abundance of birdlife, particularly waterfowl and riparian birds along the rivers and creeks, and owls and hawks around the farm country. You'll also find many animals that prefer open range to the deep woods, including red fox, muskrat, opossum, groundhogs, and shrews, as well as turtles and other reptiles and amphibians near water sources.

Much of the southeastern section of the circle consists of the **Piedmont Province,** where you will find large outcroppings of quartzite, mica, and schist. Perhaps the most distinctive part of this province is the lower Susquehanna River gorge, which begins in the area around Chickies Rock just north of Columbia at US 30. To the south, the river is fed by streams that have their headwaters in the Great Valley. As the streams have made their way to the river over the years they have carved wonderful ravines, glens, and small gorges through weaknesses in the underlying strata. Several of the hikes in Lancaster County explore these hemlock- and rhododendron-filled steep hollows. One of these, **Kellys Run,** in my eyes, is a national treasure. The Piedmont Province provides excellent opportunities for birding, with the Susquehanna River in this area being home to bald eagle, osprey, and many other birds that prefer a riparian environment.

Finally, the fourth and smallest physiographic province is **South Mountain,** which straddles the Pennsylvania–Maryland border south and west of York County. Characterized by rolling hills, many of which are capped with erosion-resistant white quartzite rock outcroppings, the lay of these mountains couldn't be more different from those found in the Valley and Ridge Province. Here, the mountains are much more irregular in shape and look more like one would expect a mountain range to look (some of the views in South Mountain remind me of northern New Mexico or New England). Unlike the hikes in the Valley and Ridge area, where you tend to have one big mile-long hill, the hikes in South Mountain tend to be rolling, with plenty of ups and downs. The region is thick with mountain laurel, the Pennsylvania state flower, and the foliage can be breathtaking in late May or early June.

All of the hikes in this book are on public lands that are administered by several different state and local agencies. Many of the hikes make use of state game lands. Although there are no regulations concerning opening and closing hours for game lands, typically camping is not allowed except by thru-hikers on the AT corridor. Most important, when hiking on game lands, respect the rights of hunters. Exercise extra caution during hunting season and consider hiking on Sundays, when hunting is not allowed. From November 15 through December 15, you must wear at least 250 square inches of blaze orange (a vest and hat are adequate). As the signs say at many of the game-land entrances, HUNTERS WEAR ORANGE, SO SHOULD YOU! Unless it is a hot day in the middle of summer and I am wearing shorts and a T-shirt, I always wear a blaze orange hat, shirt, or sweatshirt when I hike on game lands.

Many of the trails traversed by the hikes described in this book are marked with blazes, painted marks on trees indicating the path of the trail. A single named trail uses a blaze of one color. When you see blazes of multiple colors on a single tree, two or more trails are sharing a common path. Typically, a tree (or sometimes a rock) will be marked with a single blaze indicating that the trail continues basically straight. Double blazes of the same color indicate a change of direction, and you should take care to stay on track. Currently, no consistent system for blaze colors is used throughout this part of the state, with the exception of the three long-distance trails in the area: the Appalachian Trail (white blazes), the Horse-Shoe Trail (yellow blazes), and the Conestoga Trail (red blazes). So some hikes may have orange blazes, some red, some orange that look like red, some blue, pink, lavender, and so forth. (I'm not exaggerating.) Please be aware that the trail markings may change over time (indeed, the trails themselves are often rerouted) and that in spite of how good the guidebook is, travel in the backcountry still requires sound judgment and making decisions.

The area covered by this book is extremely rich in both natural and cultural history. As I worked on this guide, I found the following three books indispensable for helping me to learn about the area:

The Geological Story of Pennsylvania, by John H. Barnes and W. D. Sevon (The Pennsylvania Geological Survey, Harrisburg, PA, 2002)

Susquehanna: River of Dreams, by Susan Q. Stranahan (Johns Hopkins University Press, Baltimore and London, 1993)

Wildlife of Pennsylvania and the Northeast, by Charles Fergus and Amelia Hansen (Stackpole Books, Harrisburg, PA, 2000)

I also relied extensively on many of the nature and wildlife guides available in bookstores for helping me to identify and learn about the flora and fauna of the region.

I have tried to be as accurate as possible in my collection of information and data for this book, and in identifying what I have seen. I'm not a professional naturalist, so I may have misnamed things (the identification of trees beyond simple classifications of oak, maple, pine, spruce, hemlock, and so on continues to escape me). If you notice any errors, omissions, or changes in routes, or you have suggestions for other hikes or comments, please contact me at matt@mattwillen.com.

60 Hikes by Category

Hike Categories

✓ 1–3 Miles	✓ > 6 Miles	✓ Young Children	✓ Bicyclists
✓ 3–6 Miles	✓ Along Creeks	✓ Good Views	

REGION Hike Number/Hike Name	page	1–3 Miles	3–6 Miles	> 6 Miles	Along Creeks	Young Children	Good Views	Bicyclists
NORTHEAST								
1 Appalachian Trail: Sand Spring Loop	18			✓	✓			
2 Boyd Big Tree Preserve Conservation Area	23		✓					
3 Bullfrog Valley Pond to Shank Park	28		✓		✓	✓		✓
4 Clarks Ferry Loop	33		✓				✓	
5 Cold Spring and Rausch Gap Loop	37		✓		✓			
6 Jonathan Eshenour Memorial Trail: Bullfrog Valley Pond to Western Terminus	42	✓				✓		✓
7 Joseph E. Ibberson Conservation Area Loop	47		✓			✓	✓	
8 Middle Creek Wildlife Management Area: Conservation Trail Loop	51	✓					✓	
9 Middle Creek Wildlife Management Area: Middle Creek and Elders Run Loop	55		✓		✓		✓	
10 Ned Smith Center	60		✓					
11 Rattling Run Town Site	64			✓				
12 Rausch Gap via Gold Mine Trail	68			✓	✓			
13 State Game Land 156	73			✓				✓
14 Stony Mountain from the North	78			✓			✓	
15 Stony Mountain from the South	83			✓			✓	
16 Swatara State Park: Rail-Trail/Bear Hole Loop	88			✓	✓			✓
17 Table Rock and Peters Mountain	92	✓					✓	
18 Weiser State Forest: Greenland Road	96		✓					
19 Weiser State Forest: Haldeman Tract	100		✓				✓	
20 Wildwood Lake Loop	104	✓				✓		✓
21 Yellow Springs Loop	109		✓					

REGION Hike Number/Hike Name		page	1–3 Miles	3–6 Miles	> 6 Miles	Along Creeks	Young Children	Good Views	Bicyclists
NORTHWEST									
22	Cove Mountain and Hawk Rock Loop	116		✓				✓	
23	Darlington Trail Loop: East	120		✓					
24	Darlington Trail Loop: West	124		✓					
25	Flat Rock Overlook	128	✓					✓	
26	Flat Rock and Warner Trail Loop	132		✓				✓	
27	Frank E. Masland Jr. Natural Area Trek	137	✓			✓			
28	Hemlocks Natural Area Loop	141	✓			✓	✓		
29	Little Buffalo State Park	145	✓						
30	Tunnel Trail and Iron Horse Trail Loop	150		✓					
SOUTHEAST									
31	Conewago Trail: Elizabethtown to Old Hershey Road	158	✓			✓	✓		✓
32	Clarence Schock Memorial Park	163	✓					✓	
33	Enola Low Grade Trail	168			✓	✓	✓	✓	✓
34	Governor Dick	172	✓					✓	✓
35	Kellys Run and Pinnacle Overlook Loop	176	✓			✓			
36	Lancaster Central Park	181	✓			✓	✓		
37	Lancaster Junction Recreation Trail	186	✓			✓	✓		✓
38	Lebanon Valley Rail-Trail: Lawn to Colebrook	190	✓				✓		✓
39	Lebanon Valley Rail-Trail: Mount Gretna to Cornwall	194		✓			✓		✓
40	Money Rocks County Park	199	✓					✓	
41	Shenks Ferry Wildflower Preserve	203	✓				✓		
42	Silver Mine Park	208		✓					
43	Steinman Run Nature Preserve	213		✓		✓			
44	Susquehannock State Park	217	✓					✓	
45	Tucquan Glen Nature Preserve	221	✓			✓			

REGION Hike Number/Hike Name	page	1–3 Miles	3–6 Miles	> 6 Miles	Along Creeks	Young Children	Good Views	Bicyclists
SOUTHWEST								
46 Buck Ridge Trail	228		✓					
47 Gettysburg National Military Park	232			✓			✓	
48 Hosack Run	237			✓				
49 Kings Gap	241	✓					✓	
50 Mary Ann Furnace Trail	246	✓				✓		
51 Mount Holly Marsh Preserve	250		✓		✓			
52 Pinchot Lake	255			✓				
53 Pole Steeple and Mountain Creek	260		✓		✓		✓	
54 Rocky Knob	264		✓				✓	
55 Rocky Ridge County Park	268		✓					✓
56 Samuel S. Lewis State Park	272	✓				✓	✓	
57 Strawberry Hill Nature Preserve	276		✓					
58 Sunset Rocks	281			✓			✓	
59 White Rocks and Center Point Knob	286		✓				✓	
60 William H. Kain County Park	290			✓				

Hike Categories *(Continued)*

✓ Runners	✓ Wildlife	✓ Near Fishing	✓ Author's Favorites
✓ Bird-Watching	✓ Wildflowers	✓ Cross-Country Skiing	

REGION Hike Number/Hike Name	page	Runners	Bird-Watching	Wildlife	Wildflowers	Near Fishing	Cross-Country Skiing	Author's Favorites
NORTHEAST								
1 Appalachian Trail: Sand Spring Loop	18		✓					
2 Boyd Big Tree Preserve Conservation Area	23		✓					
3 Bullfrog Valley Pond to Shank Park	28	✓				✓	✓	
4 Clarks Ferry Loop	33					✓		
5 Cold Spring and Rausch Gap Loop	37	✓		✓				✓
6 Jonathan Eshenour Memorial Trail: Bullfrog Valley Pond to Western Terminus	42	✓						
7 Joseph E. Ibberson Conservation Area Loop	47	✓			✓			
8 Middle Creek Wildlife Management Area: Conservation Trail Loop	51		✓		✓			
9 Middle Creek Wildlife Management Area: Middle Creek and Elders Run Loop	55			✓				✓
10 Ned Smith Center	60	✓				✓	✓	
11 Rattling Run Town Site	64					✓		
12 Rausch Gap via Gold Mine Trail	68			✓				✓
13 State Game Land 156	73	✓		✓			✓	✓
14 Stony Mountain from the North	78			✓	✓			
15 Stony Mountain from the South	83			✓	✓			
16 Swatara State Park: Rail-Trail/Bear Hole Loop	88	✓	✓			✓	✓	
17 Table Rock and Peters Mountain	92	✓						
18 Weiser State Forest: Greenland Road	96			✓	✓			✓
19 Weiser State Forest: Haldeman Tract	100	✓			✓	✓		✓
20 Wildwood Lake Loop	104	✓	✓		✓			
21 Yellow Springs Loop	109			✓				

REGION Hike Number/Hike Name	page	Runners	Bird-Watching	Wildlife	Wildflowers	Near Fishing	Cross-Country Skiing	Author's Favorites
NORTHWEST								
22 Cove Mountain and Hawk Rock Loop	116							✓
23 Darlington Trail Loop: East	120			✓	✓			
24 Darlington Trail Loop: West	124				✓			
25 Flat Rock Overlook	128			✓				
26 Flat Rock and Warner Trail Loop	132			✓				
27 Frank E. Masland Jr. Natural Area Trek	137		✓	✓		✓		✓
28 Hemlocks Natural Area Loop	141				✓			
29 Little Buffalo State Park	145	✓	✓		✓	✓	✓	
30 Tunnel Trail and Iron Horse Trail Loop	150			✓				
SOUTHEAST								
31 Conewago Trail: Elizabethtown to Old Hershey Road	158	✓			✓		✓	
32 Clarence Schock Memorial Park	163							✓
33 Enola Low Grade Trail	168	✓	✓			✓	✓	
34 Governor Dick	172	✓						
35 Kellys Run and Pinnacle Overlook Loop	176		✓		✓			✓
36 Lancaster Central Park	181	✓			✓	✓	✓	
37 Lancaster Junction Recreation Trail	186	✓	✓				✓	
38 Lebanon Valley Rail-Trail: Lawn to Colebrook	190	✓	✓				✓	
39 Lebanon Valley Rail-Trail: Mount Gretna to Cornwall	194	✓					✓	✓
40 Money Rocks County Park	199			✓				
41 Shenks Ferry Wildflower Preserve	203				✓			
42 Silver Mine Park	208	✓	✓		✓	✓	✓	
43 Steinman Run Nature Preserve	213				✓		✓	✓
44 Susquehannock State Park	217	✓	✓					
45 Tucquan Glen Nature Preserve	221				✓			✓

REGION Hike Number/Hike Name	page	Runners	Bird-Watching	Wildlife	Wildflowers	Near Fishing	Cross-Country Skiing	Author's Favorites
SOUTHWEST								
46 Buck Ridge Trail	228			✓				
47 Gettysburg National Military Park	232		✓		✓		✓	
48 Hosack Run	237			✓	✓			✓
49 Kings Gap	241	✓			✓			
50 Mary Ann Furnace Trail	246	✓				✓		
51 Mount Holly Marsh Preserve	250		✓	✓	✓			✓
52 Pinchot Lake	255					✓		
53 Pole Steeple and Mountain Creek	260		✓	✓				
54 Rocky Knob	264			✓	✓			
55 Rocky Ridge County Park	268	✓	✓				✓	
56 Samuel S. Lewis State Park	272	✓						
57 Strawberry Hill Nature Preserve	276			✓	✓			
58 Sunset Rocks	281			✓				✓
59 White Rocks and Center Point Knob	286			✓				
60 William H. Kain County Park	290	✓	✓			✓		

Introduction

WELCOME TO *60 HIKES WITHIN 60 MILES: HARRISBURG.* If you're new to hiking or even if you're a seasoned trailsmith, take a few minutes to read the following introduction. We explain how this book is organized and how to use it.

How to Use This Guidebook

OVERVIEW MAP, MAP KEY, AND MAP LEGEND

The overview map on the inside front cover shows the primary trailheads for all 60 hikes. The numbers on the overview map pair with the key on the facing page. A legend explaining the map symbols used throughout the book appears on the inside back cover.

REGIONAL MAPS

The book is divided into regions, and prefacing each regional section is an overview map. The regional maps provide more detail than the overview map, bringing you closer to the hikes.

TRAIL MAPS

Each hike contains a detailed map that shows the trailhead, the route, significant features, facilities, and topographic landmarks such as creeks, overlooks, and peaks. I gathered map data by carrying a GPS unit while hiking. This data was downloaded into a digital-mapping program, Garmin BaseCamp, and processed by expert cartographers to produce the highly accurate maps found in this book. Each trailhead's GPS coordinates are included with each profile (see next page).

ELEVATION PROFILES

Most hikes contain a detailed elevation profile that corresponds directly to the trail map. This graphical element provides a quick look at the trail from the side, enabling you to visualize how the trail rises and falls. On the diagram's vertical axis, or height scale, the number of feet indicated between each tick mark lets you visualize the climb. To keep flat hikes from looking steep and vice versa, varying height scales provide an accurate image of each hike's climbing challenge. Elevation profiles for loop hikes show total distance; those for out-and-back hikes show only one-way distance. Note that hikes with an elevation gain/loss of fewer than 100 feet do not include an elevation profile.

GPS TRAILHEAD COORDINATES

As noted in "Trail Maps," on the previous page, I used a handheld GPS unit to obtain geographic data and sent the information to the cartographers at Menasha Ridge. Provided for each hike profile, the GPS coordinates—the intersection of latitude (north) and longitude (west)—will orient you from the trailhead. In some cases, you can park within viewing distance of a trailhead; other hikes require a short walk to the trailhead from a parking area.

The latitude–longitude grid system is likely quite familiar to you, but here's a refresher, pertinent to visualizing the coordinates:

Imaginary lines of latitude—called *parallels* and approximately 69 miles apart from each other—run horizontally around the globe. The equator is established to be 0°, and each parallel is indicated by degrees from the equator: up to 90°N at the North Pole, and down to 90°S at the South Pole.

Imaginary lines of longitude—called *meridians*—run perpendicular to lines of latitude and are likewise indicated by degrees. Starting from 0° at the Prime Meridian in Greenwich, England, they continue to the east and west until they meet 180° later at the International Date Line in the Pacific Ocean. At the equator, longitude lines also are approximately 69 miles apart, but that distance narrows as the meridians converge toward the North and South Poles.

In this book, latitude and longitude are expressed in degree–decimal minute format. For example, the coordinates for Hike 1, Appalachian Trail: Sand Spring Loop (page 18), are as follows:

N40° 32.270' W76° 07.403'

To convert GPS coordinates given in degrees, minutes, and seconds to degrees and decimal minutes, divide the seconds by 60. For more on GPS technology, visit usgs.gov.

Hike Descriptions

Each hike contains seven key items: an In Brief description of the trail, a key-information box, directions to the trail, GPS trailhead coordinates, a trail map, an elevation profile, and a trail description. Many hike profiles also include notes on nearby activities.

IN BRIEF

A "taste of the trail." Think of this section as a snapshot focused on the historical landmarks, beautiful vistas, and other sights you may encounter on the hike.

KEY INFORMATION

The information in this box gives you a quick idea of the statistics and specifics of each hike.

LENGTH How long the trail is from start to finish. There may be options to shorten or extend the hikes, but the mileage corresponds to the described hike. Consult the Description to help decide how to customize the hike for your ability or time constraints.

CONFIGURATION Defines the type of route—for example, an out-and-back (which takes you in and out the same way), a point-to-point (or one-way route), a figure-eight, or a balloon-and-string (a loop with an entrance or exit trail).

DIFFICULTY The degree of effort that a typical hiker should expect on a given route. For simplicity, the trails are rated as *easy, moderate,* or *strenuous.*

SCENERY A short summary of the attractions offered by the hike and what to expect in terms of plant life, wildlife, natural wonders, and historic features.

EXPOSURE A quick check of how much sun you can expect on your shoulders during the hike.

TRAIL TRAFFIC Indicates how busy the trail might be on an average day. Trail traffic, of course, varies from day to day and season to season. Weekend days typically see the most visitors. Other trail users that may be encountered on the trail are also noted here.

TRAIL SURFACE Indicates whether the trail surface is paved, rocky, gravel, dirt, boardwalk, or a mixture of elements.

HIKING TIME How long it takes to hike the trail. A slow but steady hiker will average 2–3 miles an hour, depending on the terrain.

DRIVING DISTANCE Listed in miles.

ACCESS A notation of any fees or permits necessary to hike or park at the trailhead.

MAPS Here, you'll find a list of maps that show the topography of the trail, including Appalachian Trail maps, state forest maps, and USGS topographic maps.

FACILITIES What to expect in terms of restrooms and water at the trailhead or nearby.

WHEELCHAIR TRAVERSABLE Indicates whether all or part of the hike can be enjoyed by persons with disabilities.

CONTACT Listed here are phone numbers and/or websites for checking trail conditions and gleaning other basic information.

SPECIAL COMMENTS Any extra details that don't fit into the categories above.

DIRECTIONS

Used in conjunction with the overview map, the driving directions will help you locate each trailhead. Once at the trailhead, park only in designated areas.

GPS TRAILHEAD COORDINATES

These can be used in addition to the driving directions if you enter the coordinates into your GPS unit before you set out. See previous page for more information.

DESCRIPTION

The heart of each hike. Here, the authors provide a summary of the trail's essence and highlight any special traits the hike has to offer. The route is clearly outlined, including landmarks, side trips, and possible alternate routes along the way. Ultimately, the hike description will help you choose which hikes are best for you.

NEARBY ACTIVITIES

Look here for information on things to do or points of interest: nearby parks, museums, restaurants, and the like. Note that not every hike has a listing.

Weather

With the exception of rather short-lived extremes in weather, hiking can be done year-round in south-central Pennsylvania. Each season brings its own distinctive and pleasant features, all of which are worth exploring. My favorite time of year for getting out is the fall, which tends to offer many clear and crisp days, and, for a couple of weeks, the colorful foliage. If you spend enough time trekking around, you'll notice that fall brings other events, such as the seasonal hawk migrations, the shortening of the days, and a lot of hustle and bustle around the forest as the animals prepare for winter. The fall is also accompanied by the constant crunching of leaves beneath your feet, making it very difficult to be silent as you walk. Fall can also bring wet, cold rain—perfect conditions for hypothermia—so be prepared for sudden weather changes when you go out.

Winter brings the short days, rather stark lighting as the leaves have fallen from the trees, and occasional snowfalls. A snowpack of a couple of feet is not uncommon in the higher elevations, but most years it tends to be rather short-lived. This is an especially good time of year for seeing fox, and for watching birds because it is more difficult for them to hide with the absence of foliage. Some of my nicest days out have been during the winter, though you do want to be prepared for sudden changes in weather and dips in temperature. At this time of year, you want to take special care around stream crossings, which are often icy, as a slip could have very unpleasant consequences.

Spring in south-central Pennsylvania can be a little muddy and wet, but this part of the state is home to many species of surprising and beautiful wildflowers. Wildlife becomes more active as birds and animals begin raising young, and the seasonal migrations can be extraordinary (I recommend a trip to the Middle Creek Wildlife Management Area to view the migration of snow geese). Again, be prepared for sudden changes in weather, particularly in March and April when cold rains are not atypical. This is also the time of year when streams run high, making some hikes impassable or more hazardous.

AVERAGE TEMPERATURE BY MONTH: HARRISBURG					
	JAN	**FEB**	**MAR**	**APR**	**MAY**	**JUN**
HIGH	38	41	51	63	73	81
LOW	23	25	33	42	51	61
	JUL	**AUG**	**SEP**	**OCT**	**NOV**	**DEC**
HIGH	86	84	76	64	53	42
LOW	66	64	57	45	36	28

Finally, summers are characteristically warm and can be rather humid, especially getting into August. This is a great time of year to hike along the high ridges north of Harrisburg, but take care to hike early to avoid afternoon thunderstorms and the heat of midday. Be sure to carry plenty of water with you as the humidity can deplete your strength very quickly.

Water

How much is enough? Well, one simple physiological fact should persuade you to err on the side of excess when deciding how much water to pack: A hiker working hard in 90-degree heat needs approximately 10 quarts of fluid per day. That's 2.5 gallons—12 large water bottles or 16 small ones. In other words, pack along one or two bottles even for short hikes.

Some hikers and backpackers hit the trail prepared to purify water found along the route. This method, while less dangerous than drinking it untreated, comes with risks. Purifiers with ceramic filters are the safest. Many hikers pack along the slightly distasteful tetraglycine–hydroperiodide tablets to debug water (sold under the names Potable Aqua, Coughlan's, and others). I have had some experience recently with ultraviolet-light wands. They are effective and lightweight, although they won't clear murky water like a filter will. You will also need to carry extra batteries for use with them.

Probably the most common waterborne "bug" that hikers face is giardia, which may not hit until one to four weeks after ingestion. It will have you living in the bathroom, passing noxious rotten-egg gas, vomiting, and shivering with chills. Other parasites to worry about include E. coli and cryptosporidium, both of which are harder to kill than giardia.

For most people, the pleasures of hiking make carrying water a relatively minor price to pay to remain healthy. If you're tempted to drink "found water," do so only if you understand the risks involved. Better yet, hydrate prior to your hike, carry (and drink) 6 ounces of water for every mile you plan to hike, and hydrate after the hike.

Clothing

Use common sense when dressing for a hike and be prepared for sudden changes in weather. I always check the forecast before I go out for a hike, and then I always count on it being worse than predicted. Getting caught without the appropriate clothes can be both dangerous and uncomfortable.

In the summertime, I tend to hike in shorts and T-shirt. In my pack, however, I carry rain gear (both a jacket and pants) and a wool sweater or some type of synthetic pullover (polypropylene, Capilene, Thermax, etc.). I also wear a broad-brimmed hat during the summer as the sun can be very strong. In the winter, I dress in layers and carry a Gore-Tex jacket and wind pants. I wear gloves, a wool hat, and wool socks. Because I hike alone quite often, I always ask myself, "What if?" I typically pack so that I have enough clothes to spend a night if doing so should become necessary. In the winter, I always carry an extra set of dry pile pants and top with me. Pennsylvania winters can be notoriously damp and stream crossings can be troublesome.

Footwear is something that needs to be taken rather seriously when hiking around south-central Pennsylvania. For most of the rail-trails, you can get away with a good pair of sneakers or lightweight pair of hiking books. When you get into the backcountry, you would be foolhardy not to wear a good, sturdy pair of boots, especially on the trails in the Valley and Ridge Province. Many of the trails are extremely rocky and rugged. By wearing lightweight boots, not only do you risk a sprained ankle, but you can also develop some very painful foot injuries (such as heel spurs) that take a long time to heal. I typically wear a traditional pair of one-piece leather hiking boots, and I don't have problems.

The Ten Essentials

One of the first rules of hiking is to be prepared for anything. The simplest way to be prepared is to carry the "Ten Essentials." In addition to carrying the items listed below, you need to know how to use them, especially navigational aids. Always consider worst-case scenarios such as getting lost, hiking back in the dark, broken gear (for example, a broken hip strap on your pack or a water filter that gets plugged), twisting an ankle, or a brutal thunderstorm. These items don't cost a lot of money, don't take up much room in a pack, and don't weigh much—but they might just save your life.

➢ *Extra food:* trail mix, granola bars, or other high-energy snacks.

➢ *Extra clothes:* rain gear, a change of socks, and, depending on the season, a warm hat and gloves.

➢ *Flashlight or headlamp* with extra bulb and batteries.

➢ *Insect repellent:* for some areas and seasons, this is vital.

➢ *Maps and a high-quality compass.* Don't leave home without them, even if you know the terrain well from previous hikes. As previously noted, you should bring maps in addition to those in this book, and consult them before you hike. If you're GPS-savvy, bring that device, too, but don't rely on it as your sole navigational tool—battery life is limited, after all—and be sure to check its accuracy against that of your maps and compass.

➢ *Pocketknife and/or multitool.*

➢ *Sun protection:* sunglasses, lip balm, sunscreen (check the expiration date), and sun hat.

➢ *Water.* Again, bring more than you think you'll drink. Depending on your destination, you may want to bring a container and iodine or a filter for purifying water in case you run out.

➢ *Whistle.* It could become your best friend in an emergency.

➢ *Windproof matches and/or a lighter,* as well as a fire starter.

First-Aid Kit

In addition to the preceding items, the ones that follow may seem daunting to carry along for a day hike. But any paramedic will tell you that the products listed here are just the basics. The reality of hiking is that you can be out for a week of backpacking and acquire only a mosquito bite . . . or you can hike for an hour, slip, and suffer a cut or broken bone. Fortunately, the items listed pack into a very small space. Convenient prepackaged kits are available at your pharmacy or online.

➢ Ace bandages or Spenco joint wraps

➢ Adhesive bandages

➢ Antibiotic ointment (such as Neosporin)

➢ Aspirin, acetaminophen (Tylenol), or ibuprofen (Advil)

➢ Athletic tape

➢ Blister kit (such as Moleskin or Spenco 2nd Skin)

➢ Butterfly-closure bandages

➢ Diphenhydramine (Benadryl), in case of allergic reactions

➢ Epinephrine in a prefilled syringe (EpiPen), typically available by prescription only, for people known to have severe allergic reactions to hiking mishaps such as bee stings

➢ Gauze (one roll and a half-dozen 4-by-4-inch pads)

➢ Hydrogen peroxide or iodine

Hiking with Children

No one is too young for a hike in the outdoors. Be mindful, though. Flat, short, and shaded trails are best with an infant. Toddlers who have not quite mastered walking can still tag along, riding on an adult's back in a child carrier. Use common sense to judge a child's capacity to hike a particular trail, and always count that the child will tire quickly and need to be carried.

When packing for the hike, remember the child's needs as well as your own. Make sure children are adequately clothed for the weather, have proper shoes, and are protected from the sun with sunscreen. Kids dehydrate quickly, so make sure you have plenty of fluid for everyone. To assist an adult with determining which trails are suitable for children, hike recommendations for kids are provided in the chart on pages xv–xvii.

General Safety

While many hikers hit the trail full of enthusiasm and energy, others may find themselves feeling apprehensive about possible outdoor hazards. Although potentially dangerous situations can occur anywhere, your hike can be as safe and enjoyable as you had hoped, as long as you use sound judgment and prepare yourself before hitting the trail. Here are a few tips to make your trip safer and easier:

> ➢ *Hike with a buddy.* Not only is there safety in numbers, but a hiking companion can help you if you twist an ankle on the trail or if you get lost, can assist in carrying food and water, and can be a partner in discovery. A buddy is good to bring along not only to infrequently traveled or remote areas but also to urban areas.

> ➢ *If you're hiking alone, leave your hiking itinerary with someone you trust,* and let him or her know when you return.

> ➢ *Don't count on a mobile phone for your safety.* Reception may be spotty or nonexistent on the trail, even on an urban walk—especially one embraced by towering trees.

> ➢ *Don't leave valuables unattended in your car.* If you must leave something behind, don't invite trouble: Conceal items rather than leaving them out in plain view.

> ➢ *Always carry food and water, even on short hikes.* Food will give you energy and sustain you in an emergency until help arrives. Bring more water than you think you'll need—we can't emphasize this enough. Hydrate throughout your hike and at regular intervals; don't wait until you feel thirsty. Treat water from streams or other sources before drinking it.

> ➢ *Ask questions.* Public-land employees are on hand to help. It's a lot easier to solicit advice before a problem occurs, and it will help you avoid a mishap away from civilization when it's too late to amend an error.

➤ *Stay on designated trails.* Most hikers get lost when they leave the path. Even on the most clearly marked trails, you usually reach a point where you have to stop and consider the direction in which to head. If you become disoriented, don't panic. As soon as you think you may be off-track, stop, assess your current direction, and then retrace your steps back to the point where you went awry. Using a map, compass, and this book—and keeping in mind what you've passed thus far—reorient yourself and trust your judgment about which way to continue. If you become absolutely unsure of how to continue, return to your vehicle the way you came in. Should you become completely lost and have no idea how to return to the trailhead, remaining in place along the trail and waiting for help is most often the best option for adults and always the best option for children.

➤ *Always carry a whistle.* It could become a lifesaver if you get lost or hurt.

➤ *Be especially careful when crossing streams.* Whether you're fording the stream or crossing on a log, make every step count. If you have any doubt about maintaining your balance on a foot log, go ahead and ford the stream instead. When fording a stream, use a trekking pole or stout stick for balance and *face upstream as you cross.* If a stream seems too deep to ford, turn back. Whatever is on the other side isn't worth risking your life for.

➤ *Be careful at overlooks.* While these areas may provide spectacular views, they are potentially hazardous. Stay back from the edge of outcrops, and be absolutely sure of your footing.

➤ *Standing dead trees and storm-damaged living trees pose a hazard to hikers and tent campers.* Loose or broken limbs could fall at any time. When choosing a spot to rest, camp, or snack, *look up.*

➤ *Know the symptoms of heat exhaustion, or hyperthermia.* Lightheadedness and loss of energy are the first two indicators. If you feel these symptoms coming on, find some shade, drink your water, remove as many layers of clothing as practical, and stay put until you cool down. Marching through heat exhaustion leads to heatstroke—which can be deadly. If you should be sweating and you're not, that's the signature warning sign. If you or a companion reaches this point, your hike is over: Do whatever you can to cool down, and seek medical help immediately.

➤ *Likewise, know the symptoms of subnormal body temperature, or hypothermia.* Shivering and forgetfulness are the two most common indicators of this stealthy killer. Hypothermia can occur at any elevation, even in the summer— especially if you're wearing lightweight cotton clothing. If symptoms develop, get to shelter, hot liquids, and dry clothes ASAP.

➤ *Most importantly, take along your brain.* A cool, calculating mind is the single most important asset on the trail. Think before you act. Watch your step. Plan ahead. Avoiding accidents before they happen is the best way to ensure a rewarding and relaxing hike.

Animal and Plant Hazards

TICKS Ticks like to hang out in the brush that grows along trails. Hot summer months seem to explode their numbers, but you should be tick-aware during all months of the year. Ticks, which are arachnids and not insects, need a host to feast on in order to reproduce. The ticks that alight onto you while hiking will be very small, sometimes so tiny that you won't be able to spot them. Primarily of two varieties, deer ticks and dog ticks, both need a few hours of actual attachment before they can transmit any disease they may harbor. The best way to avoid getting ticks is by wearing long pants tucked into your socks. This is not always pleasant when hiking in the summer. Alternately, or in addition, use a bug spray that contains DEET, which is very effective. I typically spray my pants, socks, and boots when I go out. Nonetheless, as I have grown older, I seem to have also grown more attractive to them. Ticks may settle in shoes, socks, and hats, and may take several hours to actually latch on. The best strategy is to visually check every half-hour or so while hiking, do a thorough check before you get in the car, and then, when you take a posthike shower, do an even more thorough check of your entire body. Ticks that haven't attached are easily removed. To remove a tick that is already embedded, use tweezers made especially for this purpose; you should be careful to remove the head as well as the body. If you suspect that an embedded tick is a deer tick, which carries Lyme disease, put it in a plastic bag and call your doctor. Many times doctors will have the tick checked for Lyme disease, so that treatment can begin before symptoms arise.

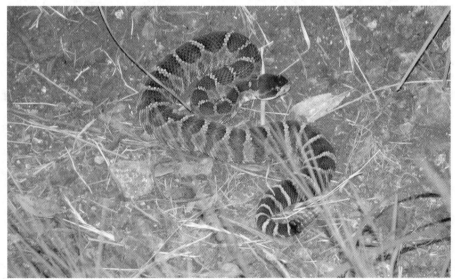

Photo: Jane Huber

Rattlesnake

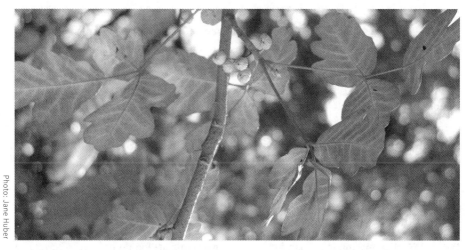

Photo: Jane Huber

Poison oak

SNAKES South-central Pennsylvania is home to two types of poisonous snakes: the timber rattler and the copperhead. Rattlesnakes are commonly encountered in the rocky, mountainous areas; the Flat Rock Trail at Colonel Denning State Park (see Hikes 25 and 26, pages 128 and 132) is the most well-known place in the area to see them. Be careful if you move rocks or when climbing around outcrops, where snakes like to sun themselves. Copperheads seem to like the woods and can be encountered just about anywhere. In the summer of 2014, I came upon one lying across the Conewago Trail outside of Elizabethtown. If you see any snake that has a diamond-shaped head (characteristic of many poisonous snakes) or have any doubts, give it a wide berth. There is no need to bother any wildlife you come across.

POISON IVY, OAK, AND SUMAC Recognizing poison ivy, oak, and sumac and avoiding contact with them is the most effective way to prevent the painful, itchy rashes associated with these plants. In central Pennsylvania, poison ivy ranges from a thick, tree-hugging vine to a shaded ground cover, three leaflets to a leaf; poison oak occurs as either a vine or shrub, with three leaflets as well; and poison sumac flourishes in swampland, each leaf containing 7–13 leaflets. Urushiol, the oil in the sap of these plants, is responsible for the rash. Usually within 12–14 hours of exposure (but sometimes much later), raised lines and/or blisters will appear, accompanied by a terrible itch. Refrain from scratching because bacteria under fingernails can cause infection and you will spread the rash to other parts of your body. Wash and dry the rash thoroughly, applying calamine lotion or another product to help dry the rash. If itching or blistering is severe, seek medical attention. To keep from spreading the misery to someone else, wash not only any exposed parts of your body but also any oil-contaminated clothes, hiking gear, and pets.

MOSQUITOES   Although it's not a common occurrence, individuals can become infected with the West Nile virus by being bitten by an infected mosquito. *Culex* mosquitoes, the primary varieties that can transmit West Nile virus to humans, thrive in urban rather than natural areas. They lay their eggs in stagnant water and can breed in any standing water that remains for more than five days. Most people infected with West Nile virus have no symptoms of illness, but some may become ill, usually 3–15 days after being bitten.

In south-central Pennsylvania, late spring and summer are the times considered to be the highest risk periods for West Nile virus. At this time of year—and anytime you expect mosquitoes to be buzzing around—you may want to wear protective clothing, such as long sleeves, long pants, and socks. Loose-fitting, light-colored clothing is best. Spray clothing with insect repellent. Remember to follow the instructions on the repellent and to take extra care with children.

WILDLIFE   The mountains around central Pennsylvania are home to a wide variety of wildlife, including white-tailed deer, black bears, bobcats, foxes, raccoons, porcupines, etc. For the most part, these animals pose little danger unless they feel threatened, cornered or harassed. If you see any wildlife, it is OK to watch from a distance, but it is neither safe nor ethically sound to approach it, feed it, or engage it in any fashion. Consider yourself a guest in its home. Black bears are probably the only mammals that may pose any sort of threat and they are common in the Valley and Ridge Province. If you encounter a bear in the woods, it will likely run off. If not, try to look large, make noise, and back away slowly. Don't run off or climb a tree.

Tips for Enjoying Harrisburg

Before you go out for a hike, do some homework to make sure things go as smoothly as possible. Check the forecast to find out what the weather is going to be like so you can plan accordingly. There is no reason not to hike when it is raining, provided you're not venturing out into a hurricane or thunderstorm. Just dress appropriately. Some of nature's finest wonders reveal themselves during foul weather. If you are like me and enjoy solitude, try to hike during the week. I do most of my hiking during the week and I never see anybody, except along the Appalachian Trail.

Review the descriptions in this book to see if you are up for the hike. In particular, you might find the elevation profiles included in each chapter to be very helpful. From them, you can get a pretty good sense of how much climbing and descending you will have to do. Also, plan plenty of time for your hike. The hiking times I provided are based on a hiking speed of about 2 miles per hour. Many people may think that is somewhat slow. Personally, I am in no rush when I get out in the woods; I want to spend as much time out as possible. If you like to look at flowers or take pictures or simply sit and relax, allow more time. This area of Pennsylvania is not a place that lends itself to the sweeping view of the landscape. Many of its treasures are small and easily overlooked. You will feel more relaxed, and you will see more things if you take your time and take a closer look at the land around you. You will be surprised by what is out there.

Topographic Maps

The maps in this book have been produced with great care and, used with the hike text, will direct you to the trail and help you stay on course. However, you'll find superior detail and valuable information in the US Geological Survey's 7.5-minute-series topographic maps. At **MyTopo.com,** for example, you can view and print free USGS topos of the entire United States. Online services such as **Trails.com** charge annual fees for additional features such as shaded relief, which makes the topography stand out more. If you expect to print out many topo maps each year, it might be worth paying for such extras. The downside to USGS maps is that most are outdated, having been created 20–30 years ago; nevertheless, they provide excellent topographic detail.

Digital programs such as DeLorme's Topo North America enable you to review topo maps on your computer. Data gathered while hiking with a GPS unit can be downloaded into the software, letting you plot your own hikes. Of course, **Google Earth** (earth.google .com) does away with topo maps and their inaccuracies . . . replacing them with satellite imagery and its inaccuracies. Regardless, what one lacks, the other augments. Google Earth is an excellent tool whether you have difficulty with topos or not.

If you're new to hiking, you might be wondering, "What's a topo map?" In short, it indicates not only linear distance but elevation as well, using contour lines. These lines spread across the map like dozens of intricate spiderwebs. Each line represents a particular elevation, and at the base of each topo a contour's interval designation is given. If, for example, the contour interval is 20 feet, then the distance between each contour line is 20 feet. Follow five contour lines up on the same map, and the elevation has increased by 100 feet.

In addition to the sources listed previously and in Appendix B, you'll find topos at major universities, outdoors shops, and some public libraries, as well as online at national map.gov and store.usgs.gov.

Trail Etiquette

Whether you're on a city, county, state, or national-park trail, always remember that great care and resources (from nature as well as from your tax dollars) have gone into creating these trails. Treat the trail, wildlife, and fellow hikers with respect.

> ➤ *Hike on open trails only.* Respect trail and road closures (ask if not sure), avoid possible trespassing on private land, and obtain all permits and authorization as required. Also, leave gates as you found them or as marked.

➢ *Please do not cut switchbacks.* Doing so leads to excessive and unnecessary erosion of the area around the trail, and will eventually lead to a trail needing to be relocated.

➢ *Leave only footprints.* Be sensitive to the ground beneath you. This also means staying on the existing trail and not blazing any new trails. Be sure to pack out what you pack in. No one likes to see the trash someone else has left behind.

➢ *Never spook animals.* An unannounced approach, a sudden movement, or a loud noise startles most animals. A surprised animal can be dangerous to you, to others, and to itself. Give it plenty of space.

➢ *Plan ahead.* Know your equipment, your ability, and the area in which you are hiking—and prepare accordingly. Be self-sufficient at all times; carry necessary supplies for changes in weather or other conditions. A well-executed trip is a satisfaction to you and to others.

➢ *Be courteous to other hikers, bikers, equestrians,* and others you encounter on the trails.

OPPOSITE: *Dense ferns along the Appalachian Trail near Toms Run (see Hike 58, Sunset Rocks, page 281)*

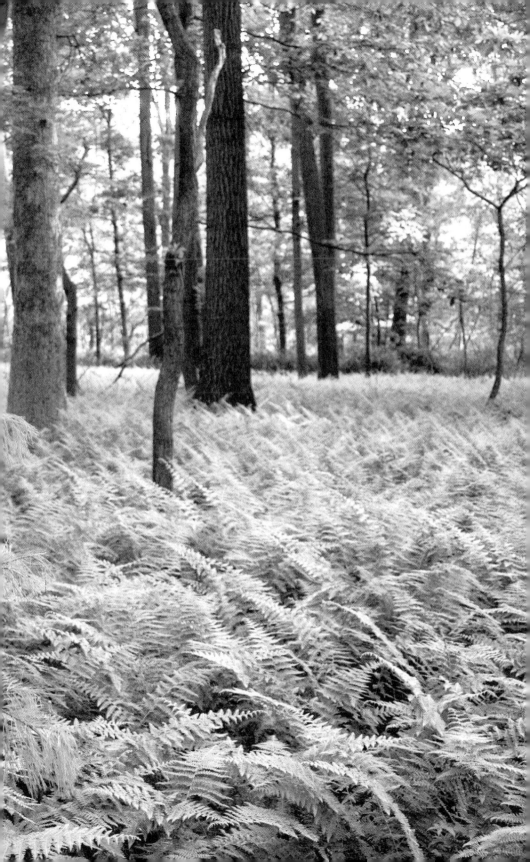

NORTHEAST

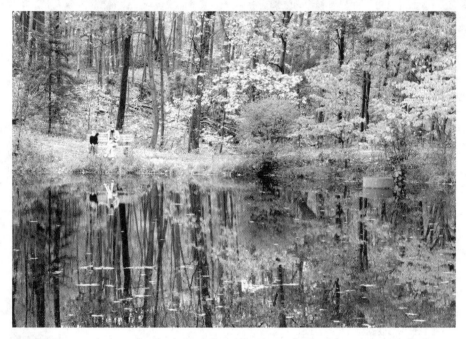

Reflection pond along the Eagle Path (see Hike 7, page 47)

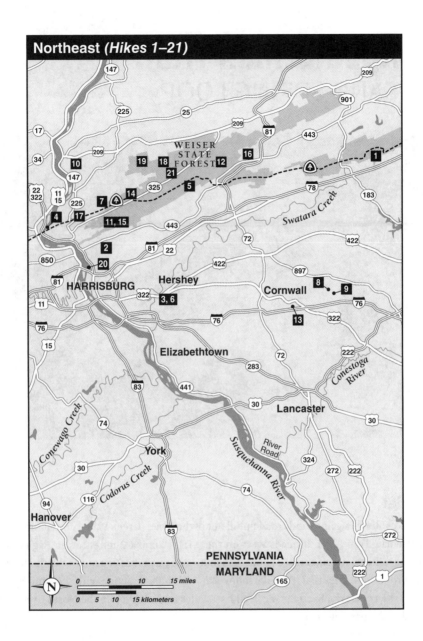

Northeast (Hikes 1–21)

1 Appalachian Trail:
SAND SPRING LOOP

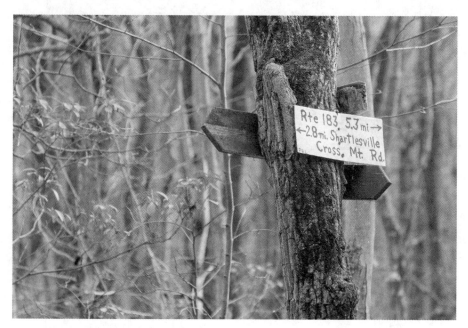

Trail sign along the AT

In Brief

This hike follows a game-lands road uphill out of the North Creek Valley until it meets the Appalachian Trail (AT). It heads west on the AT for almost 2 miles to the Eagles Nest Shelter Trail. A short side trip of about 0.25 mile each way takes you out to the shelter and back. From the shelter trail, the hike follows the AT to the junction with the Sand Spring Trail. It then takes the Sand Spring Trail for 2 miles back down into the North Creek Valley and to the parking area.

Description

Ever in search of good loop hikes along the ridges east of I-81 that don't see a lot of traffic, I discovered this hike while looking for alternatives to the Round Head hike that I wrote about in the first edition of this book. I enjoy that hike, though it had some grueling sections, and parts had become so overgrown that route finding had become increasingly difficult. Not to be dissuaded from grueling sections, this loop hike has about a mile along

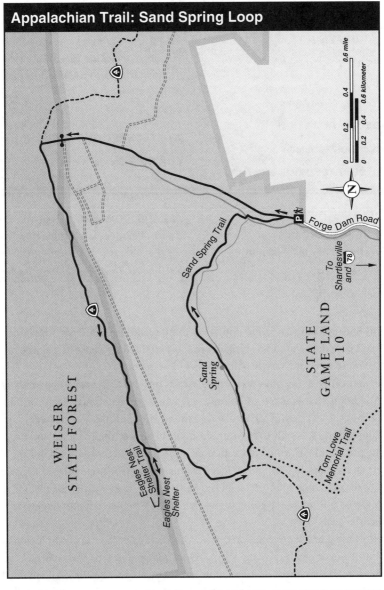

Appalachian Trail: Sand Spring Loop

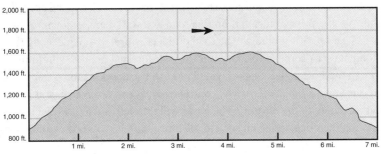

LENGTH 7 miles	**ACCESS** Open
CONFIGURATION Loop	**MAPS** USGS *Auburn;* Keystone Trail Association *Appalachian Trail in Pennsylvania, Sections 1 Through 6: Delaware Water Gap to Swatara Gap*
DIFFICULTY Strenuous	
SCENERY Eagles Nest Shelter, Sand Spring, AT environs	
EXPOSURE Mostly shaded	**FACILITIES** None
TRAIL TRAFFIC Light	**WHEELCHAIR TRAVERSABLE** No
TRAIL SURFACE Mostly dirt; rocky on Sand Spring Trail	**CONTACT** Pennsylvania Game Commission, 717-787-4250, tinyurl.com /pagamelands
HIKING TIME 3–4 hours	**SPECIAL COMMENTS** Generally this is a hike of moderate difficulty; however, the rugged and rocky Sand Spring Trail leads me to class its difficulty as strenuous.
DRIVING DISTANCE 46 miles from the junction of I-81 and I-83 north of Harrisburg	

the Sand Spring Trail that is just tough on the feet and ankles. That I hiked it with an ankle that I later discovered was broken probably affected my sense of it a little bit. Nonetheless, be sure to wear a sturdy pair of boots for this one.

Begin the hike at the obvious parking area at the end of the pavement on Forge Dam Road. You know that you are at the right one when you encounter a gate and road sign that reads STOP EXIT ONLY. The woods around the parking area are very nice, with many tall pine trees. North Creek tumbles by just west of the road. As you head up the road, the first landmark you will encounter is the trailhead for the Sand Spring Trail, on your left after a couple of hundred feet. That is where the loop will end. You could, of course, walk this loop counterclockwise; in fact, the rocky section of the Sand Spring Trail might be a little easier going doing that. I did the hike counterclockwise and will describe it as such.

Follow the game-lands road up the North Creek Valley to the north. It climbs for 1.5 miles, but it never gets especially steep. At 1.1 miles, you will pass another significant game-lands road that heads off to a saddle east of our road. Continue hiking north along the road and at 1.4 miles you will come to a gate across the road, and the open road heads to the left (west). You can turn left on this road and walk 2 miles down to the junction with the AT and pick it up there. The road offers very pretty walking along the ridge of Blue Mountain past some food plots and through forested area. If you do this and you want to visit the Eagles Nest Shelter, you'll need to backtrack on the AT about 0.25 mile to get to the shelter trail. Alternately, continue straight past the gate, and in about 0.25 mile you will come to the AT onto which you will turn left and follow that to the west. It too stays atop the ridge, though it stays in the forest until it crosses the game-lands road a couple of miles ahead.

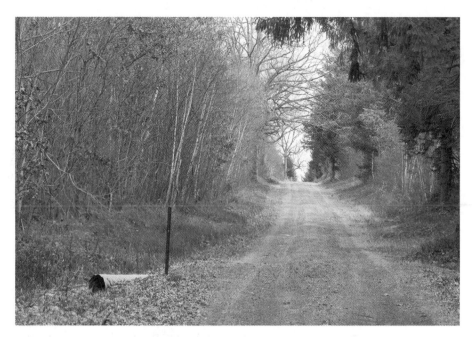

Game-land road along Blue Mountain

Stay on the AT as it traverses the ridgecrest meandering through a forest of oak and hickory trees with a few maples scattered here and there. The walking is flat along the ridge, although at times the trail gets a bit rocky. At 3.5 miles, you should see a sign for the Eagles Nest Shelter and the junction with the blue-blazed trail that will take you there. Turn right and follow the trail somewhat downhill, across a spring, and then up out of the spring to the shelter (0.3 mile). There is a picnic bench at the shelter, which makes a nice place for a break, and a privy and water source beyond. Be sure to treat the water should you fill up at the water source. After a break, head back out to the AT and continue following it to the west. The trail veers off to a more southerly direction when it crosses the forest service road, and then descends gently until it intersects the blue-blazed Sand Spring Trail at an obvious junction marked by a sign for Sand Spring and another that points in the direction of Shartlesville farther west along the AT.

Tighten your bootlaces and get ready for some rocky walking. Head left (east) on the Sand Spring Trail and follow it as it descends gently toward the valley below. The first landmarks you will encounter along this section of the hike, which are about 200 yards down the trail, are Sand Spring and the junction with the Tom Lowe Memorial Trail. Sand Spring is indeed a flowing spring of clear water that bubbles up into a pool formed by blocks of rock. Again, be sure to treat the water if you choose to drink it. The Tom Lowe Memorial Trail makes a sharp turn to the right (southwest), heads up over the ridge, and eventually traverses the ridge to the east and north to end about 100 yards downstream from the parking area below. Just beyond this location you'll find a small campsite where you want to stay left and cross the creek. The trail is well blazed and follows the drainage over and around rocks downhill for the next mile, which gets about as rocky as it is tolerable. This is quite typical geology of the Valley and Ridge Province of this part of Pennsylvania. On the ridgetops or in the valleys, the hiking is generally not quite as rugged as it is going between a ridgetop and a valley, as is the case on this trail. Along the way, 5.5 miles into the hike, you should see another sign for Sand Spring off to the right where another small pool is located.

After about a mile, or even a little less, of the rugged hiking, the trail starts to hug the left (north) side of the drainage and the walking gets considerably more pleasant as the trail becomes more dirt than rock and is even covered in sections with pine duff. For the next mile back to the road, the walking is much nicer as the path winds through lovely forest of pine and oak trees and stands of young hemlocks. After about 1.25 miles the valley becomes very steeply sided, although there are flat areas scattered between Sand Spring (which has a fair flow near the bottom of the valley) and North Creek. After the two join the flow is substantial. For the last 0.75 mile the hiking is really pleasant. The trail is smooth and relatively wide, and it rolls up and down through the woods. Just before reaching the trailhead, you'll come to a stream crossing that in low water is insignificant. I would conclude, however, that after a heavy rain, hiking along this section of trail could become hazardous. Throughout the woods are signs of some very heavy and high creek flows in the past. Beyond the crossing, the trailhead at the road is just a short distance ahead. Turn right at the road and walk back to the car.

Nearby Activities

There are gas stations and fast-food emporiums located north of I-78 at Exit 23. South of the highway you'll find the **Blue Mountain Family Restaurant,** which I recommend highly (24 Roadside Drive; 610-488-0353, bluemountainfamilyrestaurant.com). Also south of the highway on Roadside Drive is **Roadside America** (610-488-6241, roadsideamericainc.com). A classic piece of Americana, it boasts "the world's greatest indoor miniature village." Essentially a huge electric train display, it's worth seeing at least once in your lifetime.

GPS TRAILHEAD COORDINATES AND DIRECTIONS
N40° 32.270' W76° 07.403'

From Harrisburg and points west, take I-78 East to Exit 23 (Shartlesville). Turn left (north) after exiting on Mountain Road. Follow Mountain Road 0.4 mile to Forge Dam Road and turn left. Take Forge Dam Road north about 1.5 miles to the parking area at the gate and the STOP: EXIT ONLY sign.

2 Boyd Big Tree Preserve Conservation Area

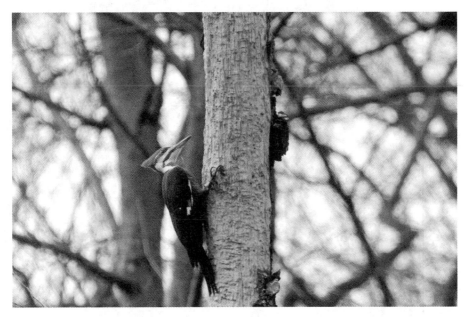

Pileated woodpecker

In Brief

From the parking area, this hike follows the Pond Loop Trail to the Creek Trail and the Coach Trail along the western edge of the conservation area. After a short climb, this hike joins the Janie Trail and follows it along the ridge to the eastern edge of the conservation area. A short stretch on the Upper Spring Trail takes you to the East Loop Trail and back to the parking lot.

Description

Located only 8 miles or so from downtown Harrisburg, the Boyd Big Tree Preserve Conservation Area is a gem of a recreation area. The park is similar in design to the Joseph Ibberson Conservation Area located two valleys to the north, with its educational pavilion on the edge of the parking area overlooking a valley to the north (see page 47). The Boyd Big Tree area was established in 1999 thanks to Alexander Boyd of the Union Deposit Corporation, who donated the land for conservation purposes. Situated mostly on the north

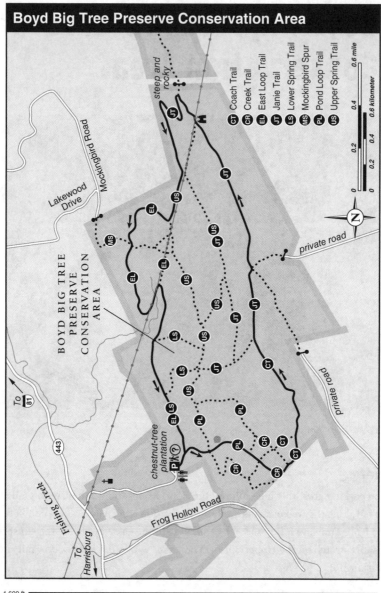

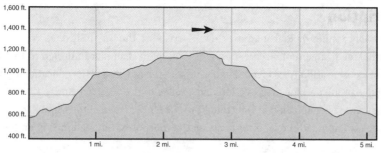

LENGTH 5.1 miles	**ACCESS** Sunrise–sunset
CONFIGURATION Loop	**MAPS** USGS *Harrisburg East;* maps of the park are available at the parking area or online at tinyurl.com/boydbigtreemap.
DIFFICULTY Moderate	
SCENERY Conservation area environs and nice views of the Lebanon Valley to the north from the Janie Trail	**FACILITIES** Water, toilets, telephone, picnic tables
	WHEELCHAIR TRAVERSABLE No
EXPOSURE More shade than sun	**CONTACT** c/o Little Buffalo State Park, 717-567-9255, tinyurl.com/boydbigtree
TRAIL TRAFFIC Light	
TRAIL SURFACE Dirt	**SPECIAL COMMENTS** This hike combines several trails, all well marked, to follow the perimeter of the conservation area. A multitude of variations to it can be made with assistance from the park map.
HIKING TIME 2.5–3 hours	
DRIVING DISTANCE 3 miles from junction of PA 443 and US 22/322 west of Harrisburg	

side of Blue Mountain, the area provides habitat to diverse species of tall trees, wildflowers, birds, and mammals. The park sports seven trails of various lengths and difficulties, providing a variety of options for exploring the terrain, viewing some of the plant and animal life, and simply getting a little bit of peace and quiet.

This hike strings together several of the park trails to create an excursion around the perimeter of the conservation area. Much of the walking is on old logging roads that have been converted to trails, so the grades are generally easy and the footing is mostly pleasant and secure. Start out by following the pink-blazed Pond Loop Trail southeast from the parking area, staying right at a junction after a couple of hundred feet. Continue uphill following the pink blazes, passing another trail junction at approximately 0.25 mile. From that junction the trail descends to the small pond, surrounded by stands of cattails and thicket on its banks. You'll find a bench at the far end of the pond and several bird boxes in the area.

As you pass the pond on the old logging road to its right, take a look off into the woods and notice the prolific signs of woodpeckers on the trees. In addition to the common downy woodpeckers, if you keep your eyes open you may also see the large pileated woodpecker, redheaded woodpeckers, and even some flickers. Follow the path uphill for a short distance to the junction with the Creek Trail, identified by its blue blazes. The Pond Loop Trail turns left here. Continue straight on the Creek Trail for 200 feet or so, at which point the main blue trail heads downhill and an old connector trail with blue blazes continues ahead. Go straight on the connector trail for 0.15 mile to the main Creek Trail again at the edge of the park and turn left, heading uphill for a short distance to a Y-intersection with the yellow-blazed Coach Trail. Turn right (south) at the Y, and follow the Coach Trail.

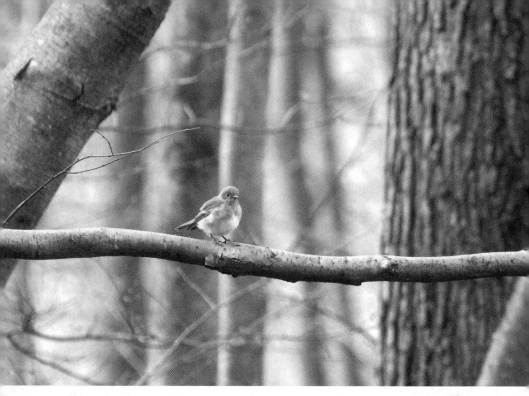

Bluebird on a winter's day

The Coach Trail follows an old coach road for 0.75 mile across the hillside through a lovely forest of mature white oak, poplar, hickory, and beech trees. At the end of the Coach Trail, you'll reach the red-blazed Janie Trail, which makes a 2.5-mile loop through the park. Turn right (east) and follow the red blazes as the trail rises gently along the side of Blue Mountain to its ridge. At the crest, you'll get a nice view of the Lebanon Valley to the south. A major geographic feature southeast of the Valley and Ridge Province, the Lebanon Valley is one section of the Great Valley, an unbroken valley that extends from New York to Georgia. A small meadow on the ridge provides habitat for many songbirds and bedding for white-tailed deer. From the crest, the Janie Trail makes a left turn and follows the ridge just south of the crest for 0.65 mile to some power lines. Along the way, you'll pass through sections of dense thicket, which provide cover for many songbirds. The clear-cut at the power lines is a great place to spot cardinals, bluebirds, and chickadees, and offers a nice view of the valleys to the south and to the north from the ridgetop.

At the power lines, follow the trail to the right back into the woods and along the ridge for a short distance. As you walk along, keep your eyes open to the left for a small cairn that marks the place where the Janie Trail leaves the old roadbed and heads over the ridge to the north. The junction is tough to spot, particularly in the fall. If you reach a gate across the roadbed, you've gone about 100 feet too far. From the junction, you should be able to spot a red blaze on a prominent silver-barked tree to the north of the road. Follow the blazes to the north side of the ridge, where the trail leads back west toward the power lines. The trail gets rocky in this area, then makes a switchback by some tall spruce trees, and descends a steep and rugged bit before reaching another old coach road at about 2.9 miles. Turn left (west) on the road and walk out to the power lines, where you'll turn right onto the Upper Spring Trail, marked by a white blaze on a post. Head downhill beneath the power lines and turn right onto the green-blazed East Loop Trail just before you reach the second tower.

Also an old roadbed, the East Loop Trail winds through a beautiful section of forest with pine trees scattered among the hardwoods. As the trail bends back to the west, it comes to a T-intersection above a hollow on the left where you will stay to the right. At about 4.2 miles, you'll regain the power line again at a pretty area where a small creek flows beneath—yet another great place for birding here. The East Loop Trail leaves the power line and heads west for just shy of a mile to the junction with the Pond Loop Trail near the parking lot.

At the parking area, be sure to take a walk to the plantation of young chestnut trees surrounded by a fence across from the pavilion. Chestnuts were all but wiped out earlier in the 20th century by blight, and this represents an attempt at redeveloping the species. The bird boxes surrounding the plantation provide homes for eastern bluebirds, which are abundant in the area.

Nearby Activities

Fort Hunter Mansion & Park (717-599-5751, forthunter.org), north of the Harrisburg city limits at 5300 N. Front St., provides an interesting historical excursion, with its museum and mansion, not to mention a view of the Susquehanna River and a nice place to picnic and walk. Follow PA 443 west to Front Street and turn left. The park is about 0.5 mile ahead on the right.

GPS TRAILHEAD COORDINATES AND DIRECTIONS
N40° 21.230' W76° 51.030'

From US 22/322 west of Harrisburg, take the PA 443/Fishing Creek exit. Follow PA 443 east 2.8 miles. Turn right onto the access road for the park (marked by a sign), just beyond Frog Hollow Road. The parking area is at the top of the hill.

3 Bullfrog Valley Pond to Shank Park

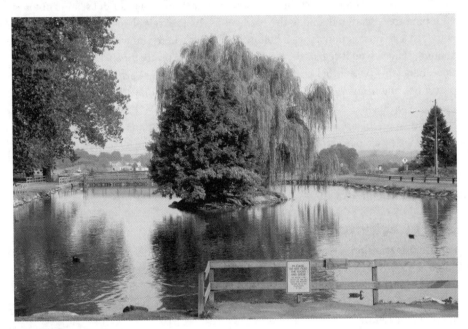

Bullfrog Valley Pond

In Brief

This hike follows the paved Jonathan Eshenour Memorial Trail beneath a canopy of tall tulip poplars into Shank Park. Upon entering the park, the nature trail departs from the Eshenour Trail and makes a loop around the perimeter of the park.

Description

The Bullfrog Valley Pond–Shank Park Nature Trail begins at the Bullfrog Valley Pond parking area and then follows a 0.85-mile section of the Jonathan Eshenour Memorial Trail south to Shank Park. At that point, the nature trail departs from the Eshenour Trail, enters the woods, and makes a 1.5-mile loop through the environs of the 90-acre Shank Park before rejoining the paved Eshenour Trail and returning to the car.

To begin this hike, walk from your car in the Bullfrog Valley Pond parking lot across the footbridge over the feeder stream to Bullfrog Valley Pond, and turn left (south) on the Eshenour Trail. A box containing a numbered "life list" of the different flora you can spot on the hike is located on the right side of the trail. The list is impressive, with

LENGTH 3.1 miles	**MAPS** USGS *Hershey* and *Middletown;* a map of the entire Jonathan Eshenour Memorial Trail is available online at tinyurl.com/eshenourtrailmap.
CONFIGURATION Balloon	
DIFFICULTY Easy–moderate	
SCENERY Bullfrog Valley Pond and creek; Shank Park environs	**FACILITIES** Portable toilet, soda/water machines, picnic pavilion at trailhead
EXPOSURE Mostly shaded	**WHEELCHAIR TRAVERSABLE** The first 0.85 mile is paved.
TRAIL TRAFFIC Moderately heavy	**CONTACT** Derry Township, 717-533-7138, tinyurl.com/derrytwpparks
TRAIL SURFACE Paved and dirt sections	
HIKING TIME 1.5 hours	**SPECIAL COMMENTS** Although the trail can get busy, within Shank Park it is always possible to find some peace and privacy at one of the many benches along the hike.
DRIVING DISTANCE 0.8 mile from US 322 in Hershey	
ACCESS Sunrise–sunset	

approximately 170 entries, more than 50 of which are broadleaf trees alone. The numbers on the list correspond to small numbered signs posted on trees or placed into the ground to make for easy identification. The variety of trees makes the hike a spectacular blaze of color during the fall.

The nature trail here follows the Eshenour Trail along the path of the old Brownstone–Middletown Railroad Grade. Originally a wagon road used for transporting brownstone blocks from quarries west of Waltonville Road, the railroad was developed along this path because breakage of the stone was too common when hauled by wagon. In 1892, a standard-gauge railroad was built that hauled the stone for approximately 3 miles to the Reading Railroad in Hummelstown. The railroad was rather short-lived, ending operations in 1939 when brick became a cheaper alternative to quarried brownstone. Nonetheless, in its heyday, brownstone was a sought-after building material, and the stone quarried in Pennsylvania was shipped as far away as Tampa, Chicago, and St. Louis.

The railroad bed is now a lovely paved walking trail that climbs gently up Bullfrog Valley, parallel to the course of the small Bullfrog Creek. On this lower section of the path, you walk beneath a wonderful canopy of tall tulip poplar trees. At 0.1 mile, the trail passes by a bench, some waste and recycling baskets, and a 7.75-mile marker, indicating the distance from the beginning of the Jonathan Eshenour Memorial Trail at the eastern boundary of Derry Township (see page 42 for a hike on the Eshenour Trail). At 0.4 mile into this hike, the trail reaches an area landscaped with a tie wall and crosses Derry Woods Drive. A bench sits in an attractively landscaped area to the right of the trail. At 0.5 mile, the trail crosses Stoney Run Road, and just past this crossing have a look at the lovely wetlands area with plenty of cattails to the right of the trail. At 0.7 mile, the trail passes over a small tributary to Bullfrog Creek and through a cut in a rocky section of the valley. The creek on the right is picturesque as it tumbles over a rough angular stone bed.

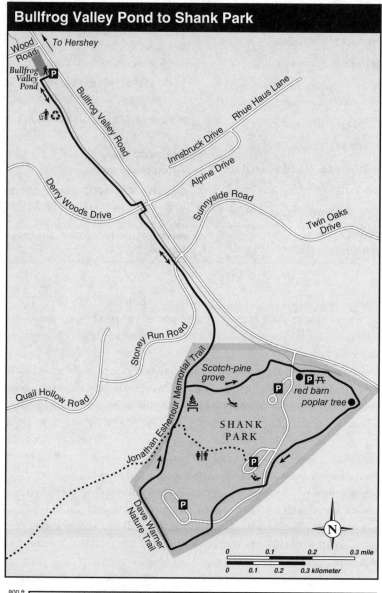

Bullfrog Valley Pond to Shank Park

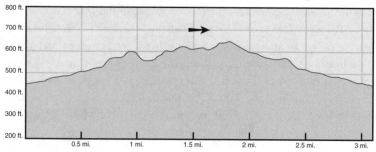

At 0.85 mile, the nature trail departs from the Eshenour Trail, entering the woods and Shank Park to the left (east) onto the Dave Warner Nature Trail. A sign marks the intersection, and the trail surface at first is mulch. Quickly the trail passes a small bench, crosses a footbridge, turns to dirt, and climbs for a short distance into a pretty and fragrant stand of Scotch pine trees, which is a great place to spot inchworms hanging around—literally!—on a warm summer day. Leaving the pines, the trail enters a high meadow and passes by several broadly scattered conifer and deciduous trees as it crosses the top of a hill. This hill serves as the local sledding area in the winter.

At 1 mile, the trail enters the woods again at a location marked by a sign indicating that you are indeed following the nature trail. Immediately, you will come to a bench and the trail splits into three forks, all heading downhill. All of the forks take you to the same location down below, though the left option is the least steep and from my best estimation the trail proper. At the bottom of the hill, the trail turns right and shortly crosses the main Shank Park road. A large red barn with restrooms and soda machines sits uphill from the trail as it passes into an open area with several picnic tables, some tall shade trees, and a few barbecue grills. Through this open area, the trail is narrow but has an asphalt surface until it reenters the woods aside Bullfrog Creek, where it becomes dirt again. The creek here is a good place to hunt for salamanders and small crawfish.

After entering the woods, the trail meanders about the creek, crossing two footbridges and passing a small bench before it bends to the right and climbs gently. Just beyond the second footbridge, keep your eyes open on the right for an enormous tulip poplar, at least 80 feet tall. It is quite a sight. As the trail levels off again, it passes soccer fields, a beautiful white oak tree (#5 on the life list), and a bench. Continue along the trail a short distance until it leaves the woods, becomes paved again, and crosses the park road at a playground and pavilion (restrooms located here). The trail enters the woods next to the pavilion and in another 0.25 mile exits the woods, makes a quick left turn, crosses the park road under some power lines, and enters the woods again. Be careful here, as two trails enter the woods from beneath the power lines. Take the right-hand trail, marked by a small sign.

Shortly, the trail passes a spur that takes off to the right to a ballfield. The nature trail descends gently to the left and meets up with a dirt road at the boundary of the park (1.9 miles). Turn right on the dirt road, which changes to grass, and continue walking downhill past a footbridge that exits the park on your left for another 150 feet. A manhole cover in the grass marks your next bit of route finding. Make a 90-degree right turn and cross the grassy hill under some power lines. Resist the temptation to walk directly downhill to the paved Eshenour Trail just below you, as the area around that trail can be rather marshy. Just past the power lines, the trail enters the woods yet again (marked by a trail sign) and meanders gently downhill past some thick woods and berry bushes. At 2.15 miles, the trail emerges from the woods in a shaded grassy area, which you walk across to the paved Eshenour Trail. Be sure to turn right on the paved trail, and when you reach the fork just ahead, stay to the left.

In just about a mile, you will return to the Bullfrog Valley Pond parking area. As a final note, about 0.1 mile past the above-mentioned fork, a small dirt spur exits the Eshenour Trail to the right that heads back to some benches and a fire ring next to the stand of Scotch pines the trail passed through earlier. That is a pleasant and serene spot to rest for a snack or simply some solitude. The benches are visible from the Eshenour Trail.

Nearby Activities

Hershey Park (800-437-7439, hersheypark.com) and **ZooAmerica** (717-534-3900, zoo america.com), both in Hershey, are popular destinations for families from the mid-Atlantic states. **The Hotel Hershey** (844-330-1711, thehotelhershey.com), on the hill to the north of town, provides some high-quality dining along with pretty views of the countryside. Across the street from the hotel is **Hershey Gardens** (717-534-3492, hersheygardens.org), which makes for a lovely walk.

GPS TRAILHEAD COORDINATES AND DIRECTIONS
N40° 15.451' W76° 41.051'

From US 322 in Hershey, head south on Bullfrog Valley Road. This is either the first light after US 322 and US 422 split coming from the west or the last light before they join coming from the east (just beyond the Penn State Milton S. Hershey Medical Center). The parking lot for Bullfrog Valley Pond is 0.82 mile ahead on the right, just past the intersection with Wood Road at the obvious duck pond.

---

4 Clarks Ferry Loop

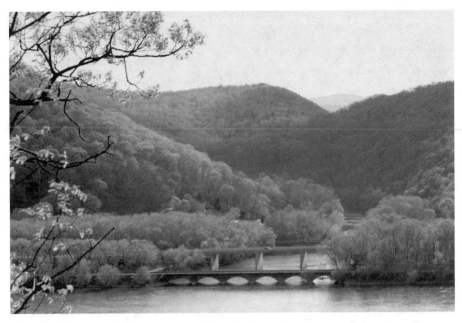

Sherman Creek from the Duncannon Overlook

In Brief

This hike follows the Appalachian Trail (AT) for a short distance uphill from the Susque-hanna River before picking up a side trail that takes you to the top of Peters Mountain near the Clarks Ferry Shelter. Upon reaching the ridge, pick up the AT and walk out to the shelter and to the ridgecrest just above. To return, this hike follows the AT back to the parking lot.

Description

The AT from Clarks Ferry on the Susquehanna River north of Harrisburg is a very popu-lar place for area hikers. Understandably so: The route up to the crest of Peters Mountain provides several excellent views of the river and side valleys. Plus, the hiking is very pleas-ant. This hike offers a little variation on the typical out-and-back excursion, allowing you to make a loop hike over Peters Mountain.

This hike begins where the AT crosses the railroad tracks across the street from the parking area. Look for the large trail sign on the shoulder of the road, make your way over the tracks, and begin traversing the steep hillside. Although the terrain is steep, the trail

Clarks Ferry Loop

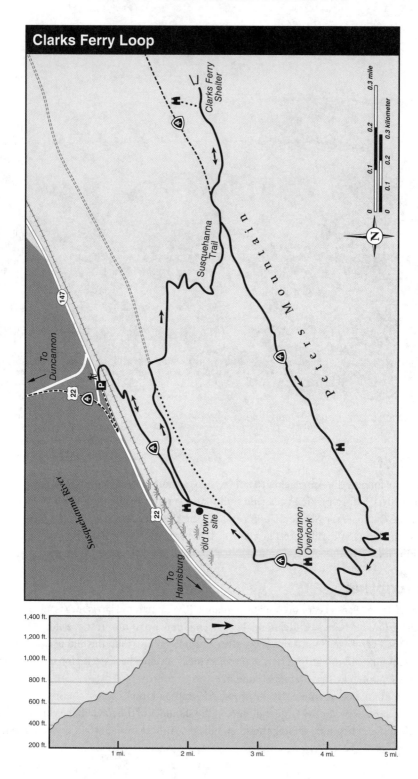

LENGTH 5 miles	**ACCESS** Open
CONFIGURATION Loop with a stretch of out-and-back	**MAPS** USGS *Duncannon* and *Halifax*; Keystone Trail Association *Appalachian Trail in Pennsylvania, Sections 7 and 8: Susquehanna River to Swatara Gap*
DIFFICULTY Moderate	
SCENERY Overlooks of Susquehanna River; nice ridge walk	**FACILITIES** None
EXPOSURE Mostly shaded	**WHEELCHAIR TRAVERSABLE** No
TRAIL TRAFFIC Moderately heavy	**CONTACT** Appalachian Trail Conservancy, 717-258-5771, appalachiantrail.org
TRAIL SURFACE Dirt and some scrambling among rocks along ridgetop	
HIKING TIME 2.5 hours	**SPECIAL COMMENTS** A fine mountain walk near Harrisburg. The rocky ridge of Peters Mountain is prime habitat for timber rattlesnakes, so exercise caution when scrambling around the area.
DRIVING DISTANCE 12 miles from intersection of I-81 and US 22/322 outside of Harrisburg	

climbs at a very pleasant grade generally toward the south. Not far beyond a rock outcrop, the terrain levels out and the blue-blazed Susquehanna Trail heads off on a northern track (about 0.5 mile).

Turn left (east) and follow the blue blazes along level ground until you reach an old dirt road heading east–west and marked with blue blazes. This old forest road leads east across the north side of Peters Mountain to a power line that you can follow up to the AT on the ridge. That is about a 5- or 6-mile trek one-way. To reach the crest of Peters Mountain directly and the Clarks Ferry Shelter, walk across the road and follow the Susquehanna Trail as it begins to climb and switchback up the side of Peters Mountain. Although the trail gets a bit rocky in a few places, it is never excessively steep. Before you know, about a mile has passed and you have reached the ridge of Peters Mountain, where you rejoin the AT about 0.3 mile west of the shelter. So this little path saves slightly more than a mile of hiking up and is no steeper than following the AT.

After joining the AT, turn left, descend for a short distance, and just before returning to the ridge you'll reach the junction with the trail for the shelter, visible about 100 yards slightly downhill. The shelter has a nearby spring (treat the water if you drink it), a picnic table, and privy. About 100 yards from the junction, the AT crosses the ridge between two rock outcrops. When the leaves aren't thick on the trees, you can get a decent view to the north from this area.

The return trip follows the AT southbound (west) along the ridge. After passing the blue-blazed side trail that you followed up, the ridge gets rather narrow in places and requires you to do a fair bit of scrambling around and over rocks. At several spots you get nice views from the rocks to the north and south, but you reach the granddaddy of them all at about 0.75 mile beyond the junction with the ascent trail. The AT passes an open area along the rocks and affords a spectacular vista of the Susquehanna River and surrounding hillsides to the south.

Not far beyond the viewpoint, the ridge widens and the trail begins to descend to the right of a rock outcrop. For the next quarter-mile or so, the trail hugs rocks near the ridge, which afford many good places to have a seat and look out over the river. As the rocks come to an end, the AT begins to switchback down the very end of the Peters Mountain ridge as it descends to the river. Just beyond the last switchback is another very pretty vantage point that affords a view of Duncannon and the mouth of Sherman Creek across the river.

From the overlook, you have about a half-mile of pleasant, mostly level walking through the woods. This section of woods was home to an old settlement, the ruins of which still remain. Just before the junction with the ascent trail, you'll notice several stone foundations to the left of the trail. If you walk over to them, you can get another nice view of the river. From there, the AT descends for a half-mile back to the parking area.

Aside from the excellent views, this hike is also a nice place for birding, especially early and late in the day when the forest is filled with birdsong. Many species common to central Pennsylvania can be found in the area, including woodpeckers, warblers, and thrushes.

Nearby Activities

See profile for the nearby **Cove Mountain and Hawk Rock Loop** (Hike 22, page 116).

GPS TRAILHEAD COORDINATES AND DIRECTIONS
N40° 23.756' W77° 00.471'

Follow US 22/322 west from Harrisburg and take the PA 147/Halifax exit (just before the highway crosses the Susquehanna River). Park on the left at the end of the exit ramp.

5 Cold Spring and Rausch Gap Loop

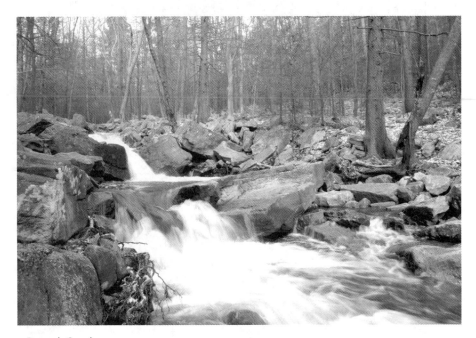

Rausch Creek

In Brief

This wonderful hike follows the Cold Spring Trail north out of the old town site of Cold Spring to the ridge of Sharp Mountain, where it joins the Appalachian Trail (AT). From there, you follow the AT east into Rausch Gap and down to the Stony Creek Trail (a.k.a. the Dauphin and Susquehanna Railroad Grade). Then follow the railroad grade west back to the parking area.

Description

This hike is one of my favorites in the area. It is neither long nor difficult, and it takes you through some wild and remote country. As you descend Cold Spring Road from the top of Second Mountain, either by car or by foot, look up the valley to the east and you'll be able to see a gap in Sharp Mountain, the ridge north of the Stony Creek Valley. That gap is Rausch Gap, the eastern extent of the hike.

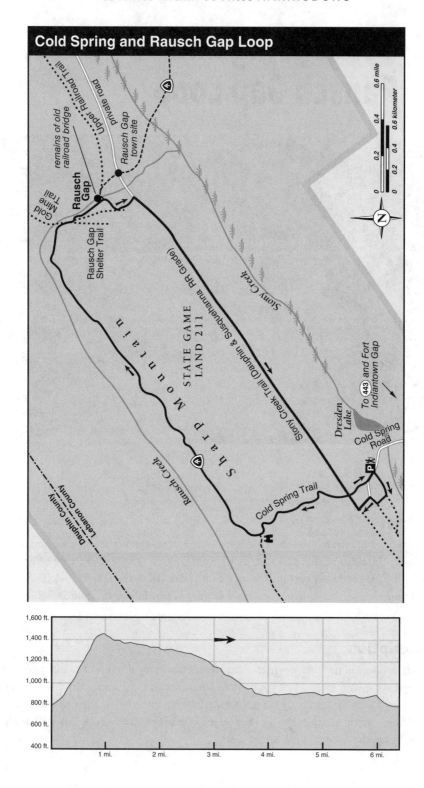

Cold Spring and Rausch Gap Loop

LENGTH 6.4 miles

CONFIGURATION Loop

DIFFICULTY Moderate except for 1 hill climb

SCENERY Cold Spring town site, upper Rausch Creek, Rausch Gap, Stony Creek Valley

EXPOSURE Shade

TRAIL TRAFFIC Light

TRAIL SURFACE Dirt

HIKING TIME 3–4 hours

DRIVING DISTANCE 6.4 miles from I-81 and PA 934 north of Harrisburg

ACCESS Open

MAPS USGS *Grantville, Tower City,* and *Indiantown Gap;* Keystone Trail Association *Appalachian Trail in Pennsylvania, Sections 7 and 8: Susquehanna River to Swatara*

Gap. The entire hike is on PA State Game Land 211, maps for which can be downloaded from the Pennsylvania Game Commission Mapping Center at tinyurl.com/pagamemappingcenter.

FACILITIES None

WHEELCHAIR TRAVERSABLE No

CONTACT Pennsylvania Game Commission, 717-787-4250, tinyurl.com /pagamelands

SPECIAL COMMENTS Cold Spring Road from the top of Second Mountain to the parking area can be very rough, with the worst bit being about 0.25 mile downhill. If you don't have a high-clearance vehicle, park at the top and walk down the road a short distance to see if it is passable. If not, park at the top of Second Mountain and walk down to the trailhead. Doing so will add about 1.6 miles to the round-trip, but may save you considerable aggravation.

This hike begins at the old town site of Cold Spring, a popular summer resort in the latter part of the 19th century. Reasonably well-preserved ruins of many of the resort buildings, including the hotel, caretaker's house, and mineral springs, still remain. After the resort closed, a water bottling company came into the area and attempted to market the spring water. And in the 1920s and '30s, a YMCA camp was located in the large meadow around what is now the parking area.

Begin this hike by walking north out of the parking lot past the large gate. After about 50 yards, turn right onto a significant (though unmarked) trail, following the path of an old logging road through a hemlock forest. This is the Cold Spring Trail. Walk uphill along the trail 0.25 mile and you'll reach the Stony Creek Trail. A sign marks the crossing of the Cold Spring Trail and another points in the direction of the AT, located just shy of a mile away on Sharp Mountain at the end of the Cold Spring Trail. Cross the rail-trail and head for the AT. Although the trail is rather rocky and climbs the entire way, it never gets excessively steep, and it makes for a rather pleasant warm-up. Just below the ridge, the trail joins a significant old roadbed and makes a couple of switchbacks up to the crest. You'll find a nice place to rest there at the junction with the AT. Enjoy the view and take a snack.

Turn right and head east now on the AT. At this point, you are traveling in the upper part of the Rausch Creek drainage, as wild and remote a country as you can find in this part of the state. To the right of the trail, the forest is rather open on the hillside up toward the ridge and consists of oak and hickory trees with some pines scattered about the rocky terrain. To the left, you'll see mountain laurel and thick brush because the creek is in that direction and the terrain is more swampy. The forest in the area provides excellent cover for all sorts of wildlife. On a December day with a couple of inches of fresh snow on the ground, I came up here and had the good fortune of spotting a bobcat sitting on the trail. I have also seen bear along the AT in this area.

The AT parallels Rausch Creek for 2 miles before both the trail and the creek make a bend to the south and cut through the Sharp Mountain ridge. This is Rausch Gap. A distinctive feature of the Valley and Ridge physiographic province of Pennsylvania, water gaps such as Rausch Gap (as well as others like the nearby Swatara and Indiantown Gaps) have uncertain origins, though many geologists believe that they may have been formed by the erosive force of glacial runoff as it found its way through weak bands of rock in the ridges many millions of years ago.

Approaching Rausch Gap, about 3 miles into the hike, you'll begin to see evidence of the coal mines that were in operation in the area late in the 19th century. Piles of culm and rock waste, now covered by ferns and trees, are an integral feature of the forest landscape. As you enter the gap, the trail passes in close proximity to the creek and at 3.25 miles, the red-blazed Gold Mine Trail (see page 68) enters from the left by a large camping area. Another 0.15 mile takes you to the junction with the blue-blazed Rausch Gap Shelter access trail (0.3 mile) to the right.

From the shelter trail, you can simply follow the AT down into the valley. I highly recommend, however, a slight deviation from that route for historic as well as aesthetic interest. At the junction with the shelter trail, look in the woods toward the creek and you'll see some red blazes. This is the lower end of the Gold Mine Trail. Although the trail is indistinct at times, the blazes are prolific as they follow the banks of Rausch Creek at its steepest and most rugged section. The creek thunders in places as it tumbles over boulders and steep drops to the Stony Creek. Follow those red blazes along the creek for 0.5 mile to the impressive ruins of an old railroad bridge across the creek. The bridge was the crossing on the upper railroad spur that used to run between Gold Mine Run and Rausch Gap. At the bridge, turn right on the old railroad grade and follow it back out to the AT (about 0.1 mile). Turn left and follow the AT down to the Stony Creek Trail, 0.25 mile farther on.

When you reach the rail-trail, take a few minutes to walk east over to the town site of Rausch Gap. The stone-arch bridge over Rausch Creek at the site is quite pretty. To complete this hike, walk 2 miles west on the rail-trail to the Cold Spring Trail. Before you head back to the car, however, be sure to visit some of the ruins of the old town site of Cold Spring. Walk another 0.2 mile west on the rail-trail and turn left onto the significant dirt road. Soon the road comes to a T. To the right will be the remains of the old hotel with its enormous spruce trees lined up across the front of it. On the left will be the foundation of the caretaker's house. If you turn left at the T, you'll come to the parking area very quickly. If you turn right and then make a quick left on the first old road, you'll come to the site of the old spring house. It is worth visiting. From there, you can pick up a red-blazed trail heading east and follow that a short distance to the parking area.

Nearby Activities

Memorial Lake State Park, in the town of Fort Indiantown Gap, has picnic and recreational facilities. The **Second Mountain Hawk Watch,** accessed by car along the ridge of Second Mountain east of Cold Spring Road, is well worth a visit, too. During the spring hawk migration, it is a popular spot for local wildlife enthusiasts. At all times of the year, it offers excellent views of Indiantown Gap, the Stony Creek Valley, and the terrain that the hike passes through.

GPS TRAILHEAD COORDINATES AND DIRECTIONS

N40° 28.638' W76° 37.548'

Take the Fort Indiantown Gap exit off I-81 north of Harrisburg. Follow PA 934 north 0.5 mile and turn left on Asher Miner Road, which eventually becomes PA 443. Follow 443 north into the water gap (Indiantown Gap). Turn left onto McLean Road (also called Ammo Road) just as you pass through the gap (there is a sign for the Second Mountain Hawk Watch on the right at the turn). Turn right on Cold Spring Road and follow it through the military reservation over the top of Second Mountain and down to the Cold Spring parking area in the Stony Creek Valley. *(See note on page 39.)*

---

6 Jonathan Eshenour Memorial Trail:

BULLFROG VALLEY POND TO WESTERN TERMINUS

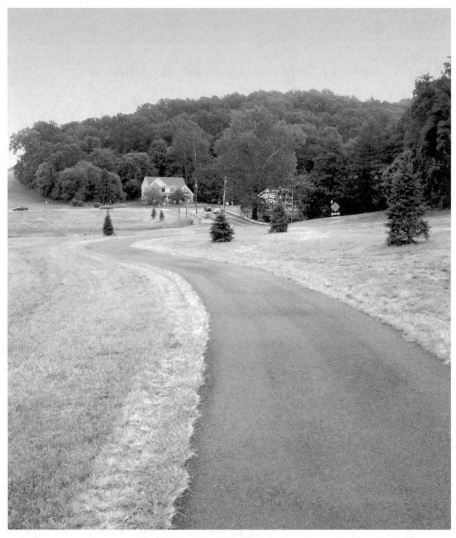

Jonathan Eshenour Memorial Trail east of Waltonville Road

LENGTH 3 miles	**ACCESS** Sunrise–sunset
CONFIGURATION Out-and-back	**MAPS** USGS *Hershey;* a map of the trail is available online at tinyurl.com /eshenourtrailmap.
DIFFICULTY Easy	
SCENERY Farmland and hills to the north of Harrisburg	**FACILITIES** Portable toilet, soda/water machines, picnic pavilion at trailhead
EXPOSURE Sunny	**WHEELCHAIR TRAVERSABLE** Yes
TRAIL TRAFFIC Light–moderate	**CONTACT** Derry Township, 717-533-7138, tinyurl.com/derrytwpparks
TRAIL SURFACE Paved	
HIKING TIME 1 hour	**SPECIAL COMMENTS** A very nice hike, though it might best be avoided on hot afternoons in the summer, as there is no shade.
DRIVING DISTANCE 0.8 mile from US 322 in Hershey	

In Brief

This pleasant hike follows the Jonathan Eshenour Memorial Trail from the Bullfrog Valley through farmland and meadows to its end west of Waltonville Road.

Description

The Jonathan Eshenour Memorial Trail is maintained by the Township of Derry and is named in honor of a young member of the Hershey community who was fatally injured in a bicycling accident in 1997. Funded in part by the Jonathan Eshenour Foundation, which sponsors the annual "Bike It–Hike It for Jon" event every year in May, the trail provides members of the community with safe recreational opportunities for walking, running, bicycling, inline skating, and wheelchair traveling throughout the township. Donations are accepted for development and maintenance of the trail, and interested parties can contact the Township of Derry Department of Parks and Recreation at 717-533-7138 for more information.

While estimations of its length vary depending on the source of information (the township map says the trail is 11.5 miles, while one website says it is 22 miles in length), my calculations show the trail to be 12.3 miles long. The primary 9-mile section extends from the eastern boundary of Derry Township at Lingle Road near Palmyra, winding its way through commercial and residential areas, and by public parks to Waltonville Road, south and east of Shank Park. An additional 1.5-mile spur heading south from the 4.5-mile mark of the trail, along with another 1.8-mile spur, the newest section of the trail, traveling west from Bullfrog Valley Pond along Wood Road, make for the rest of its mileage. Plans are under way to continue development of the trail by extending the new section west for another 3 miles to Middletown Road and the western township boundary.

This hike follows the newest leg of the trail, the 1.8-mile spur from Bullfrog Valley Pond to the western terminus of the trail and back. I chose this section for the hike because,

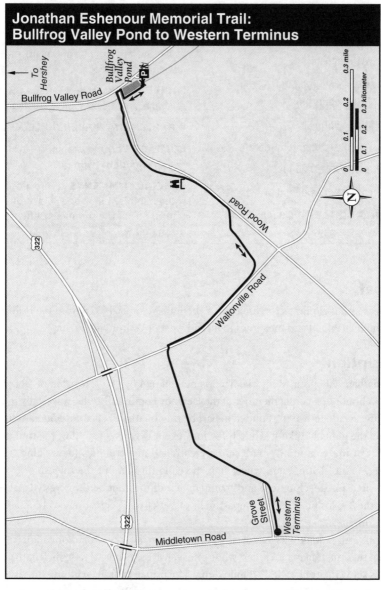

**Jonathan Eshenour Memorial Trail:
Bullfrog Valley Pond to Western Terminus**

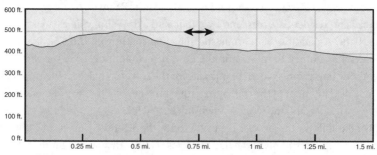

having hiked the entire trail many times, I think this section offers the nicest views of the farmland and hills to the north. It also does not appear to be as heavily traveled as other sections of the trail, and it tends to have less noise from traffic than other sections of the trail (especially that which follows alongside US 322 through town). The whole trail is nice, however, and is an enormous benefit to the community.

This hike begins at the parking lot at Bullfrog Valley Pond, located at the corner of Bullfrog Valley Road and Wood Road. The pond is a favorite fishing spot for young children having their first go at angling. In the past, the pond was also popular for feeding the geese and other waterfowl that visit the environs during the summer and fall. The constant supply of food, however, disrupted the migratory habits of the birds, and feeding them is now prohibited.

From the parking lot, cross the small footbridge over the stream and turn right onto the trail. I was impressed by the damage to Bullfrog Creek by the heavy rains that fell earlier this summer when I visited the trail to gather information for this profile. The stream had carved a new bed around a small flood dam just upstream from the bridge. Follow the trail around Bullfrog Valley Pond to where it crosses Wood Road at a stop sign, noting the spectacular sycamore tree at the northwest corner of the pond. Cross Wood Road and turn left. The trail immediately crosses the outflow from Bullfrog Valley Pond over a new footbridge, landscaped with black-eyed Susans and ornamental grasses. From the bridge, the trail climbs a grassy hill parallel to Wood Road on the left. At the top of the rise, 0.4 mile, you'll find a bench for sitting, with several young maple, oak, and fir trees planted behind it (aspiring shade trees). The view from this promontory to the north is outstanding, as it looks over large tracts of farmland dotted with stacked hay bales in the foreground and farther on to the hills north of Harrisburg.

From the top of the rise, the trail descends to the west and, at 0.7 mile, begins to make a long curve around a small farm complex at the intersection of Wood and Waltonville Roads. At 0.9 mile, the trail meets Waltonville Road, turns sharply right (north) and follows the road for 0.3 mile, where it turns left and crosses the road. Please be sure to use caution at this crossing.

Once across Waltonville Road, the trail continues directly west. On the right is a large field, planted some years with corn and other years with soybeans. On the left, the trail passes by a small stand of spruce and sumac trees. This stand is undoubtedly a resting area for white-tailed deer and red fox, as I have seen droppings from both along the trail on several occasions. The stand of trees is a good place to watch for songbirds. I have spotted bluebirds and goldfinches here in the past, as well as gray jays and grackles.

The trail continues west through farmland, offering pretty views to the south, and passes beneath power lines at 1.5 miles. At 1.8 miles the trail passes a pedestrian access point by a neighborhood cul-de-sac where a bench is located. Continue west for another 0.2 mile to the end of the trail at Middletown Road, where you will find a gazebo. From here, turn around and retrace your steps back to Bullfrog Valley.

Just a final word: While this section of the trail offers a lovely hike, it is almost entirely in the sun, and it can be very warm in the afternoon during the summer.

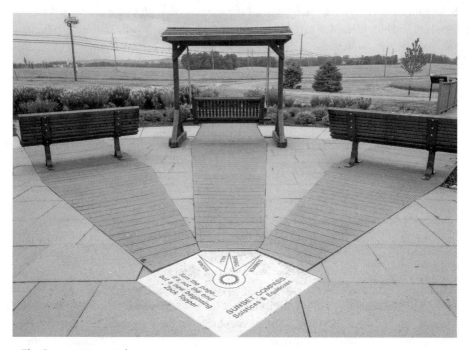

The Sunset Memorial

Nearby Activities

Hershey Park (800-437-7439, hersheypark.com) and **ZooAmerica** (717-534-3900, zoo america.com), both in Hershey, are popular destinations for families from the mid-Atlantic states. **The Hotel Hershey** (844-330-1711, thehotelhershey.com), on the hill to the north of town, provides some high-quality dining along with pretty views of the countryside. Across the street from the hotel is **Hershey Gardens** (717-534-3492, hersheygardens.org), which makes for a lovely walk.

GPS TRAILHEAD COORDINATES AND DIRECTIONS
N40° 15.451' W76° 41.051'

From US 322 in Hershey, head south on Bullfrog Valley Road. This is either the first light after US 322 and US 422 split coming from the west or the last light before they join coming from the east (just beyond the Penn State Milton S. Hershey Medical Center). The parking lot for Bullfrog Valley Pond is 0.82 mile ahead on the right, just past the intersection with Wood Road at the obvious duck pond.

7 Joseph E. Ibberson Conservation Area Loop

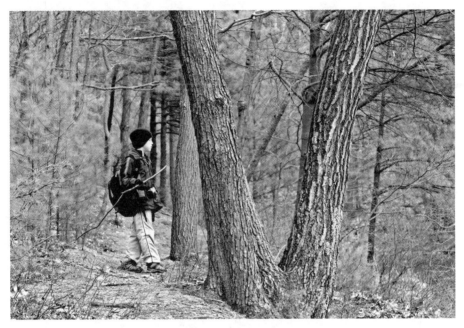

Enjoying the view from the Eagle Path

In Brief

This hike follows the Victoria Trail from just outside the parking area up to the Peters Mountain ridge. From the ridge, it backtracks the Victoria Trail for a half-mile and then follows several easy park trails back to the parking area.

Description

Located about 25 minutes north of Harrisburg, the Joseph E. Ibberson Conservation Area hosts a network of trails along the north side of Peters Mountain. Most of the trails have been created from old forest roads, so they are generally wide open and the grades gentle. The park is, consequently, a great place for an outing with the family, and it offers hikes ranging from less than a mile to several miles in length. This hike makes use of the trails around the perimeter of the 350-acre conservation area, and includes a side trip up to the Appalachian Trail on the crest of Peters Mountain.

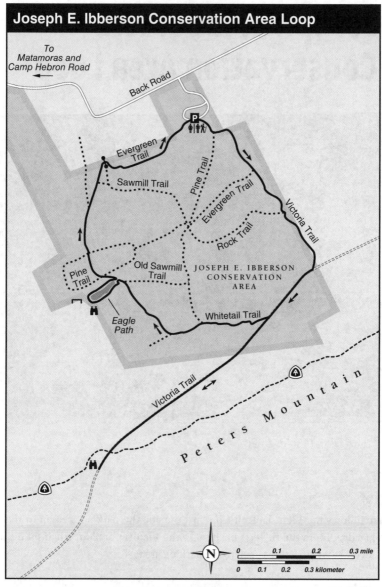

Joseph E. Ibberson Conservation Area Loop

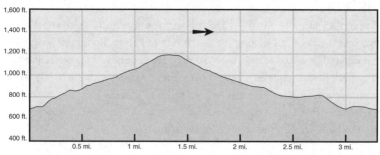

LENGTH 3.3 miles	**ACCESS** Sunrise–sunset
CONFIGURATION Loop with a section of out-and-back	**MAPS** USGS *Enders;* map available at parking area and online at tinyurl.com/ibbersonmap.
DIFFICULTY Easy–moderate	
SCENERY Nice walk in the woods; pretty views to north	**FACILITIES** Restrooms and water available at parking area
EXPOSURE Mostly shade	**WHEELCHAIR TRAVERSABLE** No
TRAIL TRAFFIC Moderate	**CONTACT** c/o Little Buffalo State Park, 717-567-9255, tinyurl.com/jibberson
TRAIL SURFACE Dirt	
HIKING TIME About 2 hours	**SPECIAL COMMENTS** This hike is a great outing with older kids in beautiful forest. If you leave out the climb to the top of Peters Mountain, it makes a good hike for the whole family.
DRIVING DISTANCE 10.75 miles from intersection of US 22/322 and PA 225 in Dauphin west of Harrisburg	

Originally purchased as a tree farm by forest manager Joseph Ibberson, the conservation area is home to a wide variety of trees, including oaks, pines, maples, poplars, and hemlocks. If you want to learn to identify trees, this is the place to do it. The forest provides habitat for many birds and deep-woods animals, including deer and black bear. A good time to visit the park to view wildlife is early in the day. The park is used primarily for recreational and environmental education purposes.

Begin this hike by walking out of the parking area from the main trailhead for the Evergreen Trail (by the restrooms) and turning left (southeast) on the first trail, following blue blazes. This is the Victoria Trail, and it runs all the way up to the ridge of Peters Mountain and then down the other side to PA 325 at the site of the old Victoria Furnace. The original trail served as a road that provided transportation of lumber to the furnace. You'll join the old roadbed in a short distance.

As you follow the blue blazes, you will pass several trails heading off left and right. None of the junctions provide any sort of route-finding difficulties. Just continue along the path following the blazes. At 0.5 mile, the trail joins the old roadbed that was the path of the original Victoria Trail. Turn right on the road and follow it for another mile up to the ridge. As you begin walking along the road, take note of the junction with pink-blazed Whitetail Trail on the right. After visiting the ridge, you'll return to this spot and head north on that trail.

The trek along the road up to the ridge is not very difficult, though it might prove to be a bit much for young children. If that is the case, you can skip the side trip and make the hike 1 mile shorter. Older kids should have no problem with it. When the leaves are off the trees, the Victoria Trail offers some nice views of the hills to the north. At the top, you'll find a gate and the junction with the Appalachian Trail. If you follow that to the west, you'll reach the Peters Mountain Shelter in about a mile (see page 92). After visiting the ridge, walk back down to the Whitetail Trail. Turn left and follow the pink blazes along a pleasant roadbed that descends at a very gentle rate. In a short distance, a yellow-blazed trail enters from the right (2 miles). Stay to the left following the pink blazes. After another 0.3 mile, you'll pass another junction with that yellow-blazed trail and then come to a pond on the left. A sign that says EAGLE PATH points to the short blue-blazed loop around the pond. Completing the Eagle Path loop is worth the effort. At the far end of the pond, you'll find a wonderful spot to sit and rest at a scenic bench. This pond is especially pretty in the fall when the leaves are changing.

After walking around the pond, turn left on the trail and walk up a moss-covered hill. At the top of the hill, you'll cross the green-blazed Pine Trail. Continue following the pink blazes downhill, and cross the Pine Trail yet again. In another 0.1 mile a trail with light blue blazes goes off to the left, and not far beyond that the Whitetail Trail (and the pink blazes) makes a sharp right turn uphill toward a small house in the woods. Continue downhill on the road from this point for a hundred feet or so to a gate across the road. At the gate, turn right onto the Evergreen Trail (red blazes) and follow that back to the car about 0.2 mile on.

Nearby Activities

Although it is not really that nearby, if you follow PA 225 north to Halifax and then pick up PA 147 north and take that to Millersburg, you can catch a ride on the **Millersburg Ferry,** the last operational ferry on the Susquehanna River. The paddle-wheel boat has room for three cars and passengers, and the trip across the river takes about 30 minutes.

GPS TRAILHEAD COORDINATES AND DIRECTIONS
N40° 26.544' W76° 51.555'

From US 22/322 west of Harrisburg, take the PA 225/Halifax exit. Follow PA 225 north over Peters Mountain 6 miles to Camp Hebron Road in Halifax. There is a sign for the conservation area at Camp Hebron Road. Turn right onto Back Road and follow it 4.75 miles to the entrance of the park, on the right.

8 Middle Creek Wildlife Management Area:
CONSERVATION TRAIL LOOP

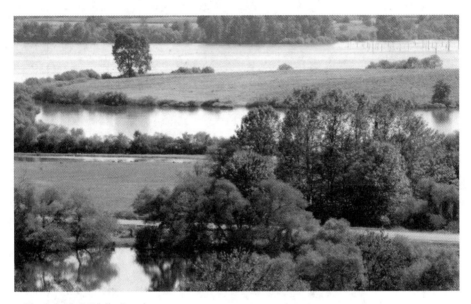

The lake at Middle Creek

In Brief

This short but pleasant hike begins by climbing a grassy hillside to a fence line that it follows to a trail in the forest. After a short level stretch, the trail descends, passes some food plots, and enters a wetlands area. After passing through the wetlands, it reaches a clearing for picnicking, and then climbs through a field of wildflowers back to the parking lot.

Description

This short hike is understandably popular with many visitors to the Middle Creek Wildlife Management Area. It provides a nice view of the management area from atop the first hill and offers the hiker exposure to various wildlife habitats, including forest, wetlands, and open fields. If you walk the loop counterclockwise (recommended), you'll reach a beautiful open area for picnicking near its end.

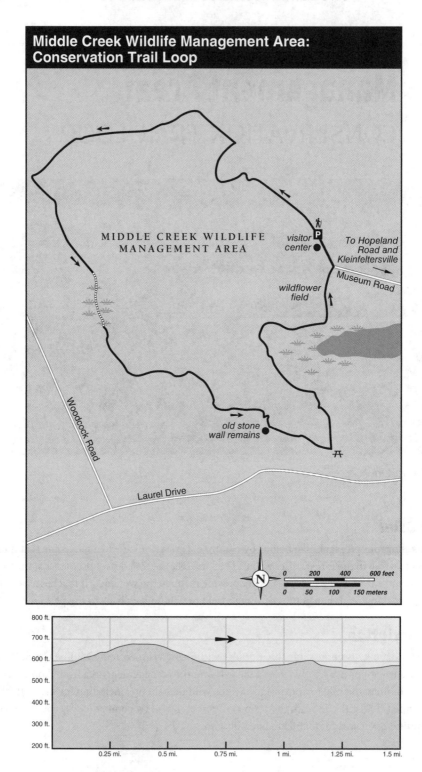

Middle Creek Wildlife Management Area:
Conservation Trail Loop

LENGTH 1.5 miles	**MAPS** USGS *Richland;* a trail map and interpretive brochure are available at the visitor center.
CONFIGURATION Loop	
DIFFICULTY Easy	**FACILITIES** Water and restrooms available at visitor center
SCENERY Views of the wildlife management area, forest, and wetlands	
	WHEELCHAIR TRAVERSABLE No
EXPOSURE Mix of sun and shade	**CONTACT** Middle Creek Wildlife Management Area, 717-733-1512, tinyurl.com/middlecreekwildlife
TRAIL TRAFFIC Moderate	
TRAIL SURFACE Dirt	**SPECIAL COMMENTS** This is a great hike for kids. It can easily be done in an afternoon along with the Willow Point Trail, which ends at a wildlife-viewing area by the lake. Information for the Willow Point Trail is available at the visitor center.
HIKING TIME 1 hour	
DRIVING DISTANCE About 13 miles from US 322 and PA 419 east of Hershey	
ACCESS Sunrise–sunset	

This hike begins at the main parking lot at the visitor center for the management area. A trip to the center is something you should do before (or after) the hike. Aside from information about wildlife management, you will find mounted examples of many of Pennsylvania's indigenous mammals and birds. Along the back of the building is a wonderful display of owls and raptors, and a picture window that offers a great view of the songbird feeding station and the main lake. The lake is a seasonal migratory resting place for Canada geese, a large variety of ducks, as well as herons and egrets and the occasional bald eagle. In early March, thousands of snow geese visit the lake during their spring migration.

The Conservation Trail leads out of the parking area from its northwest corner. From the door of the visitor center, facing the lot, it will be to your right. A sign that indicates you are indeed going in the right direction is located in the grassy field at the base of a short hill. Yellow blazes mark the route. The trail starts out as a path cut through grass and climbs the hill to the corner of a food plot by the trees. Then it heads left, following the treeline before turning right up a short steep section and out to a meadow by an old fence line. The view of the wildlife-management area here is wonderful.

After stopping to soak up the scenery, follow the trail along the fence line for 0.25 mile to where it enters the woods. The walk through the woods is pleasantly shaded on a wide-open, level path that gets a little rocky in places. After another 0.25 mile or so, the trail meets an old footpath that goes off to the right. The Conservation Trail stays left and descends 0.1 mile. The hickory and oak trees in this area are very tall, and it is a great place to watch for birds. Nesting boxes maintained by the game commission can be found on trees throughout the hike.

I've noticed when looking for birds, here and elsewhere, that you can walk for a long distance and not see any, and then suddenly you'll see several varieties clustered around the same area. I suspect that this has to do with the available food supply. But when I am looking, I tend to listen a lot, and when I hear them I'll stop for a while, wait, and watch. I've had pretty good luck spotting some unusual species this way.

After descending the short hill, from 0.5 to 0.6 mile, the trail passes three old food plots on the left. The right side of the trail has some dense thicket that provides good cover for chickadees and cedar waxwings. Just beyond the last of the food plots, the trail enters the wetlands area. I've always found this section of the hike rather enchanting. The trail crosses little creeks and marshy areas on bridges and short sections of boardwalk. The trees are very tall, and the lighting is rather subtle.

At 0.85 mile, the trail passes the remains of an old stone wall on the right, and another 0.1 mile takes you by a clearing, again on the right. The trail goes to the left at the clearing, not into it, and then enters a very rocky section before climbing to a large open field (the trail proper makes a sharp left where it meets the field). If you walk across the field toward the large trees, you'll find some picnic tables. Or just sit out on the grass.

To complete the hike, come back to the place where the trail meets the field and head downhill. Keep bearing left as the trail exits the woods along the side of a meadow and then back into the woods at a boardwalk through a boggy area. After passing the bog, the trail comes to a hillside of wildflowers and veers to the right along its bottom. Turn right, and in a short distance the trail turns left through a cut in the field toward a large oak tree at the parking area. It's worth taking your time through this meadow, as there are several nesting boxes here that provide shelter for tree swallows, eastern bluebirds, and great crested flycatchers. This is also a great spot to see butterflies in the late summer.

Nearby Activities

Both **Kleinfeltersville** and **Schaefferstown** are historic villages with a few small shops that are worth some time spent looking around. Schaefferstown is home to **The Franklin House Tavern & Restaurant** (101 N. Market St.; 717-949-2122, franklinhousetavern.com), where I have eaten several times and have been quite pleased. A little farther away, the site of the old **Cornwall Iron Furnace** (717-272-9711, cornwallironfurnace.org), a historic landmark, is just south of PA 419 in Cornwall.

GPS TRAILHEAD COORDINATES AND DIRECTIONS
N40° 16.288' W76° 15.044'

From US 322 East, turn left onto PA 419 toward Cornwall about 13 miles east of Hershey. Follow PA 419 into Cornwall, where you turn right and then make a quick left. Follow PA 419 north into Schaefferstown, where it merges with PA 897 and then turns north away from PA 897. Follow PA 897 east into Kleinfeltersville and make the first right onto Hopeland Road (11 miles from US 322). A sign for the Middle Creek Wildlife Management Area points the way. Follow Hopeland Road 2.3 miles past the lake on the left and turn right on Museum Road into the visitor center parking lot. The trail begins from the northwest corner of the lot.

9 Middle Creek Wildlife Management Area:
MIDDLE CREEK AND ELDERS RUN LOOP

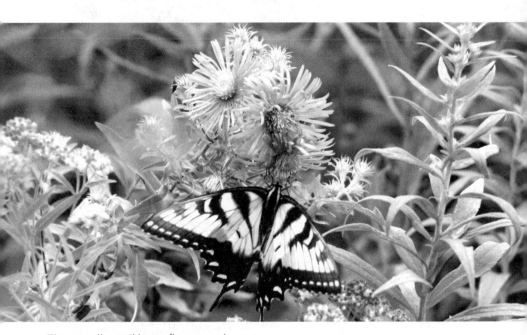

Tiger swallowtail butterfly on purple asters

In Brief

This hike follows the Middle Creek Trail along Middle Creek for just more than a mile to the junction with the Elders Run Trail, which it follows for another mile up to a ridge above the wildlife-management area. There it heads east on the Horse-Shoe Trail 1.75 miles back down to the car.

Description

This is my favorite hike in the Middle Creek Wildlife Management Area. At 3.75 miles, it is a pleasant length, and it passes through some varied terrain, each with its own rewards, including the pleasant scenery of the rocky Middle Creek, some old ruins, and nice views from the Horse-Shoe Trail along the ridge. This is a nice hike for kids, and for spotting

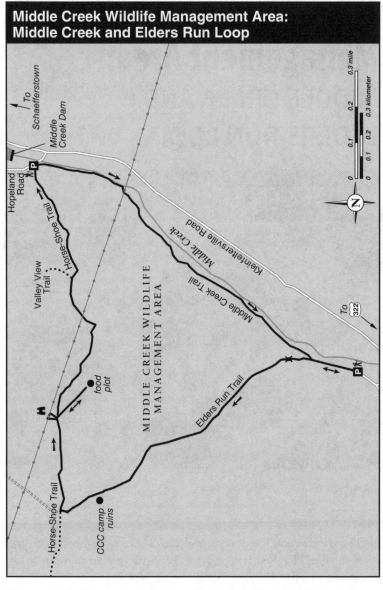

Middle Creek Wildlife Management Area: Middle Creek and Elders Run Loop

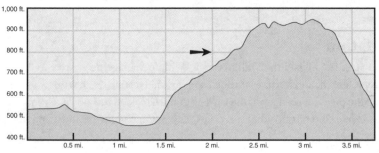

LENGTH 3.75 miles	**MAPS** USGS *Richland* and *Womelsdorf*; a map of the trails is available at the visitor center.
CONFIGURATION Loop	
DIFFICULTY Moderate	
SCENERY Middle and Elders Creeks, ruins of CCC camp, views of Lebanon County	**FACILITIES** None on trail; water and restrooms available at visitor center
EXPOSURE Mostly shaded	**WHEELCHAIR TRAVERSABLE** No
TRAIL TRAFFIC Generally light	**CONTACT** Middle Creek Wildlife Management Area, 717-733-1512, tinyurl.com /middlecreekwildlife
TRAIL SURFACE Dirt, rocky in places	
HIKING TIME About 2 hours	**SPECIAL COMMENTS** A good longer hike for kids, though slightly rough and rocky in places along Middle Creek. Be sure to wear blaze orange during hunting season.
DRIVING DISTANCE About 14 miles from US 322 and PA 419 east of Hershey	
ACCESS Sunrise–sunset	

birds if you are so inclined. I've seen plenty of wildlife on this hike and am always surprised by something. The loop can be done either direction, though following it clockwise makes for more pleasant walking.

The trailhead for this hike is found on the south side of Hopeland Road, just before it crosses over Middle Creek below the dam. You'll see a yellow road sign with a warning, BRIDGE MAY BE ICY, located right at the trailhead. Two trails go into the woods from here. Begin this hike by taking the left of the two trails, the Middle Creek Trail, which follows the creek downstream to the south for 1.5 miles. The trail to the right is a segment of the Horse-Shoe Trail that traverses the wildlife-management area, and it will be your return trail from the ridge above Elders Run.

At first, the surface of the Middle Creek Trail is dirt and mud, and it crosses over several boardwalks. The forest is full of big old birch, hickory, and beech trees in this area with the occasional huge sycamore, and you'll notice some very large recent deadfall as you walk along the creek. For all intents and purposes, the grade of the trail is level as it follows Middle Creek, but the walking can be a little tough in places where it gets rather rocky. At 1.4 miles, the trail crosses a footbridge over Elders Run, a small tributary of Middle Creek entering from the west. An ominous sign is posted on a tree to the right about 20 feet before the bridge that reads CAUTION: YELLOW JACKETS UNDER BRIDGE.

At 0.1 mile beyond the bridge, the Middle Creek Trail joins the Elders Run Trail, a wide gravel road. Whereas the Middle Creek Trail is open to foot traffic only, Elders Run is open to horse and bicycle travel as well. If you were to continue straight south after the junction, you would come to a parking area and a gate in another 0.1 mile, an alternate starting point for the hike. Here, however, turn to the right (north) and follow the Elders Run Trail through a forest that features some very tall sycamores and tulip poplars.

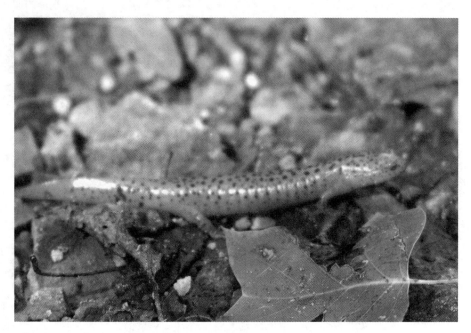

Northern red salamander

Shortly, the trail crosses Elders Run on a wide footbridge and begins to climb more steeply up the hillside for the next 0.2 mile or so before the grade becomes more gentle. In the late summer, I found a large (about 6 inches) spotted red salamander on the trail that I was very excited about, as I thought it was an endangered eastern mud salamander. From my photos, I determined later that it was a northern red salamander, which is plentiful in Pennsylvania. Nonetheless, it was an impressive and beautiful animal, especially to find just lying around on the trail.

At about 0.8 mile from the junction with the Middle Creek Trail, the Elders Run Trail passes by the ruins of an old Civilian Conservation Corps camp in the woods to the left (west) of the trail. The foundation of an old stone house with a large chimney remains, as does the stone foundation of the spring house. In another 0.2 mile, you reach the ridge at the head of Elders Run and the junction with the Horse-Shoe Trail, also an old roadbed at this point. A large clearing to the west provides browsing for deer, which I have seen frequently in this area, and another to the north provides a nice view toward Kleinfeltersville.

Turn right (east) here onto the Horse-Shoe Trail, and follow that for the next 2 miles or so back to the car. The path of the trail is marked with yellow blazes, and it climbs rather gently along the ridge from the junction. After about 0.3 mile, you'll come to a fork in the trail. The Horse-Shoe Trail continues along the right track past a large food plot. The left fork heads out to a power line and an open area that offers a nice view of the conservation area to the north. The best spot for the view is about a hundred yards along this trail and it is worth the short side trip. Another worthwhile detour is to wander around the food plot to the right of the Horse-Shoe Trail just beyond the fork. It is a great area for viewing wildlife, and a grove of large trees provides a nice spot for a break.

Not far beyond the food plot, the trail comes to a clearing. The woods on the left are home to many small songbirds, and the best time of year to view them is in November after the leaves drop. The trail is a little difficult to see as it passes through the clearing. Continue keeping the woods to the left (north) until you reach the far side of the clearing. An obvious track heads left out of the northeast corner of the clearing and very quickly meets the power lines. Tempted as you may be, don't follow it. The Horse-Shoe Trail continues directly east from the same spot, although it is a little brush covered where it exits the clearing and the blazes can be a bit difficult to spot. From this point, the Horse-Shoe Trail is a single track and it descends continuously to the car. Shortly, the trail will, itself, pass beneath the power lines, and when it reenters the woods the blazes become more obvious.

At about 2.2 miles beyond the junction with the Elders Run Trail, and about 0.4 mile from the end of the hike, the trail meets with the Valley View Trail. Marked by a sign and a yellow metallic blaze, it heads off to the left. Continue straight on the Horse-Shoe Trail, and in another 15 minutes you are back at the car.

Nearby Activities

Both Kleinfeltersville and Schaefferstown are historic villages with a few small shops that are worth some time spent looking around. Schaefferstown is home to The Franklin House Tavern & Restaurant (101 N. Market St.; 717-949-2122, franklinhousetavern.com), where I have eaten several times and have been quite pleased. A little farther away, the site of the old Cornwall Iron Furnace (a historic landmark) is located just south of PA 419 in Cornwall.

GPS TRAILHEAD COORDINATES AND DIRECTIONS
N40° 15.868' W76° 14.324'

From US 322 East, turn left onto PA 419 toward Cornwall about 13 miles east of Hershey. Follow PA 419 into Cornwall, where you turn right and then make a quick left. Follow PA 419 north into Schaefferstown, where it merges with PA 897 and then turns north away from PA 897. Follow PA 897 east into Kleinfeltersville and make the first right onto Hopeland Road (11 miles from US 322). A sign for the Middle Creek Wildlife Management Area points the way. Follow Hopeland Road 3.2 miles past the lake on the left and the visitor center on the right, and park on the side of the road just before the bridge over Middle Creek at a sign that says BRIDGE MAY BE ICY. The trailhead is by the sign.

10 Ned Smith Center

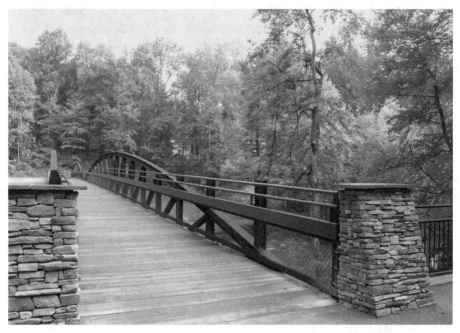

Bridge over Wiconisco Creek

In Brief

This hike follows the trail from the Ned Smith Center parking lot downhill to the bridge over Wiconisco Creek. After crossing the bridge, it climbs to the Railroad Bed Trail, where it turns to the right (west) or left (east). It follows the Railroad Bed Trail out to its end, and then back.

Description

I selected this hike because I wanted to include a nice hike that was wheelchair accessible even after a good rain and that provided reliable access to some of the beautiful Valley and Ridge scenery. I drove up to the Ned Smith Center for Nature and Art with the intention of hiking the Railroad Bed Trail, which I knew was wheelchair traversable. A new trail and bridge allows travelers to begin at the center and make their way across the river to the Railroad Bed Trail. I think that this makes a prettier and more varied excursion than simply following the Railroad Bed Trail, which is characteristic of a good rail-trail—well

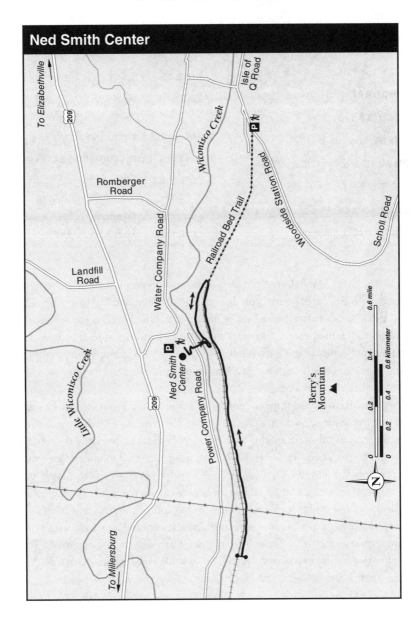

Ned Smith Center

graded, mostly straight, and accessible to bikers, hikers, and horseback riders. This hike offers more varied scenery.

The Ned Smith Center for Nature and Art is a wonderful place, and you should be sure to include a visit to its museum when you venture there to do this hike. Located just a couple of miles east of Millersburg above Wiconisco Creek at the base of Berry's Mountain, the center was founded in 1993 with the intention of promoting the relationship between nature and the arts. It is named for E. Stanley "Ned" Smith, a self-trained artist

LENGTH Either 2 miles or 3 miles, depending on which way you follow the Railroad Bed Trail	**DRIVING DISTANCE** About 2 miles from PA 147 and PA 209 in Millersburg
CONFIGURATION Out-and-back	**ACCESS** 8 a.m.–sunset
DIFFICULTY Easy	**MAPS** USGS *Millersburg;* trail map available at tinyurl.com/nedsmithtrailmap
SCENERY Wiconisco Creek	**FACILITIES** Water and restrooms
EXPOSURE More sun than shade	**WHEELCHAIR TRAVERSABLE** Yes
TRAIL TRAFFIC Moderate	**CONTACT** Ned Smith Center, 717-692-3699, nedsmithcenter.org
TRAIL SURFACE Cinder and gravel	**SPECIAL COMMENTS** An excellent excursion for wheelchair users
HIKING TIME 1.5 hours	

and naturalist from Millersburg who wrote about recreation and the environment for many years. Some of his artwork is on display at the center, and it is impressive. The gallery at the center has rotating exhibits by artists of national and regional importance. It also sponsors an annual nature and arts festival and many educational programs. One of its signature programs is the Saw-Whet Owl Research Program, which allows participants to "Adopt an Owl." For more information on the center and its programs, check its website at nedsmithcenter.org.

Begin this hike from the upper parking area at the center. From the sidewalk along the north side of the building, pick up a crushed gravel path heading into the woods toward the west. At the time of this writing, this initial section of the trail, from the center across the creek to the Railroad Bed Trail, was being completed. The trail follows gentle grades as it winds its way downhill toward the south to the bridge over Wiconisco Creek. Cross the bridge, and stop for a moment to admire the lovely chainsaw carving of regional birds on the south side of the bridge. Once across the bridge, follow the path as it winds up gentle grades through the woods. This is a beautiful forest containing a wide variety of trees, including several species of oak, maple, hemlocks, birch, beech, and pine trees. You'll find an attractive understory of mountain laurel, some wild raspberry, and sassafras. Poison ivy is abundant in the area as well, so be cautious about what you rub up against.

The trail climbs for nearly 0.5 mile, where it makes a sharp bend to the right (west) and joins the Railroad Bed Trail. Converted from an old rail line that used to carry coal from up the valley in Lykens and Wiconisco to the east to Millersburg for transport along the Susquehanna River, this trail extends for 1.75 miles through the center's property along the base of Berry's Mountain. You can go either left or right on the trail. If you turn left (east), you will pass the east trailhead for the Hemlock Trail almost immediately and then pass through pretty forest until reaching the eastern terminus of the trail after about 0.5 mile. If you are traveling after or during a rain, I would advise walking in this direction, as there are one or two places where the path gets a little muddy in the other direction.

If you head west, you'll soon pass trailheads for three different paths—the Mountain Laurel and Drumming Log Trails on your left, and then the western end of the Hemlock Trail on your right. Continue along the path to the west, taking in nice views of the creek and the surrounding countryside—and some raspberries if the season is right. I imagine that this would be a lovely walk in the fall. After about a mile, you'll reach a power line and the trailhead for the Powerline Trail. It is a gruesome-looking walk up the hillside. (If you are at all intrigued by it, have a look at the description for the Berry's Mountain hike in the first edition of this book.) The power line offers a pretty view of the countryside and the creek toward the north. It also makes for a good place to turn around. The trail continues for only another 0.2 mile to the west, to a gate by some private property. From the power line, turn around and retrace your path back to the parking area.

Nearby Activities

Be sure to visit the **Ned Smith Center for Nature and Art** on Water Company Road (717-692-3699, nedsmithcenter.org). In Millersburg, you'll find the **Wooden Nickel Bar and Restaurant** (717-692-3003, woodennickelpa.com) on the town square. The **Millersburg Ferry** is also worth a visit. It is the last operational ferry on the Susquehanna River. The paddle-wheel boat has room for three cars and passengers, and the trip across the river takes about 30 minutes. Follow signs for the ferry from the town square.

GPS TRAILHEAD COORDINATES AND DIRECTIONS

N40° 32.165' W76° 55.574'

From PA 147 in Millersburg, turn right onto PA 209 and follow it 1.85 miles to Water Company Road. Turn right. Follow Water Company Road downhill to the Ned Smith Center on the right. Park in the lot.

11 Rattling Run Town Site

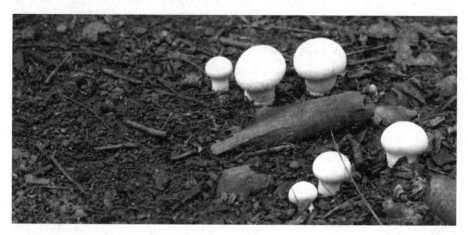

Puffballs along the Horse-Shoe Trail

In Brief

This beautiful hike follows the Stony Creek and Horse-Shoe Trails from the parking area at the gate on Ellendale Road up to the abandoned town site of Rattling Run. Most of the walk is along the old railroad grade in the bottom of the Stony Creek Valley.

Description

I have probably hiked along this section of trail above the Stony Creek more than any place else around Harrisburg. Although popular with cyclists on weekends, the trail is wide and long and encounters with other hikers tend to be infrequent. This out-and-back hike can be as long or as short as you like. It is approximately 6.5 miles from the trailhead to Rattling Run, the site of the first coal shafts in the Stony Valley (1825–1850), all but a mile of which (5–6 miles) is generally flat walking on a smooth cinder-and-dirt path. Your hike will be twice the distance you walk from the car.

The rewards of this hike are subtle. You won't find expansive views, but you'll see things such as mushrooms growing aside the trail, the contrast of fallen leaves against the brown of the trail, reflections on pools of water, shades and details and shapes of things in the woods. A few historical sites and landmarks can be found on the way. All of this against the sound of the creek flowing south of the trail.

Beginning at the Ellendale gate in the Stony Creek Valley, this hike begins by following the old Dauphin and Susquehanna Railroad Grade, which is referred to variously on maps and locally as the Stony Creek Trail or the Stony Valley Rail-Trail. About a mile along the

Rattling Run Town Site

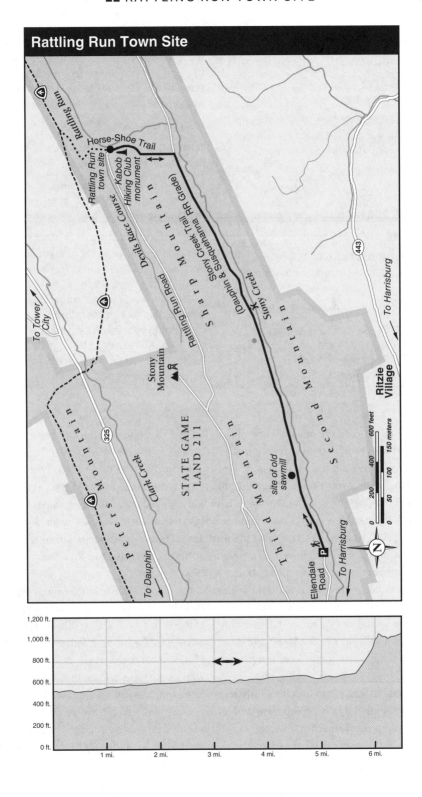

LENGTH 13 miles (or less)

CONFIGURATION Out-and-back

DIFFICULTY Easy–strenuous, depending on how far you go

SCENERY Stony Creek Valley, historic railroad, abandoned town site of Rattling Run, Kabob Hiking Club memorial

EXPOSURE Shade

TRAIL TRAFFIC Light

TRAIL SURFACE Dirt and cinders

HIKING TIME 5–6 hours

DRIVING DISTANCE About 9 miles from US 22/322 at the Dauphin Boro/Stony Creek exit west of Harrisburg

ACCESS Open; on state game land

MAPS USGS *Enders* and *Grantville*; Keystone Trail Association *Appalachian Trail in Pennsylvania, Sections 7 and 8: Susquehanna River to Swatara Gap.* The

entire hike is on PA State Game Land 211, maps for which can be downloaded from the Pennsylvania Game Commission Mapping Center at tinyurl.com/pagame mappingcenter.

FACILITIES None

WHEELCHAIR TRAVERSABLE For the first couple of miles, if dry

CONTACT Pennsylvania Game Commission, 717-787-4250, tinyurl.com /pagamelands

SPECIAL COMMENTS This hike can be made as long or as short as you like because it is out-and-back. The walk through the woods along the Stony Creek Valley is beautiful for the entire distance. Because this hike crosses state game land, care should be taken during hunting season. From November 15 through December 15, you must wear at least 250 square inches of blaze orange.

trail, you'll pass the site of an old sawmill on the right that operated during the late 1800s. Little remains now, with the exception of a flat area and a disused road cut that heads back to the creek. Beyond that, at just about 2 miles into the hike, the Water Tank Trail departs uphill to the left toward Third Mountain and the Stony Mountain Lookout Tower (see page 78). This was the site of a wooden water tank that supplied engines during the days of the railroad. If you keep your eyes open to the left of the trail along these first 2 miles, you might spot pairs of T-shaped concrete posts in the ground. These were used for storing track sections for the railroad. Track damages were frequent occurrences, and these storage areas provided the railroad crews with repair materials on the spot.

Many side paths lead down to the banks of Stony Creek. Fishing in the boulder-strewn Stony is good, and it is a pleasant stream for wading in and picnicking along. An especially nice spot on the creek is located directly south of the Water Tank Trail trailhead. It is boulder strewn with large pools. I've found the area to be good for spotting common birds such as nuthatches and woodpeckers, not to mention brook trout in the creek.

At nearly 3 miles, a small spring emerges from a steel pipe in the ground north of the trail about 20 feet. It can be a little difficult to locate but is worth looking for. It is a lovely spot surrounded by lush green ferns and mosses, and plenty of mushrooms if the time of year is right. In another 0.3 mile, the trail forks with a prominent roadbed heading right and down to the creek where it crosses over a hefty wooden logging bridge. Along the railroad grade beyond this fork the Stony Creek and Horse-Shoe Trails share the same path. The Horse-Shoe Trail east-bound turns right and crosses the creek via the bridge. The creek is quite pretty here, and if you walk upstream along its north shore, you'll find pleasant places to relax.

Continuing straight up the valley beyond the fork, the next significant landmark is the junction of the railroad grade with the end of the Rattling Run Road, entering from the north. The railroad grade continues east for another 19 miles to the Lebanon Valley Reservoir. The Horse-Shoe Trail turns left here and climbs to the Rattling Run site, 1.5 miles along the road. The first 0.8 mile provides a stiff climb before the grade becomes gentle again. If you decide to go the rest of the way, take note of the hillside to the left of the road as you climb. It is an expansive and rugged talus field in the forest all the way up.

As you approach the town site, you'll notice some ruins (mostly foundations) of old buildings on the right. Soon you'll find the monument commemorating the founding of the Kabob Hiking Club of Harrisburg and Vicinity here on October 21, 1934. I understand the club still exists, but information on their activities is difficult to come by. The turnaround for this hike is about 100 yards beyond the monument, where the Horse-Shoe Trail departs from Rattling Run Road and turns right across the Devils Race Course, the name of the drainage entering from the west. The terrain is extremely rugged and the stream here flows beneath the rocks. After a good rain, you can hear it coursing below. This boulder field is a geological formation created by the effects of erosion and freeze–thaw cycles.

If you are into very long hikes, this trek can be combined with sections of both Stony Mountain hikes in this book (see pages 78 and 83) to create a loop of about 16 miles or so back to the parking area in Ellendale. I've walked it, and it takes 8 or 9 hours. This is a popular excursion for mountain bikers.

Nearby Activities

Stony Creek is a very good fishing creek, especially in the area of the trailhead. The **Stoney Creek Inn** (717-921-8056, thestoneycreekinn.com), at the intersection of Erie Street and Stony Creek Road in Dauphin Boro, is a nice place to grab a bite after the hike.

GPS TRAILHEAD COORDINATES AND DIRECTIONS

N40° 24.385' W76° 49.106'

From Harrisburg, follow US 22/322 west to the Dauphin Boro/Stony Creek exit. Exit the highway and cross the creek. You are on Allegheny Street. Turn right on Schuylkill Street and then right on Erie Street (at stop sign). Signs point to Stony Creek. At the end of Erie Street, turn left on Stony Creek Road. Follow Stony Creek Road approximately 5 miles where it turns to dirt and is called Ellendale Road. Follow another 1.85 miles until the road ends at a gate with a large parking area.

12 Rausch Gap via Gold Mine Trail

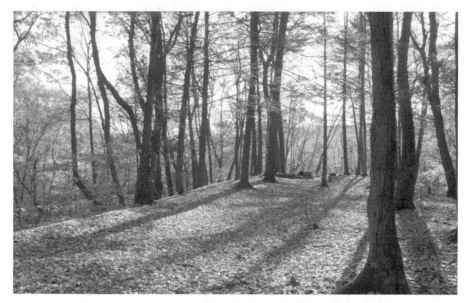

A campsite near Rausch Gap Shelter in fall

In Brief

This wonderful hike follows the Gold Mine Run drainage and makes a circuit around Sharp Mountain to its north. From the head of Gold Mine Run, descend into Rausch Gap, a water gap through Sharp Mountain, and join the Appalachian Trail (AT) near the Rausch Gap Shelter. From the shelter trail, follow the AT down to the Susquehanna Railroad Grade at the old town site of Rausch Gap, and then follow the grade east for 3 miles back to the car.

Description

This hike is one of my favorite outings in central Pennsylvania. It is a rather long hike in the hills, but with the exception of a few short rocky sections, the trails are smooth and pleasant to walk on. All along this hike you pass through remote terrain inhabited by bear and deer, as well as wild turkeys, grouse, and even the occasional bobcat. In the fall, when the leaves are changing, it can't be beat. In the winter, the light is stark and the scenery enchanting.

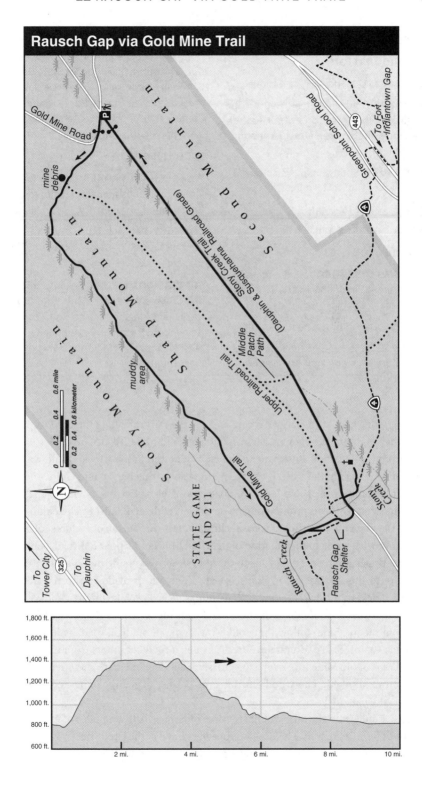

Rausch Gap via Gold Mine Trail

LENGTH 10 miles	*Appalachian Trail in Pennsylvania, Sections 7 and 8: Susquehanna River to Swatara Gap.* The entire hike is on PA State Game Land 211, maps for which can be downloaded from the Pennsylvania Game Commission Mapping Center at tinyurl .com/pagamemappingcenter.
CONFIGURATION Loop	
DIFFICULTY Moderately strenuous	
SCENERY Gold Mine Creek, Rausch Gap Shelter on the Appalachian Trail, Rausch Gap town site and cemetery, remnants of old coal mines	
	FACILITIES None
EXPOSURE Shady for first 7 miles, mostly sunny for last 3 miles	**WHEELCHAIR TRAVERSABLE** No, although the Susquehanna Railroad Grade would be when dry.
TRAIL TRAFFIC Light	
TRAIL SURFACE Dirt	**CONTACT** Pennsylvania Game Commission, 717-787-4250, tinyurl.com /pagamelands
HIKING TIME 5–6 hours	
DRIVING DISTANCE About 8 miles from the intersection of I-81 and PA 72 north of Harrisburg	**SPECIAL COMMENTS** Because this hike crosses state game land, care should be taken during hunting season. From November 15 through December 15, you must wear at least 250 square inches of blaze orange.
ACCESS Open; on state game land	
MAPS USGS *Tower City* and *Indiantown Gap;* Keystone Trail Association	

Begin this hike at the large parking area for the rail-trail along the old Dauphin and Susquehanna Railroad Grade on the west side of Gold Mine Road. The trail stretches 24 miles from the Lebanon Reservoir to the east along the Stony Creek all the way to the Ellendale trailhead in the west. From the parking area, walk back out to Gold Mine Road, turn left, and follow the shoulder of the road across the bridge over a creek. Just beyond the bridge, you will see a prominent gate on the left with an old dirt track behind it. Walk around the gate and follow the track as it climbs gently through an open forest of hemlock and oak for a half-mile to the junction of the Gold Mine and Upper Railroad Trails.

The Upper Railroad Trail heads to the left (west), traversing the south face of Sharp Mountain to the AT just below Rausch Gap. That trail provides a shorter alternative (about 8 miles) to this hike, though I think not as nice. This hike on the Gold Mine Trail goes around Sharp Mountain to the north and joins the AT above Rausch Gap.

From the junction, follow the Gold Mine Trail, an old haul road, as it heads north through a gap on Sharp Mountain. After 0.1 mile, a road cut enters from the right. Stay left and cross Gold Mine Run over a log crossing that demands care and attention to keep from getting dunked. The woods in this area consist of many young hemlocks interspersed with oak, hickory, and maple trees.

At 1.1 miles into the hike, you'll see some old mine shafts and piles of mine debris in the woods just off the trail. This area was heavily mined in the late 19th century, though as far as I am able to ascertain the mining was only for coal and not gold, as the name of the creek and trail might suggest. Deposits of gold have been found in streams in Pennsylvania, notably in York County, but mostly in the form of flakes rather than the nuggets that will make anyone wealthy.

Just beyond the mine remnants, the trail reaches a flat area and veers left, passing through a beautiful stand of pine trees. The path is marked by red blazes that become more abundant at this point. After passing the pine grove, continue in a southwest direction along a quiet and secluded old road, through beautiful forest for several miles. You are walking now along the north flank of Sharp Mountain, the crest of which is not far above you on the left. If you start early in the morning, the sun coming over the ridge is quite striking.

At approximately 3 miles into the hike, the trail gets rather muddy and at places less distinct as it passes through hemlocks (the state tree) and mountain laurel (the state flower). At this point, you have reached the wetlands forming the headwaters of Gold Mine Run, flowing east, and East Branch, flowing west. Shortly the trail becomes more distinct as it descends to the southwest. At 3.8 miles, it reaches a cut in the forest, a path for a pipeline. This is a nice spot for a break. From here you can see the ridge of Sharp Mountain just uphill to the south, and Stony Mountain to the north. The trail goes directly across the cut and enters the woods at a spot marked by several red blazes on the trunks of a few small maple trees.

After entering the woods, the trail becomes more of a footpath, dropping into Rausch Gap. Some attention to route finding is necessary as the trail approaches the AT. The blazes are plentiful for some distance and then become less so. The trail, though, is obvious, following an old logging track to the south and west as it descends into the gap. As the hemlock trees become more abundant, the trail reaches a flat spot with the remains of an old fire ring and then drops down a very short steep section. At the bottom, the trail appears to continue left across the hillside, but the red blazes call you directly downhill. Follow the blazes down to the creek. The red blazes guide you into an area where Rausch Creek is braided, and rather than making one big crossing you'll cross several small tributaries over rocks.

If you should miss the blazes, don't worry. Ultimately, whatever way you go, you'll end up at Rausch Creek rather quickly and the AT is just on the other side of it. The issue, however, is getting across the creek. The farther downstream you go, the more difficult it is to cross because its banks get steeper as it flows into the gap. If you find that's the case, head upstream until you find a suitable place to cross.

In the area of the braided stream, the blazes become more difficult to follow. But if you simply continue straight across the creek at the most convenient spot, and then veer to your left when you reach the far bank, you'll shortly reach a spot with lots of campsites above the creek. Here, the Gold Mine Trail joins the AT, with its ubiquitous white blazes that you follow south through the gap.

Not far beyond the junction of the two trails, a side trail marked by blue blazes heads off to the Rausch Gap Shelter. It is 0.3 mile out to the shelter along a broad, flat old railroad grade. The side trip is worth the effort. The shelter is actually built into an outcropping of rocks on the hillside. You'll find an outhouse and a spring at the shelter, plus a nice view to the east about halfway down the path.

From the junction with the shelter, follow the AT south down to the obvious Dauphin and Susquehanna Railroad Grade at 5.75 miles. Along the way, you will pass the junction with the Upper Railroad Trail, which began back at the east end of Sharp Mountain. Turn left (east) on the Susquehanna Railroad Grade, and follow the AT along it until the old stone arch bridge (built in 1850) over Rausch Creek. Just beyond the bridge, the AT leaves the railroad grade and heads south into the woods.

Historically, this is a very interesting area. Just north of the bridge you'll see the first limestone diversion well built in the United States (1986), which serves to reduce the acidity of Rausch Creek caused by drainage from old mines and acid rain. Upstream from the bridge, there are no fish, while downstream you'll find healthy native brook trout. Because Rausch Creek is the largest tributary of Stony Creek, the effect of the diversion well is significant for the pH levels as well as fish populations all the way down to the Susquehanna River.

Additionally, a sign on the south side of the trail at the bridge marks this as the site of the village of Rausch Run (1828–1910), whose major industries were coal mining and railroad repair. Although little remains of the town today, a side trip to the site of the Rausch Run cemetery is worthwhile. Follow the AT south from the railroad grade 0.3 mile to a trail junction marked by a wooden sign that reads CEMETERY. Turn left on the trail and follow it to the old cemetery among hemlock trees. There are several marked resting places of townspeople, and likely several other unmarked interments.

From the stone arch bridge, the remainder of the hike follows the railroad grade for another 3.5 miles back to the parking area. It's a wonderful walk with long sections through pine and hemlock forest that has a very intense bluish-green color to it.

GPS TRAILHEAD COORDINATES AND DIRECTIONS

N40° 31.456' W76° 32.462'

From I-81 north of Harrisburg, exit at Lickdale and follow PA 72 north 3.3 miles to PA 443. Turn right on PA 443 and follow it north 1.75 miles to Gold Mine Road. Turn left and follow Gold Mine Road 2.8 miles over the top of South Mountain to the parking area for the Susquehanna Railroad Grade on the left. A large cement slab is visible on the right across the road from the entrance to the parking area. Park near the gate across the railroad grade.

13 State Game Land 156

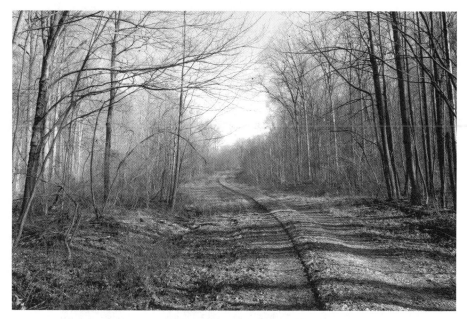

Beginning the ascent from the lowest point on the trail

In Brief

This hike follows the main state-game-lands road (snowmobiles and ATVs ridden by hand-icapped hunters are the only motorized vehicles allowed) west into the heart of the game lands. At the second major T-intersection next to a large clearing on the left, the route goes to the north (right) and makes a 3-mile loop descending down to the level of the Pennsyl-vania Turnpike before climbing back to the clearing.

Description

At nearly 10 miles in length, this is a rather long hike. Yet the entire excursion follows good dirt roads that are closed to vehicular traffic. The grades are all very reasonable, so the walking is pleasant. This excursion provides a wonderful outing through the Furnace Hills area of Lancaster County, the largest tract of forested land in the county. The region was so named because of the numerous coal furnaces and forges in operation in the area during the 19th century. Just 3 miles to the south, Speedwell Forge in Lancaster County is the coal forge closest to this hike. The Cornwall Iron Furnace in Lebanon County is also located nearby.

State Game Land 156

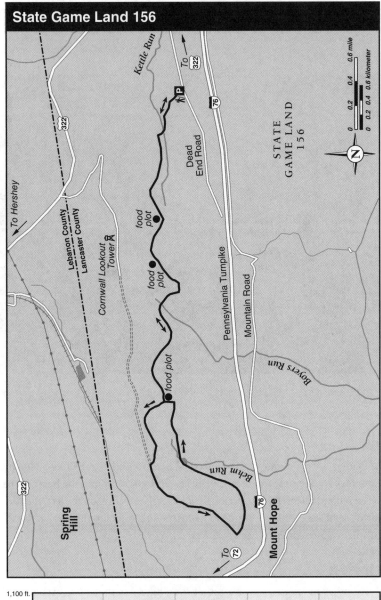

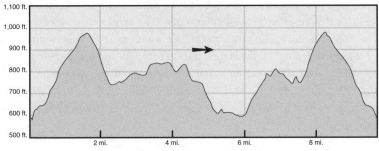

LENGTH 9.7 miles	**ACCESS** Open; on state game land
CONFIGURATION Balloon	**MAPS** USGS *Manheim* and *Lititz;* the entire hike is on PA State Game Land 256, a map of which can be downloaded from the Pennsylvania Game Commission Mapping Center at tinyurl.com/pagame mappingcenter.
DIFFICULTY Strenuous because of length	
SCENERY Furnace Hills environs; nice views of Lancaster County to southwest; pretty forest of mature white ash	
	FACILITIES None
EXPOSURE About half sun and half shade	**WHEELCHAIR TRAVERSABLE** Some sections, if trail is dry
TRAIL TRAFFIC Generally light	**CONTACT** Pennsylvania Game Commission, 717-787-4250, tinyurl.com /pagamelands
TRAIL SURFACE Dirt; trail follows old roadbeds.	
HIKING TIME 5–6 hours	**SPECIAL COMMENTS** The entire hike is on state game land. Wear blaze orange during hunting season and consider hiking on Sundays.
DRIVING DISTANCE About 8 miles from the PA 72 (Lancaster/Lebanon) exit off I-76, the Pennsylvania Turnpike	

This entire hike is on state game lands that provide habitat for white-tailed deer, red fox, rabbit, ruffed grouse, wild turkey, migrating warblers, wrens, and vireos among other species of wildlife. One of the most interesting aspects of the terrain is the abundance of mature white ash throughout the area. You will also find butternut trees along the lower, most distant stretch of the path.

Begin the hike by following the dirt road past the access gate in the back of the parking area. Climb a gentle grade through the woods and into an open area with quite a bit of thicket with several birdhouses along the road. After it passes the clearing, the trail enters the woods and then climbs a steady grade, passing several small clearings for a mile. Along the way, you'll pass many staghorn sumac trees, which in the winter present a stocky scarlet cluster of seedpods pointing upward. They are quite attractive, especially against a blue sky. At the top of the rise, about 1.25 miles, you'll come to a large clearing identified by a small stand of spruce trees near a junction with a road heading off to a food plot on the left. The clearing offers a pretty view to the north of the main ridgeline of the Furnace Hills, topped by radio towers and a lookout tower. The Horse-Shoe Trail traverses that ridge, and it may be accessed from Pumping Station Road by US 322 to the north.

The walking is flat for the next 0.25 mile and then the trail begins to descend near another food plot. The expansive view of Lancaster County to the southwest from here is quite lovely. Soon you enter the woods and shortly thereafter (2 miles) you reach a significant T-intersection in the road. The road to the left is marked by a small, triangular green equestrian sign and several large game-lands signs indicating that the area is closed to all motor vehicles and snowmobiles. Turn right here and descend into a large hollow, crossing a concrete bridge–culvert over the creek after a short distance. The forest consists of

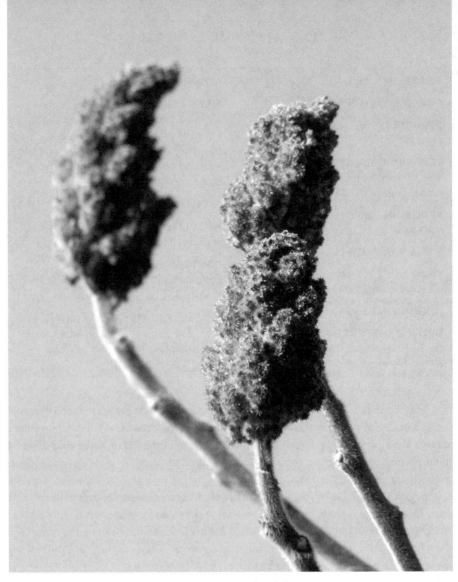

Staghorn sumac

mature birch trees and white ash. White ash is identified best by its thin seedpods about 2 inches long. They cover the ground during the fall and winter. Taller than the related black ash, which reaches only about 40 feet in height, white ash can reach 80 feet. Many of the trees in this area are nearly that tall.

At approximately 3.2 miles, you come to another T-intersection at a large food plot on the left that lies in a valley between two ridges. This is the beginning of a 3-mile loop through the lower, western section of the preserve. The food plot on the left provides a wonderful location for a break before and after completing the loop. Pull up a seat on an old log near the edge of the plot, and watch for birds in the bushes here. Turn to the right and traverse the hillside for another 0.75 mile past the access road to the radio towers on the north ridge. Continue walking straight along the road as it follows the ridgetop to the southwest. As you proceed you'll pass some timber sale areas that have been recently clear-cut.

At about 5 miles, the trail curves back to the east and descends for a little distance farther before beginning the climb back to the end of the loop. The Pennsylvania Turnpike is nearby, just a couple of hundred yards through the woods to the south, and its din is omnipresent. Before reaching the lowest elevation of the hike, you'll pass some ash saplings as well as some mature trees. Along the road are butternut trees, identified by the straggly branches and their bunches of seedpods. They are distinct from the other trees, and the contrast is enough to make them easily recognizable.

Continue along the road heading up a small valley, passing a tiny pond surrounded by cattails on the right. A birdhouse and a waterfowl box have been constructed here, though neither was occupied when I passed through in the winter. The remaining 0.4 mile from the pond back to the food plot and the end of the loop passes through a very scenic area, with the road rising ahead of you beneath a tree-covered ridge. As you enter the food plot, take notice of the propagation area on the right defined by a wire fence. A forest management site, the fence is designed to keep deer from browsing on the bark of young trees within the area.

From the end of the loop, you have another 3 miles of walking back to the car, much of which is downhill. With the trek being mostly on good dirt roads, I imagine that this route would make for a nice mountain biking trip.

Nearby Activities

Speedwell Forge County Park is about a mile south on Speedwell Forge Road from Dead End Road. The parking area is on the right just over Hammer Creek at a bend in the road. A short walk takes you to the site of the old forge. If you don't feel like hiking anymore (which wouldn't be surprising) but are still interested in taking in some of the history, the **Cornwall Iron Furnace** in Cornwall is less than 6 miles away (717-272-9711, cornwallironfurnace.org). It has a museum with several exhibits and informative programs. The grounds are also nice for picnicking. From Pumping Station Road, head east on US 322 2.9 miles. Turn right on Granite Road and follow it for another 2 miles to the furnace.

GPS TRAILHEAD COORDINATES AND DIRECTIONS
N40° 14.035' W76° 20.958'

From I-76 (the Pennsylvania Turnpike), follow PA 72 north to US 322. Drive east on 322 about 5.75 miles. Turn right on Speedwell Forge Road and, just before the turnpike overpass, turn right on Dead End Road, very obviously marked with a sign. Follow 0.75 mile to the large state-game-lands parking lot on the right, marked by a sign on the road.

14 Stony Mountain from the North

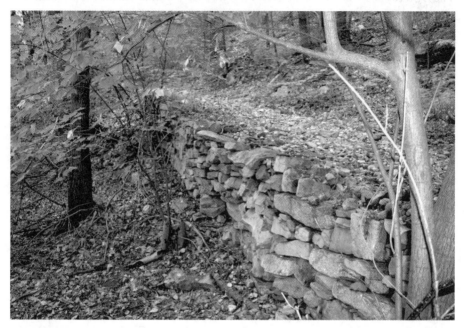

Old haul road on Stony Mountain

In Brief

This wonderful hike follows the Appalachian Trail (AT) as it traverses the north side of Stony Mountain to the ridgeline, where it joins the Horse-Shoe Trail at its western terminus. After descending the Horse-Shoe Trail for 0.6 mile, it joins Rattling Run Road at the Devils Race Course and the old town site of Rattling Run. From here, the hike follows Rattling Run Road up to Third Mountain, where it picks up the northern extension of the Water Tank Trail and descends the mountain, concluding the loop. A short (1.2 miles round-trip) side trip brings you to the site of the Stony Mountain Lookout Tower.

Description

The first 3 miles of this long and beautiful hike follow the AT up to Stony Mountain on Pennsylvania State Game Land 211. From the parking area, cross Clark Creek on a

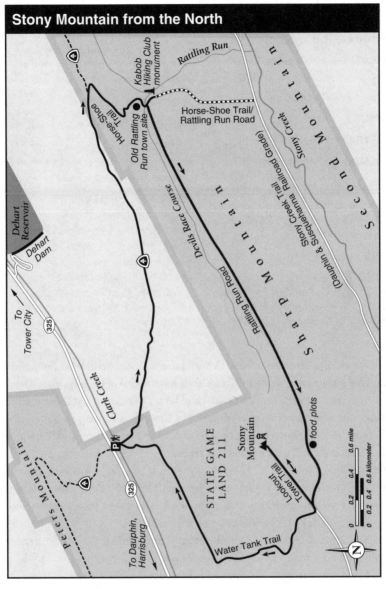

Stony Mountain from the North

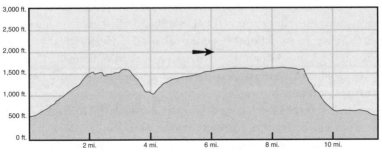

LENGTH 11.5 miles	hike is on PA State Game Land 211, maps for which can be downloaded from the Pennsylvania Game Commission Mapping Center at tinyurl.com/pagame mappingcenter.
CONFIGURATION Loop	
DIFFICULTY Very strenuous	
SCENERY Appalachian Trail; Rattling Run town site; Devils Race Course	
	FACILITIES None
EXPOSURE Mostly shaded	**WHEELCHAIR TRAVERSABLE** No
TRAIL TRAFFIC Light	**CONTACT** Pennsylvania Game Commission, 717-787-4250, tinyurl.com /pagamelands
TRAIL SURFACE Dirt and rocky	
HIKING TIME 6 hours	
DRIVING DISTANCE About 12.5 miles from the intersection of US 22/322 and PA 225 west of Harrisburg	**SPECIAL COMMENTS** A beautiful long walk in the woods, though best to allow a full day. The descent could be a little treacherous if wet. Because this hike crosses state game land, care should be taken during hunting season. From November 15 to December 15, you must wear at least 250 square inches of blaze orange.
ACCESS Open; on state game land	
MAPS USGS *Enders* and *Grantville;* Keystone Trail Association *Appalachian Trail in Pennsylvania, Sections 7 and 8: Susquehanna River to Swatara Gap.* The entire	

footbridge, passing a gate. Just beyond the bridge, you'll see two blue blazes marking a forest road. That is the end of the Water Tank Trail and the end of the loop hike. The junction with the AT is marked at this spot by two white blazes indicating that the trail turns left.

At first the AT follows a small tributary of Clark Creek along an old roadbed. The forest here is one of the prettiest places I have been in Pennsylvania, with hemlock trees along the creek, and tall hickory and oak trees stretching up the rocky and rugged hillside. The roadbed continues all the way to the crest of Stony Mountain, traversing the side of the mountain and providing nice views of the Clark Creek Valley during the fall and winter. As you progress, the trail becomes a little steep, though never too bad. It does, however, get quite rocky after the first 0.5 mile or so.

At about 2 miles, the trail descends rather significantly for a short distance. In this area you'll notice remnants of old switchbacks and retaining walls of one of the old coal roads that used to climb the mountain. Just shy of 3 miles, the trail climbs for a short distance and then tops out on the ridge. At the ridgecrest, two yellow blazes on a birch tree to your right indicate the beginning of the Horse-Shoe Trail. It extends for approximately 142 miles to Valley Forge National Historic Park outside Philadelphia. Just ahead, the Horse-Shoe Trail and the AT part ways at a stone memorial dedicated to Cyril C. Sturgis Jr., an active member of the Horse-Shoe Trail Club during the 1960s. A yellow horseshoe is nailed to the tree next to it.

After a well-deserved break here, follow the Horse-Shoe Trail past a trail register, down the south side of the ridge contouring to the west. You are now entering a region known as St. Anthony's Wilderness, one of the largest open and wild areas in the state.

The Horse-Shoe Trail descends rather steeply for the next half-mile before leveling out by the old town site of Rattling Run. Rattling Run was the location of the Stony Valley's first coal shafts, named Reliance and Perseverance, which were mined from 1825 to 1850. Just left of the trail you can find the ruins of old buildings. One look at the terrain makes obvious the sorts of hardships people went through to mine coal. The forest floor is nothing but an expansive talus field that the main creek, the Devils Race Course, flows beneath.

Just past the town site, the trail joins the old Rattling Run Road. The Horse-Shoe Trail turns to the left here and descends into the Stony Creek Valley. This hike follows Rattling Run Road uphill and west along the Devils Race Course to the head of the drainage at the junction of the ridges that form Sharp Mountain (to your left as you are walking) and Stony Mountain (to the right). A large flat rock on the right provides a comfortable spot to rest about 100 feet up the road from the trail junction. Before heading uphill, however, be sure to walk downhill about a hundred yards to have a look at the monument commemorating the founding of the Kabob Hiking Club of Harrisburg and Vicinity.

From its junction with the Horse-Shoe Trail, Rattling Run Road climbs rather steeply at first, but it soon levels out and for the next several miles climbs at a gentle grade. The hiking here through a forest of birch and hickory trees is pleasant, as the path is sandy and grassy. The occasional yellow blazes indicate that this was the old path of the Horse-Shoe Trail, now rerouted.

This hike follows Rattling Run Road for approximately 3.5 miles from the junction to the trail spur that leads to the Stony Mountain Lookout Tower. On the way, you'll pass a significant road cut on the right at 6.1 miles (the Henry Knauber Trail), and two large food plots numbered 5 and 6 (7.1 miles). These food plots provide food and shelter for wildlife on the game lands, and they are often planted with grasses or feed corn.

Another 0.6 mile beyond the plots and you arrive at the junction with the spur to the lookout (7.75 miles). No sign marks the spur, though it is easily identifiable because it is a dead straight and flat dirt road with a swath of brush and brambles about 100 feet wide on each side of it. You'll undoubtedly feel a bit tuckered out when you reach the junction, but it is a flat, easy walk out to the lookout. An old fire tower, it's a large steel structure, 150 or so feet high, with a platform and small shelter on top.

Note: Climbing the tower is illegal, and a gate around the bottom is typically locked, but the clearing at the lookout's base is a nice place to rest and offers nice views to the north and east.

After the side trip to the lookout, you'll next head to the north extension of the Water Tank Trail. It can be a little difficult to locate. From the junction of Rattling Run Road and the road to the lookout tower, walk west for 100 feet or so until you reach a small clearing to your right. Follow the road to the end of the clearing. On your left will be a tall oak with a blue blaze that marks the path of the Water Tank Trail as it enters the woods heading south. A small cairn is located on the right side of the road marking the path of the north extension, though the path is indistinct through the clearing. If you look into the woods, you should spot a blue blaze on a tree. Keep in mind that the Water Tank Trail crosses directly perpendicular to Rattling Run Road. If you don't spot the blaze, follow the edge of the clearing until you reach the woods. The trail is obvious when it enters the woods and is well marked with blue blazes all the way down the mountain. Significant deadfall obstructs the trail in several places and requires a little circumnavigation. Make sure that you get back on the trail and see the blazes before wandering too far.

After about 0.2 mile of walking through the woods along rather level terrain, the trail descends abruptly and drops left from a prominent cairn. Although steep, the trail surface is mostly dirt and offers good footing through a pretty forest of fir trees. After a while, the footing gets more rocky and rugged, demanding attention, but is manageable. At 8.9 miles, you'll reach a flat area on the hillside where you'll find a maple tree with a bunch of blazes. The trail bends to the right here.

The walking gets considerably more rocky for the next 0.8 mile from the bend, but is not as steep as above. In spots it is rather brushy and heavily eroded, appearing to be little more than a watercourse. But it is always well marked. At just about 10 miles into this hike, you emerge from the woods at a significant logging road. Turn right here (east) and follow the road for 1.5 miles to the end of the Water Tank Trail at its junction with the AT. Along the way, you'll pass a large clearing (10.5 miles) to the south of the trail with some very tall trees. This is a great place to spot hawks.

At about 11.1 miles, the road enters an area that has been recently cleared of trees, with a new road cut heading into the woods to the east. The Water Tank Trail and the original roadbed make a left here, heading downhill toward the creek. A blue blaze marks the way on a tree just downhill from the clearing.

You could, of course, reverse the route (I think it walks better in a clockwise direction), or simply hike from the Clark Creek parking area up the Water Tank Trail to visit the lookout tower (a popular and much shorter hike of about 3.3 miles each way). If you choose that route, be certain to pick up the Water Tank Trail where it begins to climb at the right place (about 1.5 miles). Heading west, you'll pass three decent-sized meadows, all of which have an old logging road heading up the side of the mountain. The Water Tank Trail is obviously a footpath where it departs from the road, although there is no sign, just a few blue blazes on a tree to the left.

Nearby Activities

Clark Creek, which parallels PA 325, offers wonderful fishing for both bait and fly anglers.

GPS TRAILHEAD COORDINATES AND DIRECTIONS
N40° 27.100' W76° 46.571'

Follow US 22/322 west from Harrisburg to the PA 225/Halifax exit. Follow PA 225 north 2.5 miles to PA 325. Turn right on PA 325 and follow it 9.9 miles to the Appalachian Trail crossing. The AT is well marked. Park on the right behind the little hill next to the road.

15 Stony Mountain from the South

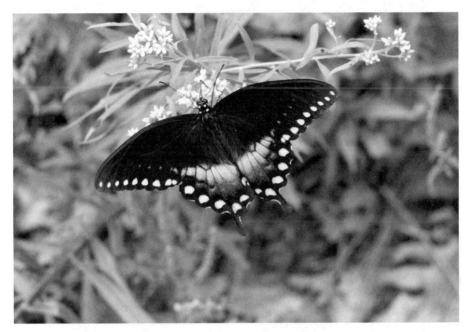

Black swallowtail butterfly

In Brief

This lovely hike begins by following the multiuse Dauphin and Susquehanna Railroad Grade for 2 miles along the Stony Creek Valley. At 2 miles, it picks up the Water Tank Trail and climbs steeply to the ridge of Stony Mountain, where it meets with Rattling Run Road. A short (1.2 miles round-trip) detour takes you to the Stony Mountain Lookout Tower. The descent follows Rattling Run Road down the south side of Third Mountain and back to Ellendale Road.

Description

Begin this hike at the Ellendale gate at the old Dauphin and Susquehanna Railroad, also known as the Stony Creek Trail. In operation during the early 1800s, the railroad was used to support coal-mining operations in and around the Stony Creek Valley. Now the

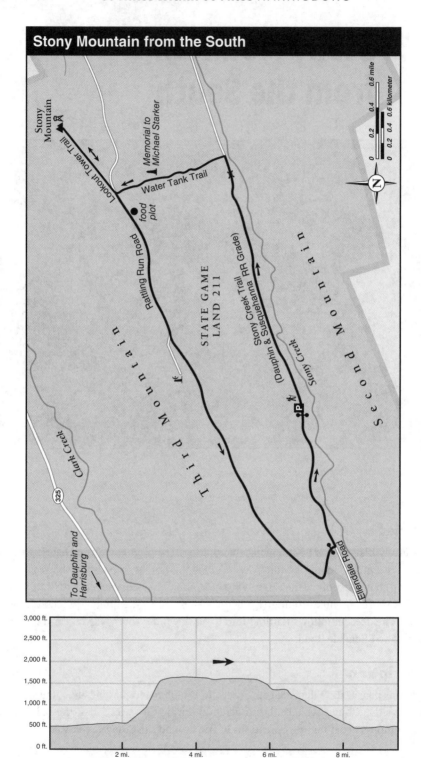

Stony Mountain from the South

LENGTH 9.5 miles

CONFIGURATION Loop

DIFFICULTY Very strenuous

SCENERY Stony Creek Valley and ridge of Stony Mountain

EXPOSURE About half sun and half shade

TRAIL TRAFFIC Light

TRAIL SURFACE Dirt and rock

HIKING TIME 4.5–5.5 hours

DRIVING DISTANCE About 9 miles from US 22/322 at the Dauphin Boro/Stony Creek exit west of Harrisburg

ACCESS Open; on state game land

MAPS USGS *Enders* and *Grantville*; Keystone Trail Association *Appalachian Trail in Pennsylvania, Sections 7 and 8: Susquehanna River to Swatara Gap.* The entire hike is on PA State Game Land 211, maps for which can be downloaded from the Pennsylvania Game Commission Mapping Center at tinyurl.com/pagame mappingcenter.

FACILITIES None

WHEELCHAIR TRAVERSABLE No

CONTACT Pennsylvania Game Commission, 717-787-4250, tinyurl.com /pagamelands

SPECIAL COMMENTS With the exception of the third mile of the hike, which ascends 1,000 feet along a rough and rocky path, all of the walking is on good roadbeds with easy or moderate grades. The Water Tank Trail is subject to flooding and may be impassable during and after heavy rains. Because this hike crosses state game land, care should be taken during hunting season. From November 15 through December 15, you must wear at least 250 square inches of blaze orange.

railroad grade serves as a path for hikers, bikers, and horseback riders, and it extends for 24 miles to the Lebanon Reservoir in Schuylkill County. This hike follows the grade for the first 2 miles to the junction with the Water Tank Trail on the left.

Locating the junction with the Water Tank Trail can be difficult, as it is marked only by three blue blazes on a small maple tree on the left of the railroad grade. There is no sign. The trailhead is just beyond a spot where a small creek passes underneath the railroad grade creek via a stone aqueduct identified by two metal poles (one on each side of the trail) painted white on the bottom and red on the top (1.9 miles). The Water Tank Trail takes off left 0.1 mile farther on from a point about 100 feet before a tree on the right marked with multiple signs: a large blue-and-white sign with a disability symbol, mounted just above a smaller green triangular sign with an equestrian symbol, mounted just above a yellow blaze. The tree sits at the far end of what appears to be an old parking pull-out to the side of the trail under some hemlock trees. This was the site of Water Tank, where a wooden storage tank that provided water for the engines passing through the valley was located.

Once you gain the Water Tank Trail, the route-finding difficulties are finished, although the difficult hiking is just beginning. Over the next mile, the trail climbs just about 1,000 feet over very rough terrain. For the first 0.25 mile, the trail climbs moderately, and it is easy to follow through the woods with plenty of blue blazes. Then it joins what appears to be an old

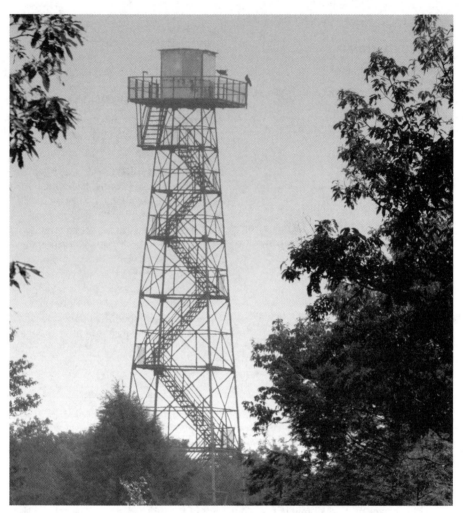

Stony Mountain Lookout Tower

haul path for lumber and takes a direct route up the mountain. Soon you meet the course of a significant creek, and just beyond that point you pass a memorial marker for Michael Starker, a hiker who went missing in the area in the fall of 2000 (2.54 miles). From here the trail gets very wet, rugged, and steep, sometimes absurdly so, for a half-mile, as it passes by some rocky outcrops and a trail marked by orange blazes to the right. At times the path crosses back and forth through the creek. At times it goes straight up it.

If this sounds unpleasant enough to make you consider walking the loop in reverse, keep two things in mind: First, the climb is short and is over with soon enough; and second, the only thing more unpleasant than walking up this path would be walking down it, especially with 7 miles of hiking behind you. A mile from the railroad grade (3 miles), the trail levels out abruptly, curves decisively to the right and then back to the left, and after about 0.1 mile tops out on the ridge at the Rattling Run Road, a wide-open and generally flat road.

From here, turn right on the road and then left at the fork just ahead. The Stony Mountain Lookout Tower is 0.6 mile from the fork. Note that the tower is closed to the public, but from the clearing at its base, you can take in a decent view of the Dehart Reservoir to the east and of the Clark Creek Valley to the north.

After visiting the tower, return to the junction with the Water Tank Trail and continue hiking west along Third Mountain. After the mile-long hill climb, the flat ridge road could not be more pleasant. Thick brush and berry bushes line the road. Tall hickory, oak, maple, and pine trees make up the woods on either side. Occasionally, you pass by wildlife food plots. In the fall, the colors are beautiful. In late summer, you can find hundreds of butterflies, frogs, praying mantises, and snakes along the trail. I discovered a 4-foot-long black rat snake in August sunning itself on the trail.

The trail is mostly level for 1.2 miles as it follows the ridge, and then it reaches a gate at a hairpin turn on the access road to the radio towers atop Third Mountain. I've never felt compelled to walk up the road to see the towers. With the exception of one just above the gate, they remain pleasantly hidden from view. This hike follows the road downhill for 2.5 miles back into the Stony Creek Valley. You'll have wonderful views of the valley and Second Mountain along the way. The road is, however, south facing and is not especially shaded for a good bit of the walk, so it can be rather hot and dry in the summertime. At just about 8 miles into this hike, you'll reach Ellendale Road, where you turn left and walk another 1.25 miles back to the car at the trailhead.

Nearby Activities

Stony Creek is a nice fishing creek, especially in the area of the trailhead. The **Stoney Creek Inn** (717-921-8056, thestoneycreekinn.com), at the intersection of Erie Street and Stony Creek Road in Dauphin Boro, is a nice place to grab a bite after the hike.

GPS TRAILHEAD COORDINATES AND DIRECTIONS
N40° 24.385' W76° 49.106'

From Harrisburg, follow US 322 west to the Dauphin Boro/Stony Creek exit. Exit the highway and drive over the creek. You are on Allegheny Street. Turn right on Schuylkill Street and then right on Erie Street (at stop sign). Signs point to Stony Creek. At the end of Erie Street, turn left on Stony Creek Road. Follow Stony Creek Road approximately 5 miles, where it turns to dirt and is called Ellendale Road. Follow for another 1.85 miles until the road ends at a gate with a large parking area.

16 Swatara State Park:
RAIL-TRAIL/BEAR HOLE LOOP

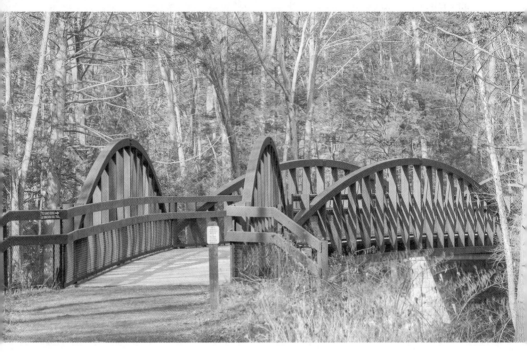

Sand Siding Bridge

In Brief

After a short walk along Swopes Valley Road, this hike picks up the Swatara Rail-Trail and follows it northwest for 3 miles to the Sand Siding Trail. Here the hike heads to the west, crossing the new bridge over Swatara Creek. After crossing the creek, the hike picks up the Bear Hole Trail and follows it for 3 miles back to the parking area.

Description

Located in Lebanon and Schuylkill Counties, the 3,520-acre Swatara State Park is a mostly undeveloped park that provides opportunities for a variety of activities, including hiking, biking, fishing, canoeing, and hunting. An 8-mile section of Swatara Creek flows the length of the park, exiting at its southern boundary in Swatara Gap, a large water gap through the flank of Blue Mountain. Interstate 81 passes through the gap directly above the creek, as does the Appalachian Trail (AT) directly beneath I-81. A significant tributary of the Susquehanna

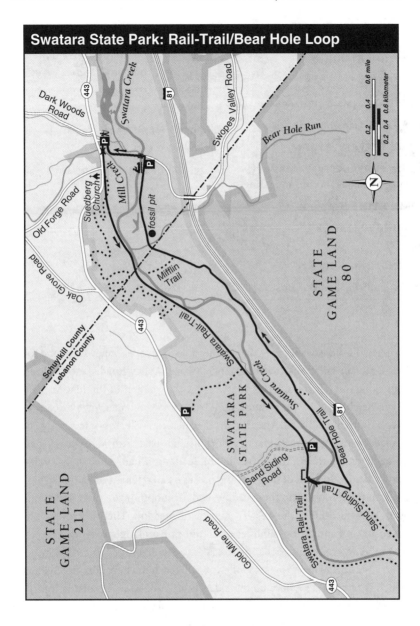

Swatara State Park: Rail-Trail/Bear Hole Loop

River, the Swatara Creek watershed encompasses a large area of the high country north and east of I-81. The creek through the park is part of the Swatara Creek Water Trail, which extends from Pine Grove to Middletown and the Susquehanna River to the southwest. The parking area for this hike, in fact, is at one of the boat access areas along the creek. Only non-motorized boats are allowed on the creek. A map of the water trail indicating all the points of interest is available at the parking area and others throughout the park.

LENGTH 7.3 miles	and *Pine Grove;* Keystone Trail Association *Appalachian Trail in Pennsylvania, Sections 1 Through 6: Delaware Water Gap to Swatara Gap.* A park map is available online at tinyurl.com/swataraspmap.
CONFIGURATION Loop	
DIFFICULTY Moderate	
SCENERY Swatara Creek and environs	
EXPOSURE Mostly shade	**FACILITIES** Portable toilets at parking areas
TRAIL TRAFFIC Medium	
TRAIL SURFACE Cinders and dirt; suitable for hiking, biking, and skiing	**WHEELCHAIR TRAVERSABLE** Yes, in most sections
HIKING TIME 3–4 hours	**CONTACT** Swatara State Park, 717-865-6470, tinyurl.com/swatarasp
DRIVING DISTANCE 2.5 miles from I-81 at Pine Grove	
ACCESS Sunrise–sunset	**SPECIAL COMMENTS** The trails used for this hike are shared with horseback riders.
MAPS USGS *Indiantown Gap, Tower City,*	

To begin this hike, walk out of the parking area to Swopes Valley Road and follow the shoulder for a half-mile back toward PA 443. Swopes Valley Road sees very little traffic, but keep along the left shoulder as you traverse this section of the hike for safety. Just before you reach PA 443, the Swatara Rail-Trail crosses Swopes Valley Road. Turn left (northwest) onto the rail-trail. After a short distance you will cross a footbridge over Mill Creek, a feeder stream to the Swatara. A short distance past the bridge you will pass by the pretty Suedberg Church on the north side of Suedberg Road. After the church the trail drops down below the level of the road and passes by an open meadow on the left. A path departs from the rail-trail into the meadow, and as an option you can follow that path; it rejoins the rail-trail again at the western edge of the meadow. There are several bird boxes among the grasses, and the possibilities for birding are pretty good in this area.

At 1 mile, the rail-trail reaches an intersection with a horse trail. Continue straight along the rail-trail, and in another 0.5 mile you will reach the Lebanon–Schuylkill County line, which is marked by a post on the side of the trail. You are walking into Lebanon County at this point. At 2 miles, a red-blazed horse trail enters from the right. At 3.5 miles into the hike, you will come to a parking area at Sand Siding Road. There is easy access to the creek from the parking area by following any of a number of trails that head in its direction. Several nice spots to rest, fish, or take in the scenery can be found in this area.

At 0.2 mile beyond the parking area, you will pass a bench and a junction with the Sand Siding Trail. Turn left onto the Sand Siding Trail and cross the Sand Siding Bridge. Made of steel with a wooden boardwalk surface, the bridge was constructed during the past five years in order to provide better access to different areas of the park. In effect, it makes possible two separate loops of the park: the one described in this profile and another loop north of this bridge that crosses the creek at the AT over the Waterville Bridge. Together, the two loops make for a 12-mile-long excursion.

After crossing the bridge, the Sand Siding Trail continues for a short distance before it ends at the Bear Hole Trail, which, in effect, follows the path of Old State Road. Turn left (east) here. The walking is very pleasant and the scenery nice along this road, although for a short distance beyond a side road on the right that heads back to a park cabin it parallels I-81 pretty closely and is a bit noisy for a mile. At 6.4 miles, a side road departs to the left; continue walking straight. At 6.5 miles, you reach the county line again, this time walking back into Schuylkill County. And another 0.1 mile beyond that brings you to the site of the old fossil pit on the right-hand side of the trail. A short hiking trail takes you above the area and provides access to the site from above. I haven't spent the time digging around for fossils here, though I have been told that they are easy enough to find. You are allowed to keep what you find here. Continuing beyond the fossil pit, the trail returns you to the car at the parking area after 7.3 miles.

Nearby Activities

There is a nice picnic area on Swopes Valley Road just across from the trailhead parking. You'll find a picnic table, a clearing, and a small pond surrounded by reeds and cattails. Swatara State Park has several mountain bike trails at its northern end. The town of Pine Grove has gas and restaurants.

GPS TRAILHEAD COORDINATES AND DIRECTIONS
N40° 31.348' W76° 28.187'

Follow I-81 north to Exit 100 (PA 443/Pine Grove). Turn left onto PA 443/Suedberg Road. Follow PA 443 for 2 miles and turn left onto Swopes Valley Road. The parking area for the trailhead is 0.5 mile ahead, on the right.

---

17 Table Rock and Peters Mountain

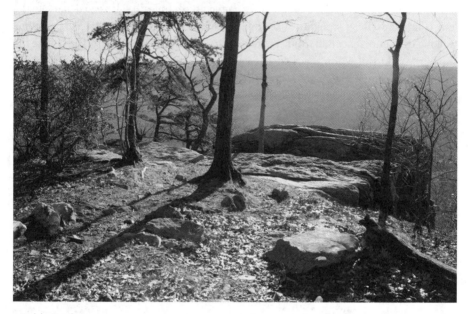

Table Rock

In Brief

This hike heads east out of the parking area along the Appalachian Trail (AT), along the Peters Mountain ridge to Table Rock, a wonderful sunny overlook. From there, you can follow the AT to the Peters Mountain Shelter, and from there to the Victoria Trail near the boundary of the Joseph E. Ibberson Conservation Area (see page 47).

Description

The first section of this hike, to Table Rock and back, is deservedly popular. The walking is easy, the distance is not too long, and the view from the rock is spectacular. Beyond Table Rock, the trail can still be busy, as a trip to the Peters Mountain Shelter and back makes for an easy overnight excursion. Beyond the shelter, you'll see fewer people, mostly folks exploring the AT.

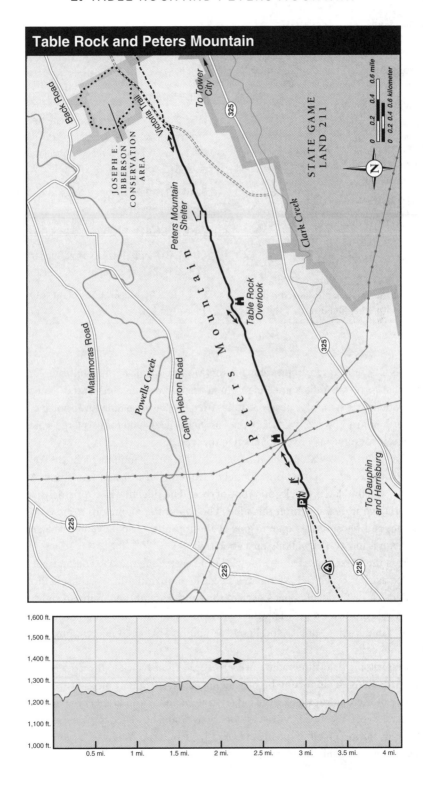

LENGTH 2 miles to Table Rock; 3.1 miles to Peters Mountain Shelter; 4.15 miles to Victoria Furnace Trail. Double the distance for return.	**DRIVING DISTANCE** About 10 miles from the intersection of I-81 and US 22/322 outside of Harrisburg
CONFIGURATION Out-and-back	**ACCESS** Open
DIFFICULTY Easy–moderate	**MAPS** USGS *Halifax* and *Enders*; Keystone Trail Association *Appalachian Trail in Pennsylvania, Sections 7 and 8: Susquehanna River to Swatara Gap*
SCENERY View of Clark Creek Valley, Peters Mountain Shelter; very nice ridge walking	
EXPOSURE Mostly shaded	**FACILITIES** Spring and privy at Peters Mountain Shelter
TRAIL TRAFFIC Moderate–heavy on weekends	**WHEELCHAIR TRAVERSABLE** No
TRAIL SURFACE Dirt	**CONTACT** Appalachian Trail Conservancy, 717-258-5771, appalachiantrail.org
HIKING TIME 2 hours for Table Rock, 3 hours for Peters Mountain Shelter, 4 hours for Victoria Furnace Trail	**SPECIAL COMMENTS** A pleasant hike year-round

This hike offers pretty views along Peters Mountain, one of the significant long, level ridges that form the Valley and Ridge physiographic province of central Pennsylvania. Peters Mountain extends for nearly 30 miles from the Susquehanna River north of Harrisburg northeast to Tower City. Across the Susquehanna, which forms a large water gap in the ridge, it continues as Cove Mountain to the west.

The top of Peters Mountain, like many of the other mountains in the Valley and Ridge Province, is composed of extremely hard, erosion-resistant sandstone. All along its crest you'll find large, blocky outcrops of rock. The ridgeline is surprisingly narrow in places, though not so much on this hike. The top of the mountain varies very little in elevation, and because this hike begins at the top of the ridge, you'll have very little climbing. It is mostly flat walking on a good trail.

From the parking area above PA 225, head east along the AT. You may get slightly confused as you leave the parking area because an inviting dirt road leads directly up the ridge. The AT actually heads over to the south side of the mountain right away to bypass the radio towers to which the road leads. Look for the white blazes and a trail sign for Table Rock (2 miles) and Peters Mountain Shelter (3 miles) pointing the way over some rocks.

After passing below the radio towers, the trail climbs back to the ridge, crosses over the top, and joins an old roadbed. The walking here is extremely pleasant. You'll begin to see some of the outcrops along the ridgetop here and if you are feeling ambitious you might scramble to the top of one or two for a view. Soon, however, the trail passes beneath a power line dropping off to the north from a large outcrop. You'll get a great view of the Susquehanna River and the valley to the north up toward Halifax from here.

Continue along the trail, which quickly becomes more of a footpath through the woods. At 2 miles, you'll reach Table Rock. Although there is no sign, it is hard to miss. It is a large sandstone outcrop that forms a cliff on the south side of the ridge, offering an incredible view of Clark Creek and the ridge of Stony Mountain. Surrounded by Table Mountain pine trees that add to the beauty of the setting, I would have to say that this is one of the prettiest views along the ridges east of the Susquehanna River. If you scan the ridge to the east across the valley, you should be able to spot the Stony Mountain Lookout Tower 4 or 5 miles distant.

After you've had your fill of the view, continue east along the AT. Just past Table Rock, you'll pass a junction with an orange-blazed trail dropping off the north side of the ridge. That is a private path, according to my AT map. Continue along the ridge for another mile to the Peters Mountain Shelter, constructed in 1994 by the Susquehanna Appalachian Trail Club. You'll find a privy here and a spring on the north side of the mountain (follow the sign from the shelter). Be sure to treat the water before drinking it.

From the shelter, continue east through more oak trees along the ridge, and descend into a saddle via some rock steps at 4.15 miles. At the saddle, the AT continues along the ridge, crossing a dirt road rising from the south and descending to the northeast. This is the Victoria Trail, an old road used for hauling lumber to the Victoria Furnace in the Clark Creek Valley from the Powell Creek Valley to the north. Below the ridge to the north is the Joseph E. Ibberson Conservation Area. This is a nice place to rest before completing the trip by retracing your steps.

A suggestion for an alternate hike: If you have two cars, you can run a shuttle, leaving one car at the parking area at the conservation area lot and the other at the AT lot at PA 225 on Peters Mountain. If you do that, you can follow this hike across Peters Mountain and then take the Victoria Trail down to the parking area at the conservation area (see page 47). Doing so will give you a one-way hike of about 6 miles.

GPS TRAILHEAD COORDINATES AND DIRECTIONS
N40° 24.715' W76° 55.795'

Follow US 22/322 north from Harrisburg to PA 225 North toward Halifax. Follow PA 225 about 4 miles to the crest of Peters Mountain. Just before the footbridge over the road, the entrance road to the AT parking area departs to the right. Park there.

18 Weiser State Forest:
GREENLAND ROAD

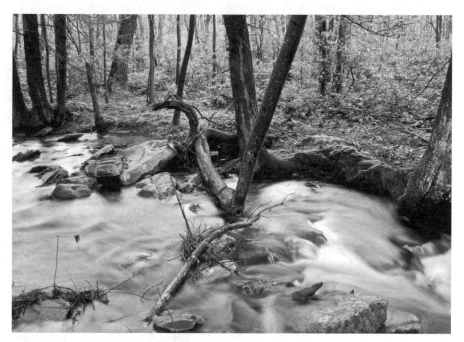

East Branch Rattling Creek

In Brief

This hike makes a circuit through Pennsylvania State Game Land 210, following open trails to the south before heading to the north. At about 6 miles, the open trails give way to a small footpath that descends into East Branch Rattling Creek. The hike follows an old path along the creek for a mile and then follows a good trail back south along Nine O'Clock Run. It finishes with a couple of miles of gentle walking on Greenland Road.

Description

I found this hike several years ago on the old "Our Favorite Hikes" list on the website of the Susquehanna Appalachian Trail Club (satc-hike.org), where it is referred to as the "Nine O'Clock Run Circle Hike." The description sounded interesting, so I figured I would give it a shot. I am glad I did. At more than 11 miles, it is a long hike; however, all of the grades are

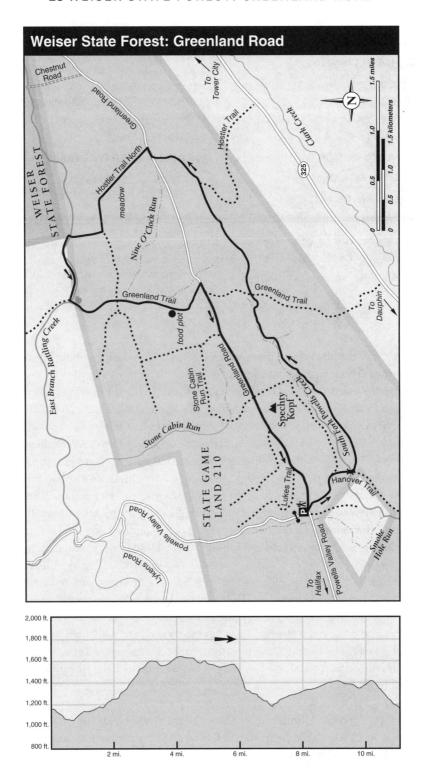

Weiser State Forest: Greenland Road

LENGTH 11.1 miles

CONFIGURATION Loop

DIFFICULTY Strenuous because of length

SCENERY Beautiful fields, forests, and streams

EXPOSURE Half sun, half shade

TRAIL TRAFFIC Light

TRAIL SURFACE Dirt

HIKING TIME 5–6 hours

DRIVING DISTANCE 22.5 miles from US 22/322 and PA 225 west of Harrisburg

ACCESS Open; state-game-land regulations apply.

MAPS USGS *Lykens* and *Tower City*; Keystone Trail Association *Appalachian Trail in Pennsylvania, Sections 7 and 8: Susquehanna River to Swatara Gap.* A state forest map is available online at tinyurl.com/weisersfmap.

FACILITIES None

WHEELCHAIR TRAVERSABLE No

CONTACT Weiser State Forest, 570-875-6450, tinyurl.com/weisersf

SPECIAL COMMENTS This entire hike is on wide-open trails with the exception of about 2 miles at its northernmost edge, where it passes through some dense stands of mountain laurel. This is a great hike for viewing wildlife.

gentle, most of the hiking is on game-land roads, and it is a really beautiful hike through varied terrain. This is an excellent hike for seeing wildlife and for birding.

Begin the hike from the gate on Greenland Road next to the parking areas for State Game Land 210. Pass through the gate and make an immediate right (south) onto the Hanover Trail, a dirt road. Follow this trail downhill for a half-mile, past a couple of large food plots and then across a wooden bridge over South Fork Powell Creek. Beyond the bridge the trail bends left and climbs to a fork near a fenced area. Veer left at the fork and follow the grassy road east. For the first mile or so the trail heads up a hollow filled with pine and oak trees. After passing a small creek flowing across the road, the path climbs out of the hollow and passes through some lovely, generally open, high country. Plenty of low brush and mountain laurel provide cover for turkey, grouse, deer, and fox. I discovered several sets of bear tracks along this stretch of road, and I suspect that they are abundant here as well.

At just shy of 3 miles, you'll reach the crossing with the Greenland Trail, a footpath that extends from PA 325 in the south almost to Wiconisco to the north. About a mile beyond that, the Hanover Trail ends at the Hostler Trail by a very large pine tree with a very large bird box. At the junction, turn left (north) and walk downhill for 0.6 mile to Greenland Road. The birding along this stretch of trail is excellent. Turn right (east) on Greenland Road and follow it for 100 yards to the junction with the Hostler Trail North. Turn left (north) and follow the grassy road as it continues its descent.

About 0.5 mile from Greenland Road, the trail passes a beautiful meadow on the left— a perfect spot for a lunch break. At 5.5 miles, the grassy road ends and the Hostler Trail becomes a small, unmarked footpath winding through thick mountain laurel. Continue straight from the end of the road. The path is obvious, and the trail a bit rocky, but after

0.2 mile, the trail comes to a T-intersection at a place that was once referred to as Carl's Crossing. Turn right and follow the north-to-south-running trail downhill (still the Hostler Trail) for a mile to the crossing over East Branch Rattling Creek (6.25 miles). Depending on the flow, crossing the creek may require you to get your feet wet, but a large flat rock on the north side beneath a tall pine tree provides a good spot to rest and dry out.

The walking for the next 0.75 mile gets rather intense. From the creek, follow the trail about 100 feet up a small incline and turn left (west) on a small, rather overgrown trail that begins just before the Hostler Trail climbs a short, steep hillside. Although the trail is not blazed, it follows East Branch Rattling Creek right along the north bank of the creek and is easy to keep track of. At times the mountain laurel is extremely dense. Plan on getting wet if you pass through this hollow after a rain. In a couple of places you'll need to negotiate some deadfall (downed trees). The trail must have been used more extensively at some time, as the hollow is filled with old bird boxes.

At 6.9 miles, you'll reach a little hunting camp with benches and a fire ring on the shore of the creek. Beyond the camp, the trail improves dramatically. A few minutes beyond the camp, you'll reach a small pond formed by a concrete dam. Cross the creek just downstream from the dam and pick up the Greenland Trail heading south up a hollow. Follow that trail up Nine O'Clock Run for a mile to a large clear-cut and food plot. If you have time to hang around for a while, this is a great spot for birding. I saw several scarlet tanagers and green herons here.

The trail eventually makes a hard left turn and heads southeast to Greenland Road at about 8.5 miles. Turn right (west) on Greenland Road and follow it for 2.5 miles back to the parking area, passing two significant trails that head to the north on the way. As you get closer to the trailhead, you'll see some great scenery off to the south.

Nearby Activities

Known for its steaks, the **Carsonville Hotel** (717-362-9379) has a pub with a deck and would be a good place to refresh after a long hike. It's in Carsonville on Powells Valley Road, where the road makes a 90-degree right turn.

GPS TRAILHEAD COORDINATES AND DIRECTIONS

N40° 31.099' W76° 41.341'

Take US 22/322 west from Harrisburg to the PA 225/Halifax exit. Follow PA 225 north 10 miles to the intersection with PA 147 (on the left). Make the first right turn north of the intersection of PA 225 and PA 147 onto Powells Valley Road (PA 4013 or Enterline Road on some maps). Follow Powells Valley for 12 miles to the large parking areas located at a sharp bend in the road, where Powells Valley (signed as Lykens Road here on some maps) begins to climb the ridge to the north.

19 Weiser State Forest:
HALDEMAN TRACT

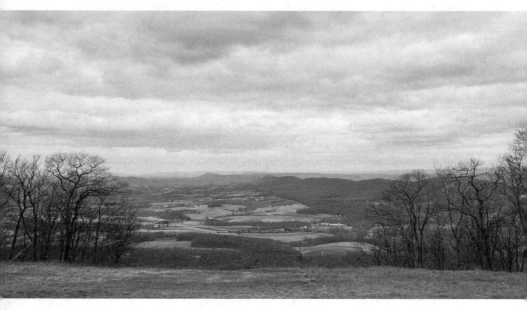

Powells Valley from the hang-glider launch

In Brief

This great hike follows several of the multiuse trails through the Haldeman Tract of the Weiser State Forest. It begins at the Minnich Hit Picnic Area and follows the Minnich Hit Trail northwest to the Matter Trail. Heading west, the Matter Trail takes you to the end of Wolf Pond Road, where you can walk out to the hang glider launch area for an outstanding view. The hike then continues south and east near the boundary of the Haldeman Tract for several miles until it reaches the Grimm Trail, about a half-mile south of the trailhead.

Description

When I was working on the first edition of this book, I discovered the Greenland Tract of the Weiser State Forest, and I really enjoyed the scenery and terrain of that hike. I thought that for this edition it would be nice to see more of that area, and so I checked out several maps and discovered that the 5,355-acre Haldeman Tract, located just a couple of miles from the Greenland Tract, would be worth some time exploring. That was a good choice.

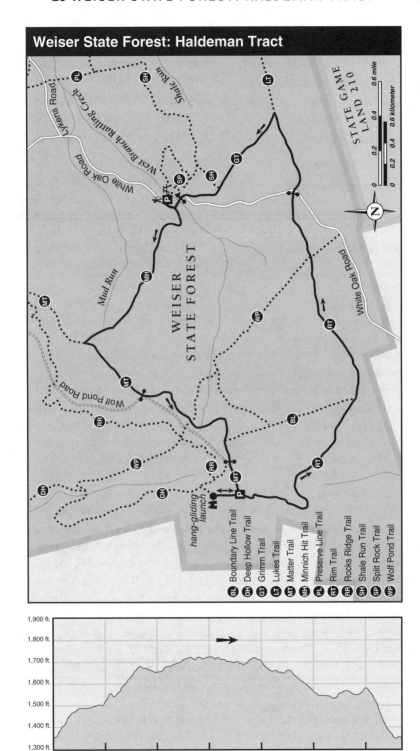

Weiser State Forest: Haldeman Tract

STATE GAME LAND 210

WEISER STATE FOREST

Lykens Road
White Oak Road
West Branch Rattling Creek
Shale Run
Mud Run
Wolf Pond Road
White Oak Road
hang-gliding launch

BL Boundary Line Trail
DH Deep Hollow Trail
GT Grimm Trail
LT Lukes Trail
MT Matter Trail
MH Minnich Hit Trail
PL Preserve Line Trail
RT Rim Trail
RR Rocks Ridge Trail
SH Shale Run Trail
SP Split Rock Trail
WP Wolf Pond Trail

1,900 ft.
1,800 ft.
1,700 ft.
1,600 ft.
1,500 ft.
1,400 ft.
1,300 ft.

1 mi.   2 mi.   3 mi.   4 mi.   5 mi.   6 mi.

LENGTH 6.7 miles	**ACCESS** Open
CONFIGURATION Loop	**MAPS** USGS *Elizabethville* and *Lykens*; a state forest map is available online at tinyurl.com/weisersfmap.
DIFFICULTY Moderate	
SCENERY Rattling Creek, Powells Valley from hang-glider launching site	
	FACILITIES Pit toilet at picnic area
EXPOSURE Mostly shade	**WHEELCHAIR TRAVERSABLE** No
TRAIL TRAFFIC Light	**CONTACT** Weiser State Forest, 570-875-6450, tinyurl.com/weisersf
TRAIL SURFACE Dirt and grass, some gravel	
	SPECIAL COMMENTS The hang-glider launching site at the end of Wood Pond Road provides a spectacular view of the surrounding terrain and makes an excellent spot to plan a long lunch break.
HIKING TIME 3–4 hours	
DRIVING DISTANCE About 12 miles from Elizabethville, PA	

This hike has become one of my favorite hikes in the area. Aside from the fact that the walking for the entire distance is along well-maintained multiuse trails, and that you get a spectacular view about halfway through the hike, I was really impressed by the quiet that I encountered along this trek. I would characterize it as a very peaceful hike.

Park at the Minnich Hit Picnic Area, located on White Oak Road. There is a trail from the picnic area that is designed for access by disabled persons and which extends to the footbridge over the west branch of Rattling Creek. Beyond the bridge you can make a short loop of about a mile, though the trail is indistinct and takes a fair amount of care to keep track of. It is marked by blue blazes, but they are very old and oftentimes spaced very far apart.

You'll begin this longer loop from the picnic area. Walk across the road and head toward the bridge over the creek just beyond the picnic area. On your right, you'll see a gated dirt road and a sign for the Minnich Hit Trail. Head up that road as it climbs gently to the east. The trail is wide open and easy to follow for the whole hike, with obvious signposts at each junction. Follow this trail for a mile up to the junction with the Matter Trail, and turn left (west). Once you are on the Matter Trail you have done most of the climbing for the hike, and the trail levels out and passes through some pretty forest of pine trees with oak and hickory scattered about. Continue along this pleasant path for 0.5 mile until you come to a gate at Wolf Pond Road. Pass the gate and head past a second gate on your left. This is the continuation of the Matter Trail, and it parallels Wolf Pond Road in the woods until it joins Wolf Pond Road again at about 2.5 miles into the hike. The walking along this path couldn't be nicer. The trail is grassy for a long way and then becomes dirt at the junction with the Wolf Pond Trail. Beyond that it gets grassy again until you reach a wide cleared area at the junction with the Boundary Line Trail. The Boundary Line Trail runs roughly north–south, and you will pass it and the Wolf Pond Trail again after you pick up the Rim Trail on the return.

About a hundred yards or so beyond the Boundary Line Trail, the Matter Trail ends at a gate on Wood Pond Road. Walk out to the road and turn left, and when you reach its end at a kind of cul-de-sac, turn right and pass a gate onto another dirt road. This path takes you out to a large clearing at the hang-glider launch area. The elevation here is about 1,700 feet above sea level, and the clearing drops off nearly a thousand feet to the west to the valley below. You are looking here across the Powells Valley as it extends to the Susquehanna River. The view is spectacular, and I highly recommend planning to spend some time at this location soaking it up.

After you have taken a break, walk back out to Wolf Pond Road and follow the obvious dirt path across the road to the south. The trail passes a large open field on the left, and if you have the inclination, you can just as easily walk through the field as along the path. At the southern end of the field, you'll find a small weather station. If you choose to wander around the field, walk back out the dirt road on an obvious path at its southwest corner; here, you will see a sign indicating that you are on the Rim Trail. This Rim Trail traverses the ridge above Wolf Run to the west for a couple of miles, taking you roughly back in the direction of the Minnich Hit Picnic Area. At 4.1 miles into the hike you will pass the Boundary Line Trail and at 4.9 miles the Wolf Pond Trail.

At 5.3 miles, the Rim Trail ends at a gate at White Oak Road. You could follow White Oak Road north back to the picnic area from here. It is about a mile along the road. Instead, I recommend crossing the road, passing the gate, continuing along Lukes Trail for 0.5 mile to the intersection with the Grimm Trail, marked by an obvious signpost. Turn left (northwest) and follow the trail downhill for 0.6 mile to White Oak Road, where it crosses the west branch of Rattling Creek. Turn right and the picnic area is 100 yards down the road, on your right.

Nearby Activities

The nearby town of **Lykens** has food and stores. Known for its steaks, the **Carsonville Hotel** (717-362-9379) has a pub with a deck and would be a good place to refresh after a long hike. It's in Carsonville on Powells Valley Road, where the road makes a 90-degree right turn.

GPS TRAILHEAD COORDINATES AND DIRECTIONS
N40° 31.361' W76° 44.852'

From Elizabethville on PA 225 north of Harrisburg, follow PA 209 east 6.4 miles to the stoplight in Lykens. Turn right at the light onto Market Street and then left after crossing the creek onto Glen Park Road. Follow that 2 miles to the intersection with Lykens Road, which is easily identified by a sign indicating that this area is part of a National Wild Turkey Federation habitat-restoration project. Turn right onto Lykens Road and follow it west 3.2 miles to White Oak Road. Turn left and continue on White Oak Road 1 mile to the Minnich Hit Picnic Area, on the left.

20 Wildwood Lake Loop

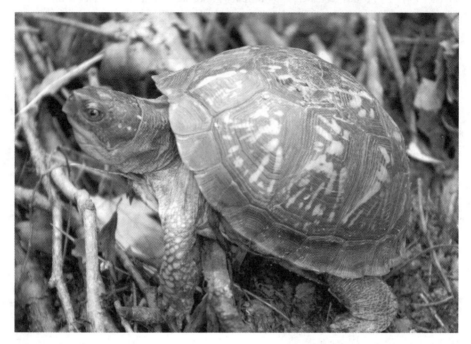

Painted turtle

In Brief

This 4.4-mile loop hike follows boardwalks and some of the lesser-used paths around the perimeter of Wildwood Lake.

Description

Formerly known as Wetzel's Swamp, the Wildwood Lake Sanctuary was constructed in 1907 as part of a movement to enhance recreational opportunities in urban areas and in order to control flood runoff from Paxton Creek, its main watershed. Located in northern Harrisburg, the sanctuary has a distinctly urban character. Industrial Road, which parallels the lake to the west, is lined with warehouses and distribution centers and sees plenty of truck traffic. To the south, the sanctuary is bordered by I-81, with US 322 forming its eastern and northern boundaries. The drone of traffic is a pervasive element of a hike around the lake.

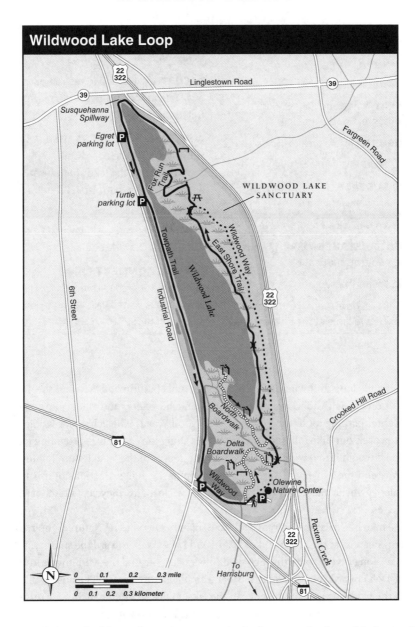

Nonetheless, the lake and its environs are looked upon quite favorably by an abundance of wildlife that make it their permanent home or that use it as a layover on their migratory routes. Every time I visit the lake, I am amazed by the variety of wildlife I see. On a single trip in August, my sons and I saw osprey, herons, egrets, several varieties of turtles and frogs, a snake, and a woodchuck, whose sudden appearance on the trail made us all jump. The variety of flora is impressive, particularly the abundance of American lotus plants, which cover the surface of the lake by late summer.

LENGTH 4.4 miles	or online at wildwoodlake.org /lake-sanctuary/map.aspx.
CONFIGURATION Loop	
DIFFICULTY Easy	**FACILITIES** Water and restrooms available at the nature center; portable toilets en route
SCENERY Wildwood Lake Sanctuary and environs; great bird-watching	
EXPOSURE Mix of sun and shade	**WHEELCHAIR TRAVERSABLE** Wildwood Way and the boardwalks on the east side of the lake are traversable as far as the Towpath Trail, 0.1 mile beyond the Susquehanna Spillway.
TRAIL TRAFFIC Moderately heavy	
TRAIL SURFACE Varies among paved, dirt, boardwalk, and gravel	
HIKING TIME 1.5–2 hours	
DRIVING DISTANCE About 4.5 miles from downtown Harrisburg	**CONTACT** Friends of Wildwood Lake, 717-221-0292, wildwoodlake.org
ACCESS Sunrise–sunset	**SPECIAL COMMENTS** Although subject to considerable road traffic noise, the sanctuary is visited year-round by many species of birds.
MAPS USGS *Harrisburg West;* a map of the park is available at the nature center	

A 3.1-mile loop following the main lakeside trails (Wildwood Way and the Towpath Trail) is popular with local walkers, joggers, and bicyclers, and the section from the nature center parking lot to the north on Wildwood Way is wheelchair accessible. At 4.4 miles, however, our hike follows the boardwalks along the east shore, providing nice side excursions to wildlife-viewing stations out in the center of the lake, before joining Wildwood Way and the Towpath Trail for the remaining 1.2 miles. Sections of this hike are accessible to wheelchairs, and the boardwalks are closed to bicycles, skateboards, and inline skates.

This hike begins at the entrance to the Benjamin Olewine III Nature Center, located at the parking area at the south end of Wildwood Lake. Walk toward the southeast corner of the lake along a paved path through wildflowers. Just beyond the wildflowers, turn right onto the Delta Boardwalk. It begins 360 feet from the nature center. The boardwalk passes through the wetlands area on the edge of the lake, and you'll find benches for resting and wildlife-watching frequently along its length. This is a good area for spotting egrets and herons, both of which frequent the open water at the south end of the lake.

At 0.25 mile, a short spur takes you to viewing scopes about 50 feet or so to the left. The boardwalk is surrounded by waterfowl nesting areas. In addition to looking for birds, keep your eyes trained on the ground along the edge of the boardwalk where you'll likely find frogs and perhaps a turtle. Beyond the spur, the boardwalk meanders along Paxton Creek, passing another short spur to the left at 0.45 mile, just before it ends at the junction with Wildwood Way.

Turn left (north) on Wildwood Way and cross over Paxton Creek via a large footbridge. After you cross the bridge, the trail will come to a T-intersection. To the right, the trail passes under US 322, exiting the natural area. Turn left and continue along Wildwood Way for 100 feet or so to the intersection with the North Boardwalk on the left (0.55 mile). Turn left onto the dirt path and left again onto the boardwalk. The trek along the North Boardwalk is 0.7 mile long (out-and-back) through wetlands to a viewing area situated among the lotuses in the middle of the lake. It is worth the walk just to see the lotuses.

Along the way, you'll encounter plenty of swamp rose mallow (purple flowers), cattails, and common arrowhead (yellow flowers) among other flowering plants. About 0.15 mile along, a short spur leads to a bird-watching station on the right. A bird-identification guide is located on the trail at the spur. Just beyond the spur, another spotting scope is located on the right. At the end of the boardwalk, you'll find another bird-watching station situated amid a landscape of lotus plants, which are not especially common in Pennsylvania. I've seen herons out in this area, though patience is necessary since they can be tough to spot among the foliage.

After a break at the end of the boardwalk, return to its beginning. Rather than going back to Wildwood Way, turn left at the end of the boardwalk onto the dirt path that follows the shore of the lake through the forest of oak, sycamore, tulip poplar, and hickory trees. This is the East Shore Trail, and you'll follow it for 0.9 mile back to Wildwood Way. Although the path can be a little damp in places, its proximity to the shore of the lake and its distance from the main path make it ideal for spotting wildlife. Along the way, it crosses a couple of short boardwalks through especially marshy areas and crosses two footbridges before joining the main trail.

Turn left at the junction with Wildwood Way, which is wide and paved in this area. A picnic table sits aside the path just after you join it. From the junction, continue north for 0.15 mile to the junction with the Fox Run Trail on the left. This 0.25-mile loop through wooded wetlands is another good place to spot wildlife, as it is also off the main path. It is the location of our famed woodchuck encounter. If you'd prefer to stick to the paved path, the Fox Run Trail joins Wildwood Way again about 50 feet from where it departs.

Upon completing the Fox Run loop, turn left on Wildwood Way and follow it over a hill and down to the north end of the lake at the Susquehanna Spillway, just below Linglestown Road. This is a rather noisy section of trail. After another 0.1 mile, Wildwood Way ends at the Egret parking lot off Industrial Road, where you'll find a picnic pavilion and portable restrooms.

From the lot, you'll want to pick up the Towpath Trail and follow it along the west shore of the lake for a mile or so to its southern edge, passing another small parking area at 0.3 mile (the Turtle lot) with no facilities. The Towpath Trail is wide, surfaced with mulch and dirt, and not wheelchair accessible. Watch the lake through the trees as you walk this path, and you may see herons or egrets or other waterfowl in the small areas of open water. To the right of the trail are the remains of the old Pennsylvania Canal, which ceased operations in 1854. It is a good place to watch for turtles and waterfowl.

At the end of the Towpath Trail, turn left onto the paved road at the southern end of the lake and walk back toward the parking area and nature center. Near the end of the hike, you'll see the Morning Glory Spillway, so named because its funnel-shaped overflow channel resembles a morning-glory flower. It was constructed by the Harrisburg Department of Public Works in 1908 to regulate the height of the water in the lake.

Nearby Activities

The **Benjamin Olewine III Nature Center** (100 Wildwood Way; 717-221-0292, wildwood lake.org/nature-center) provides interpretive information about the flora and fauna of the lake and surrounding wetlands. It's open daily from 10 a.m. to 4 p.m. except on Thanksgiving, Christmas, and New Year's Days. **The State Museum of Pennsylvania** (300 North St.; 717-787-4980, statemuseumpa.org), next to the state capitol in downtown Harrisburg, is definitely worth a visit as well.

GPS TRAILHEAD COORDINATES AND DIRECTIONS
N40° 18.410' W76° 53.020'

From I-81, take Exit 66 for Front Street. Head north on Front Street to the first traffic light and turn right onto PA 39 (Linglestown Road). Turn right at the next traffic light onto Industrial Road. Follow Industrial Road for a mile. Turn left onto Wildwood Way at a sign that says nature center. If you go underneath I-81, you have gone too far. Follow the road to the parking lot.

21 Yellow Springs Loop

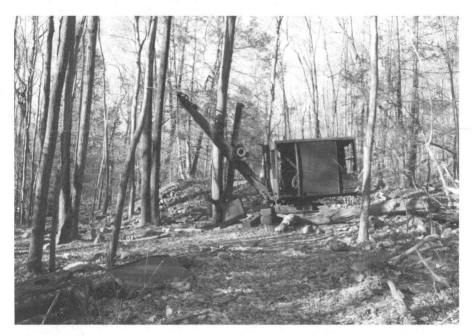

"The General"

In Brief

Cross Clark Creek just out of the parking area. Follow the Stone Tower Trail a short distance to an old roadbed and connector trail. Turn left and follow the road for a mile to the Sand Spring Trail. Head south, cross over Stony Mountain, and descend into upper Rausch Creek. A short side trip takes you to the site of "The General," an iron excavator used for digging gravel in the late 19th century. From Rausch Creek, follow the Appalachian Trail (AT) west to the Yellow Springs Trail. Head north to the Stone Tower ruins on Stony Mountain. Follow the Stone Tower Trail back to the parking area.

Description

This hike traverses the rugged and remote upper reaches of Rausch Creek in the St. Anthony's Wilderness. The terrain is prime habitat for white-tailed deer, black bear, and bobcat, all of which I have encountered along sections of this hike. A variety of birdlife, including flycatchers, warblers, thrushes, bluebirds, and tanagers, inhabits the area during the spring, summer, and fall. The riparian habitat along Rausch Creek is home to frogs,

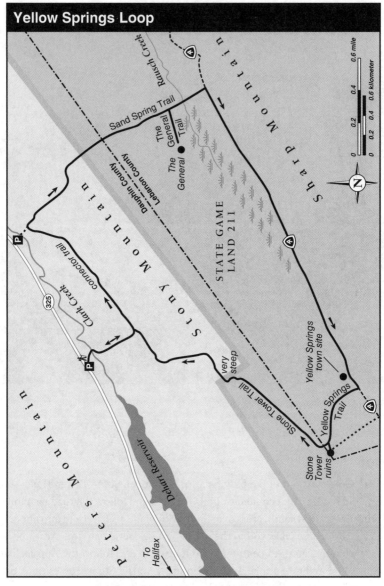

Yellow Springs Loop

STATE GAME LAND 211

Sharp Mountain

Stony Mountain

Peters Mountain

Rausch Creek

Sand Spring Trail

The General Trail

The General

Dauphin County

Lebanon County

Clark Creek connector trail

325

Dehart Reservoir

To Halifax

very steep

Stone Tower Trail

Yellow Springs town site

Yellow Springs Trail

Stone Tower ruins

0.6 mile
0.4
0.2
0
0.2   0.4   0.6 kilometer
0

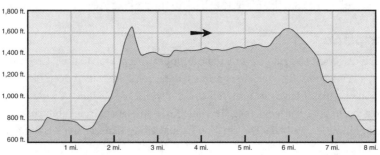

LENGTH 8 miles	**MAPS** USGS *Grantville* and *Lykens*; Keystone Trail Association *Appalachian Trail in Pennsylvania, Sections 7 and 8: Susquehanna River to Swatara Gap*. The entire hike is on PA State Game Land 211, maps for which can be downloaded from the Pennsylvania Game Commission Mapping Center at tinyurl.com /pagamemappingcenter.
CONFIGURATION Loop	
DIFFICULTY Strenuous	
SCENERY Upper Rausch Creek; "The General" (an abandoned excavator); ghost town of Yellow Springs; and the Stone Tower ruins, an old mine-ventilation shaft	
EXPOSURE Shade	
TRAIL TRAFFIC Light	**FACILITIES** None
TRAIL SURFACE Mostly dirt and rather rocky on the ascent and descent	**WHEELCHAIR TRAVERSABLE** No
	CONTACT Pennsylvania Game Commission, 717-787-4250, tinyurl.com /pagamelands
HIKING TIME About 5 hours	
DRIVING DISTANCE About 19.2 miles from the PA 225 exit off of US 22/322 west of Harrisburg	**SPECIAL COMMENTS** Take care descending the Stone Tower Trail, which is rocky and has a very steep section.
ACCESS Open; on state game land	

salamanders, and snakes, as well as a variety of ferns and mosses. I highly recommend getting an early start on this hike, not because of its length but because the quality of morning light on the Stony Mountain ridge is quite stunning.

Begin the hike by following red blazes directly south out of the parking area. You'll come to the crossing at Clark Creek in no time. Consisting of a thin log with flat boards nailed to it and a steel cable for your hands, the crossing can be tricky if wet or covered in frost. Once over the creek, you'll see a sign pointing to the Stone Tower Trail. Veer right and follow red blazes through the mountain laurel, across a couple of small streams, and uphill for 0.6 mile to a roadbed. The Stone Tower Trail continues to the right, and a pink-blazed connector trail to the Sand Spring Trail follows the roadbed to the left (east). Turn left on the connector trail and walk east for 1 mile to the Sand Spring Trail, marked by two prominent blue blazes on a tree.

Turn right onto the footpath and begin the ascent of Stony Mountain through a forest of hemlock and mountain laurel. Given that this trail, like many others in the area, was originally developed to move coal and lumber down the hillside, its direct route up the mountain is not surprising. Gravity was a big help moving the loads downhill; here it works against you on the ascent. I've never considered the climb to be too rugged or steep, but several people have disagreed with my assessment; hence, the designation of the difficulty of this hike is strenuous. The trail is steepest and rockiest at about 0.6 mile from the junction. Just beyond the steep section, you'll come to the flat ridge of Stony Mountain.

Cross over the ridge and begin the descent into Rausch Creek down a short, steep, and slippery section with uncertain footing. At the end of this section, you'll come to a pair of blazes where the trail bends right near a large boulder. The Appalachian Trail (AT) map indicates that a yellow-blazed trail traverses east from this area to a lookout below the ridge, though I've not been able to locate it. Continue into the drainage to a pair of blazes on a birch tree next to a hemlock. Here a side trail heads off to the right. The sign that used to mark the trail is no longer there, although a piece of metal is lodged into the crook of the hemlock. The GPS coordinates for the trailhead, however, are **N40° 29.342' W76° 38.332'.** Turn right and follow it for 0.25 mile. At the end of the trail, you'll find "The General," a large steel excavator dating to the early 1900s (GPS: **N40° 29.294' W76° 38.555'**). It was likely used for removing gravel from the pit on the hillside behind it. Considering the remote location, the presence of this piece of heavy machinery is rather remarkable, and it causes you to realize the extent of change this area has undergone since the heyday of mining operations more than a hundred years ago.

From "The General," return to the main trail, turn right, and walk over to Rausch Creek. The easiest crossing is just right of where the trail meets the creek. The area surrounding the creek is a serene wetlands, populated by hemlocks, mountain laurel, and carpets of moss and fern. A couple of hundred yards beyond the creek, the Sand Spring Trail ends at the AT. Turn right and walk west through oak and hickory forest for 2 miles to the Yellow Springs town site and the Yellow Springs Trail. I had my first bear encounter in Pennsylvania along this section of the AT. A large old black bruin, I mistook it for a stump in the woods, until it stood up and began sniffing the air. Then it turned and sauntered off into the woods.

The junction with the Yellow Springs Trail is identified by a white mailbox containing a trail register and by a campsite used by AT hikers. This hike turns right onto the Yellow Springs Trail and follows it back up to the crest of Stony Mountain. Like the nearby settlements of Rausch Gap and Rattling Run, Yellow Springs was a coal mining town that operated during the 1800s. Along the Yellow Springs Trail, you'll find the stone foundations of many of the original buildings. Most of the ruins are visible from the trail, though if you wander around a little bit you'll notice that this was an extensive community. The most interesting ruin is the Stone Tower near the crest of Stony Mountain about 0.7 mile along the Yellow Springs Trail. Standing about 30 feet tall, the tower is located at the head of several old coal shafts extending into Stony Mountain. When in use, it served to ventilate the deep mines by channeling air out of the shafts via a cast iron pipeline, the remains of which can be seen near the opening of the shaft. Please use caution in this area, as people die each year in Pennsylvania from accidents in abandoned mines. Beyond the tower lies the junction of the blue-blazed Yellow Springs and red-blazed Stone Tower Trails. If you follow blue blazes into the woods a short distance, you'll soon come to the remains of an old incline used for moving coal down the mountain to the Dauphin and Susquehanna Railroad in the Stony Valley.

From the ridgecrest above the tower, follow the red-blazed Stone Tower Trail to the north and then to the east as it descends from the ridge. At first the walking is rocky, but not too steep because the trail traverses the hillside. About 0.8 mile from the trail junction, however, the trail takes a rather illogical path straight down a steep but short section of hillside over large boulders. Use extra caution in this area; it is as good a place to break an ankle as any place I have been. Just before reaching the bottom of the hill, red blazes lead off to the east over the rocks. Soon the path joins an old roadbed and turns right. Follow the roadbed for 0.3 mile, keeping your eyes open for the point where the Stone Tower Trail drops down to the crossing at Clark Creek and the road turns into the pink-blazed connector trail. The junction is easy to miss, even though you passed by it a few hours earlier. Follow the trail back to the creek crossing and to the car.

Nearby Activities

Because the Dehart Reservoir is a watershed, the area immediately around it is closed to all public use. Above and below the reservoir, however, Clark Creek provides some wonderful fishing on public land.

GPS TRAILHEAD COORDINATES AND DIRECTIONS

N40° 29.761' W76° 40.076'

Exit US 22/322 West from Harrisburg on PA 225 North toward Halifax. Follow PA 225 1.8 miles, then turn right (east) on PA 325. Follow PA 325 16.4 miles. A small parking area is located on the right just beyond the end of the Dehart Reservoir. It is identified by two large red blazes on a tree above a large area of fluorescent pink spray paint on the same tree. Space is available for six or seven cars. Parking for an additional two or three cars is located a mile up the road on the right. You can cross the creek and pick up the Sand Spring Trail there.

NORTHWEST

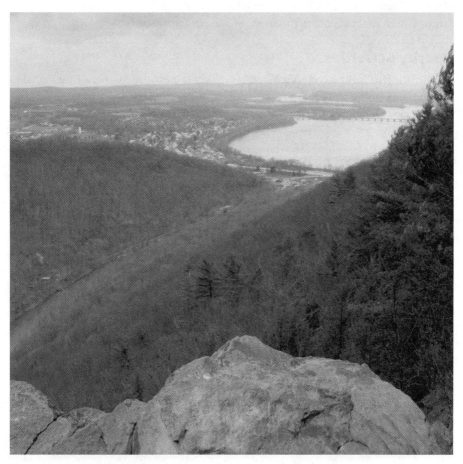

Looking northeast to the Susquehanna River from Hawk Rock (see Hike 22, page 116)

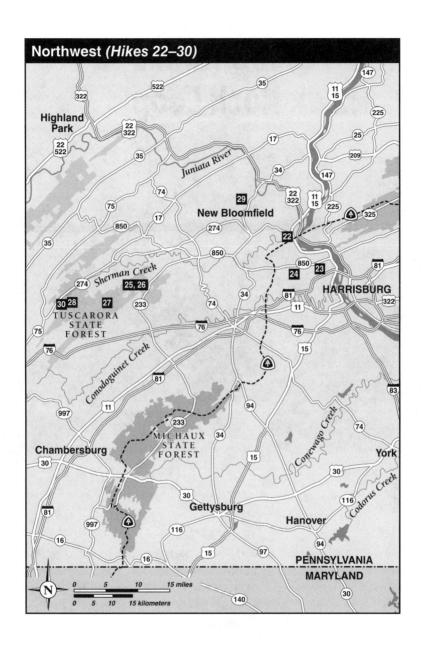

Northwest (Hikes 22–30)

147
35
522
11
15
322
225
Highland
Park
22
322
25
22
522
17
209
35
Juniata River
34
147
74
22
322
11
15
225
29
75
325
17
New Bloomfield
850
274
22
850
850
23
Sherman Creek
274
24
81
25, 26
HARRISBURG
30 28
27
233
74
34
81
322
TUSCARORA
STATE
FOREST
75
76
11
76
15
Conodoguinet Creek
81
83
997
11
94
233
74
MICHAUX
STATE
FOREST
Chambersburg
34
30
15
Conewago Creek
York
30
30
116
Codorus Creek
Gettysburg
81
997
Hanover
116
94
16
15
97
PENNSYLVANIA
16
MARYLAND
N
0   5   10   15 miles
0   5   10   15 kilometers
140
30

22 Cove Mountain and Hawk Rock Loop

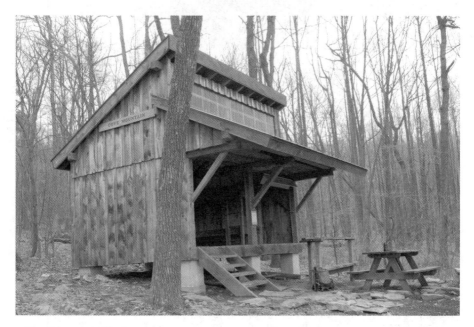

Cove Mountain Shelter

In Brief

This hike ascends Cove Mountain to the Hawk Rock Overlook via the Appalachian Trail (AT). From the overlook, it traverses Cove Mountain, makes a brief side trip to the Cove Mountain Shelter, and picks up a side trail that descends to the north. At the bottom of the trail, this hike heads east on a dirt road along a tributary of Sherman Creek and joins Sherman Creek proper about a mile from the end.

Description

Although the first mile of this hike up to Hawk Rock is a popular outing, the rest of it sees relatively little traffic. I pieced the loop together after studying a couple of maps and thought it would make for a pleasant trip. You'll get a great view from Hawk Rock, some wonderful ridge walking through the woods along Cove Mountain, and then a walk along a wildlife-management road through more of a wetlands terrain on the return.

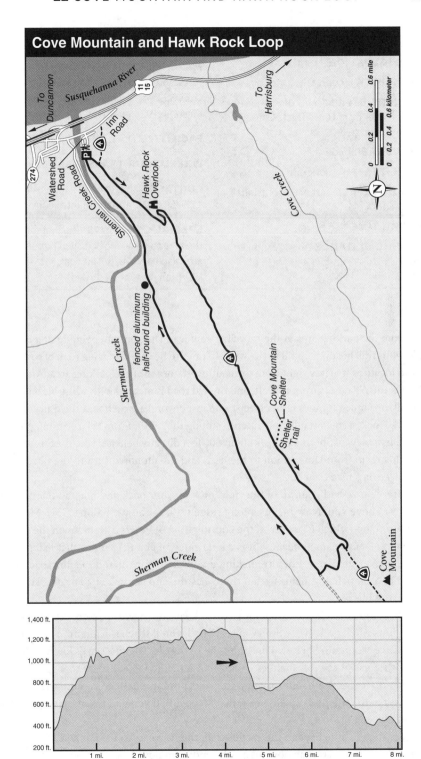

Cove Mountain and Hawk Rock Loop

LENGTH 8.1 miles	**ACCESS** Open
CONFIGURATION Loop	**MAPS** USGS *Wertzville* and *Duncannon*; Keystone Trail Association *Appalachian Trail, Susquehanna River to PA Route 94 (Sections 9, 10, and 11)*
DIFFICULTY Moderately strenuous	
SCENERY Beautiful view of Susquehanna River from Hawk Rock; Cove Mountain ridge	
	FACILITIES None
EXPOSURE Shade	
TRAIL TRAFFIC Moderate	**WHEELCHAIR TRAVERSABLE** No
TRAIL SURFACE Dirt with occasional rocky spots	**CONTACT** Appalachian Trail Conservancy, 717-258-5771, appalachiantrail.org
HIKING TIME 4–5 hours	**SPECIAL COMMENTS** The first mile of the hike to Hawk Rock is very popular and also very steep. The walk across Cove Mountain is quite secluded.
DRIVING DISTANCE About 2.2 miles from US 22/322 and PA 849 north of Harrisburg	

From the parking area at the recycling center in Duncannon, begin hiking uphill on an obvious trail heading uphill to the west. It looks to be an old logging road of sorts and is easy to locate as it leaves right from the southwest corner of the parking area. After about 0.2 mile, the AT enters from the left, and the old road is marked with white blazes. Follow it uphill for a mile (at times rather steep), and just beyond a switchback the trail comes out to Hawk Rock, a small sandstone outcrop among the pines. From this location, you'll get an excellent view of Sherman Creek about 600 feet directly beneath you, the Susquehanna River upstream from Duncannon to the east, and the mountains off to the north. It is a great place on a nice clear day.

After you've had your fill of the view, pick up your pack and hike up the AT to the ridge just above you. Now begins a long ridge walk to the west along Cove Mountain. The mountain—which is, in effect, the continuation of Peters Mountain on the east side of the river—is so named because it is a long ridge of about 12 miles that extends west from the river for 5 miles before making a complete U-turn and heading back to the river. The valley that remains within the U has the appearance of a large isolated cove just west of the river.

After about 2 miles of walking along a beautiful, wide, oak-covered ridge with many mountain laurels (very pretty in late May), you'll reach the junction with the trail to the Cove Mountain Shelter. This is the site of the old Thelma Marks Shelter. As is the case with most of the AT shelters, you'll find a picnic table, access to a spring, and a privy there. It is also a haunt for a mischievous porcupine. Bear in mind that the 0.25-mile walk to the shelter is all down a rather steep hill. If you don't want to walk back up, stay on the ridge.

Just about a mile beyond the shelter trail, the AT veers to the left and over the crest of the ridge at the head of an obvious north-tending hollow. Just after you pass the hollow, an unnamed, but well-marked, blue-blazed trail heads off to the north. Turn right and follow this trail into the valley below. The descent is rather steep at times, though for the most part the footing is good. Soon it levels out in the bottom of a small valley where it ends at a dirt road onto which you will turn right (east).

If you look at a map, you'll notice that this is an interesting valley, topographically speaking. Even though you've descended a good bit, the valley is still about 300 feet in elevation above Sherman Creek, which flows on the other side of the low ridge (Pine Ridge) to your north. The creek flowing through the woods to your left will actually exit the valley through a small water gap in Pine Ridge just east of the junction. You can see this gap if you keep your eyes on the ridge as you head east.

Follow the road for 3.5 miles back to your car. It climbs to a small saddle first and then begins the descent to Sherman Creek, which will appear from the north after about 2.7 miles. To gauge your progress, at 2.3 miles you will pass a large, half-round aluminum building surrounded by a chain-link fence. When Sherman Creek is in view, you'll pass another road that follows it to the north. Stay to the right here.

If you are hiking during April, keep your eyes open on the forest floor for Dutchman's-breeches, clusters of small yellow-and-white flowers that appear early in the spring. These pretty (if not unusually shaped) flowers grow in abundance along the side of the road above the creek.

Nearby Activities

Duncannon is a prominent layover for thru-hikers on the AT. The town has restaurants, pubs, and hotels, all of which are quite accommodating to hikers. The **Doyle Hotel** (7 N. Market St.; 717-834-6789) is a common haunt for hikers. Just outside of town at the end of Main Street and Inn Road, about 0.2 mile south of Little Boston Road, is **Tubby's Night Club,** on the left (717-834-4700). The food is good and the proprietors very friendly.

GPS TRAILHEAD COORDINATES AND DIRECTIONS
N40° 22.975' W77° 02.006'

From Harrisburg, follow US 22/322 west. Cross the Susquehanna River over the Clark Ferry Bridge and take the first exit (on the left) for PA 849/Duncannon. Follow PA 849 over the Juniata River and, when it bears to the right, make a left onto Market Street. Follow Market Street through Duncannon and follow signs for US 11/15 South. Once through town, pass beneath US 11/15 and make the first left onto Main Street. Go past the on-ramp for US 11/15 South—don't get on the highway!—and continue straight until the road crosses Sherman Creek. Turn right onto Little Boston Road and make the first right onto Watershed Road. Follow the signs to the recycling center and park on the left.

23 Darlington Trail Loop:
EAST

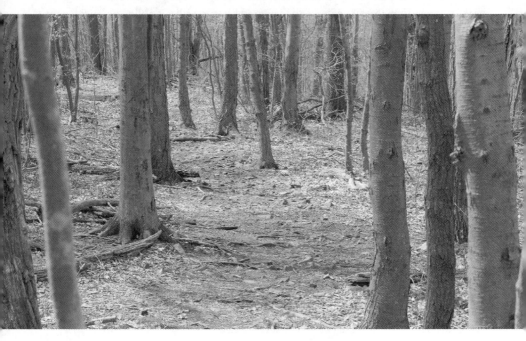

Along the Darlington Trail

In Brief

From the parking area on Tower Road, follow the Darlington Trail west into a hollow. In the hollow, pick up an old logging road and follow that south to another logging road that you'll follow west to junction with the Darlington Trail. Continue along the Darlington Trail to a junction of five trails where you pick up another logging road heading west to Lambs Gap Road. Follow a path parallel to Lambs Gap Road up to the Darlington Trail at Lambs Gap. Follow the Darlington Trail back to the parking area at Tower Road.

Description

Looking for something other than an out-and-back hike on the Darlington Trail, my son Jackson and I decided to piece together a couple of loops along the easternmost stretch of the Darlington one Saturday in April. The hike turned out to be a little rugged, but interesting for two reasons. First, it allowed us to explore some of the forest along the north side of Blue Mountain that probably very few hikers get to see (most stick to the Darlington Trail

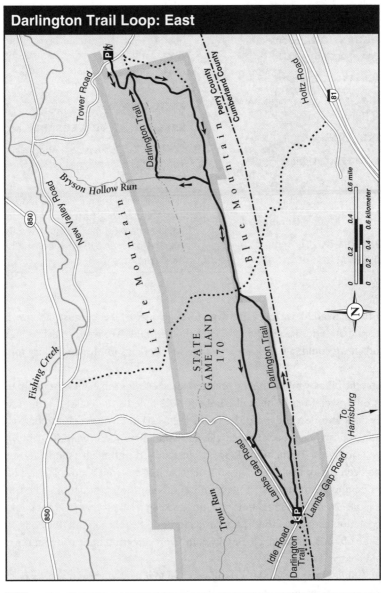

Darlington Trail Loop: East

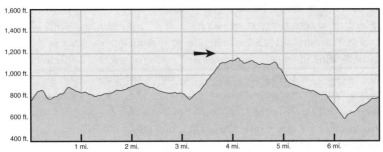

LENGTH 6.9 miles	**ACCESS** Open
CONFIGURATION 2 loops joined by a section of out-and-back	**MAPS** USGS *Wertzville* and *Harrisburg West*; a map of the entire Darlington Trail is available online at satc-hike.org /documents/darlmap.pdf.
DIFFICULTY Moderate	
SCENERY Old logging roads and forest; Bryson Hollow	**FACILITIES** None
	WHEELCHAIR TRAVERSABLE No
EXPOSURE Shaded	**CONTACT** Susquehanna Appalachian Trail Club, satc-hike.org
TRAIL TRAFFIC Light	
TRAIL SURFACE Dirt, very rocky in places	**SPECIAL COMMENTS** This is a rough hike with sections on the east loop that may be too overgrown to be feasible in the summer. It is easily completed as an out-and-back hike of 6.6 miles staying on the Darlington Trail.
HIKING TIME 3.5–4.5 hours	
DRIVING DISTANCE About 10 miles from the PA 11/15 exit on I-81	

out-and-back). Second, we had a pretty good laugh on the hike, because Jackson, being 16 years old and athletic, ate all of our food in the first mile. We were famished on the way back, and all we could talk about was driving to Wegmans in Mechanicsburg for tamales and ginger beer.

Begin the hike by following the orange-blazed Darlington Trail west out of the parking area on Tower Road. The trail climbs for 0.2 mile to the crest of a ridge where it switches back and descends into the valley below. When you reach the bottom of the hollow, the trail switches back to the west, and immediately afterward (0.3 mile) you will leave the Darlington Trail and pick up an old roadbed to the left (south) by some logs that have been cut to make the side trail accessible. This trail is not blazed. Follow the trail as it climbs gently uphill in a generally south-southwest direction. The trail is not obvious in places and requires some scouting to keep track. It may be impossible to find if the vegetation is thick. If that is the case, either do the Darlington Trail out-and-back or continue up the hillside in a generally southwest direction until you join the roadbed described below.

At 0.75 mile the trail reaches a significant old logging road that traverses the hillside. Turn right and follow this to the west. The trail stays level for most of its length, so it isn't very challenging in terms of gaining elevation. It is, however, frequently obstructed by fallen trees and marshy areas that require you to venture out and back into the woods to circumnavigate difficulties. Although only about three quarters of a mile long, this stretch of the hike can be quite time-consuming. At 1.5 miles, the logging road joins the Darlington Trail, the familiar orange blazes appear again, and the most difficult section of the hike is over. Continue along the Darlington Trail for another 0.6 mile to a junction with trails heading off in five directions. The Darlington Trail heads uphill in a generally southwest direction. Instead of following that, continue straight west on the level track ahead of you. That path provides some easy walking for a mile to a gate where the path ends at Lambs Gap Road. From the gate you want to make your way up to the Darlington Trail, where it passes through Lambs Gap. Do not hike along the paved road. Instead, from the gate look uphill to your left (south) and you should be able to make out a path that climbs the hillside parallel to the road. Head for that. The farther along the path you walk, the more distinct it becomes, and after a short, steep section it joins the Darlington Trail at a flat area near the crest of Blue Mountain above the parking lot at Lambs Gap (3.6 miles). Turn left on the Darlington Trail and follow it east as it traverses just below the crest of Blue Mountain. The trail follows the ridge for what seems like a very long time before descending. The duration of the trek along the ridge seems longer in part because the hiking in this section is very rocky. A good pair of boots is in order here. When the trail begins to descend, it does so very quickly and it only takes about 5–10 minutes to get from the ridgecrest back to the junction of the five trails.

Continue along the Darlington Trail, heading east. When you pass the logging road you took earlier the Darlington Trail veers to the north and drops into Bryson Hollow, a steep-sided water gap through the ridge. As you reach the hollow's namesake creek, Bryson Hollow Run, keep your eyes open for a pine tree with two orange blazes painted one above another with an arrow beneath them (6 miles). The trail makes a sharp U-turn here and heads upstream for a short distance before crossing the creek at some rocks. After a heavy rain this crossing may be impassable. The trail continues up Bryson Hollow for another 0.7 mile back to the switchback that climbs out of the hollow and crosses the ridge before descending to the parking. This upper section of Bryson Hollow is remarkable for the devastation caused by a significant wind event (a wind shear or perhaps a tornado) in recent years. Huge trees have been uprooted all along the trail, which would be impassable except for the efforts of the Susquehanna Appalachian Trail Club, which maintains this stretch of trail.

GPS TRAILHEAD COORDINATES AND DIRECTIONS

N40° 19.316' W76° 57.781'

From I-81 get off at the US 15/US 11 North exit toward Marysville. Follow US 11 north 2.5 miles to Marysville. Turn left onto PA 850 and follow it west 2 miles to Heisley Lane. Turn left and then right (west) onto New Valley Road. Tower Road is 0.6 mile farther on the left. Turn left onto Tower Road. The parking area is 0.8 mile up Tower Road, the last 0.4 mile of which is particularly rough. Parking is on the right on a steep hillside with enough room for three or four cars.

24 Darlington Trail Loop:
WEST

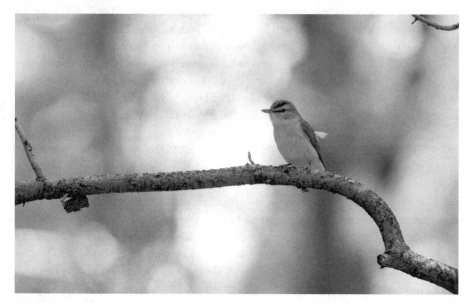

Yellow-eyed vireo

In Brief

From the parking area, follow Idle Road to the Darlington Trail at Lambs Gap. Walk the ridge west along the Darlington Trail to Millers Gap Road. The hike follows Millers Gap Road downhill to the north, where it picks up a game-lands road and footpath that leads back to the car.

Description

I discovered this hike on the "Our Favorite Hikes" page of the Susquehanna Appalachian Trail Club website (satc-hike.org). Over the years, it has become one of my favorite excursions in the area, especially during the fall, when the trees are quite colorful, and during the spring before the leaves have sprouted, when you can get some nice views. The hike makes a loop between Lambs Gap and Millers Gap on Blue Mountain west of Harrisburg. It uses the Darlington Trail across the ridgetop and a game-land trail below. Two sections of dirt road connect the two. You can park at any one of four parking areas that the route passes by, but my experience suggests that the hike walks best in a clockwise direction beginning from the parking area on Idle Road below Lambs Gap.

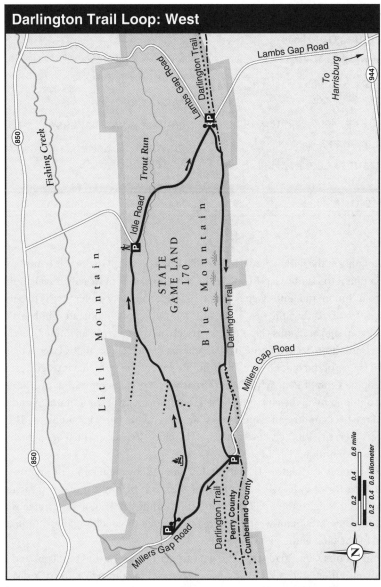

Darlington Trail Loop: West

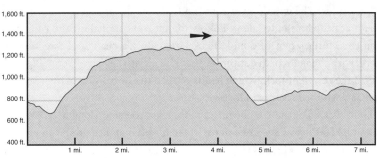

LENGTH 7.3 miles	**DRIVING DISTANCE** 3.75 miles from I-81 and PA 944
CONFIGURATION Loop	
DIFFICULTY Moderate	**ACCESS** Sunrise–sunset
SCENERY Beautiful wooded ridge walk, remote game lands	**MAPS** USGS *Wertzville*
	FACILITIES None
EXPOSURE More shade than sun	**WHEELCHAIR TRAVERSABLE** No
TRAIL TRAFFIC Light	**CONTACT** Susquehanna Appalachian Trail Club, satc-hike.org
TRAIL SURFACE Dirt, short sections of dirt road	
	SPECIAL COMMENTS One of my favorite hikes in the area
HIKING TIME 4 hours	

Beginning at the parking area, follow Idle Road downhill to the south into Trout Run and then uphill to Lambs Gap Road. While not unpleasant or heavily traveled, the climb from Trout Run up to Lambs Gap is about 0.75 mile long. My preference is to get this out of the way first, and then the rest of the hike has only short, moderate climbs. When you reach the stop sign at Lambs Gap Road, turn right and then make an immediate right turn onto the Darlington Trail, identified by a game-lands gate and orange blazes. The Darlington Trail is one of the older hiking trails in this part of the state, having been established by the Alpine Club of Pennsylvania in the early 1900s. An organization of conservation-minded outdoorsmen, the club established routes up many of the mountains and through much of the backcountry all around the state. Several libraries, including the Pennsylvania State University Library, have copies of the club's journals, which are entertaining to read at least for antiquarian interest.

The original Darlington Trail extended along Blue Mountain east and west of the Susquehanna River, although now much of that path belongs to the Appalachian Trail corridor. According to the SATC website, the Darlington Trail today stretches for 7.75 miles along Blue Mountain west of Harrisburg, much of which is along a footpath constructed by the club in the past ten years.

From Lambs Gap Road, pass the gate to get on the Darlington Trail and climb a short hill until the trail levels out and traverses the ridge through a pretty forest of birch and hickory trees. The wildflowers are abundant here during the spring, and the area is prime habitat for white-tailed deer. Follow the pleasant trail along the ridge for 2 miles until you encounter a pair of double blazes indicating a change of direction. The trail forks here, with the main path continuing straight along the ridge eventually into private property. Take the right fork, which heads over to the north side of the ridge through a more densely wooded section of forest.

In about 0.3 mile, the trail begins a long, level traverse along a very steep hillside about 50 or 60 feet below the crest of the ridge on what appears to be an old stone road grade. At 2.7 miles from Lambs Gap Road, you'll reach Millers Gap Road. Turn right and follow Millers Gap Road downhill for 0.75 mile to a trailhead with a gate across a state-game-lands track. A sign indicates that this is State Game Land 170, encompassing 9,092 acres. There is a triangular sign on the gate indicating that this is a bicycle and horse path.

Follow the grassy track east for a mile, past a small meadow and over a culvert, to a small clearing with a fire ring. The trail enters the woods on the other side of the camp and becomes more of a footpath than a road. Keep your eyes open for occasional blazes consisting of black with a white bull's-eye wherever the path joins others. At about 1.5 miles from Millers Gap Road, you'll reach a swampy area—the headwater of Trout Run—and pass a trail entering from the right and not long afterward a trail entering from the left.

Climb out of the swampy section along a hillside to a junction with a significant trail entering from the left. Stay to the right and follow this old roadbed through a long section of beautiful and fairly open pine and hardwoods back to the parking area at Idle Road.

GPS TRAILHEAD COORDINATES AND DIRECTIONS
N40° 18.866' W77° 02.008'

From I-81, south of the Susquehanna River, take Exit 61 (PA 944). Follow PA 944 west 1 mile to Lambs Gap Road. Turn right on Lambs Gap Road and follow it over the top of the mountain. Just beyond the parking area at the top, turn left onto Idle Road. The trailhead is at a large parking area 1.25 miles along on the left, where the road bends right after climbing out of Trout Run.

25 Flat Rock Overlook

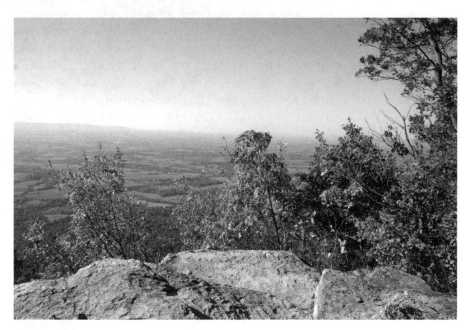

The Cumberland Valley from Flat Rock

In Brief

Departing from the Environmental Classroom at Colonel Denning State Park, follow the Flat Rock Trail uphill for 1 mile to the Wagon Wheel, a junction of five trails. From here, the Flat Rock Trail follows the path of the Tuscarora Trail for another mile out to the Flat Rock Overlook. Retrace the route back to the state park or continue following the Flat Rock and Warner Loop through Wildcat Hollow (see next hike).

Description

The first thing you will encounter when you do this hike is a sign that says you may encounter rattlesnakes along this trail. Then the trail climbs moderately for a half-mile before it gets really steep for another half-mile. You should not, however, allow these two facts to dissuade you from doing this hike. The rattlesnakes are not hanging from trees and hiding beneath every rock (though you do need to be aware that this is timber rattler country and exercise appropriate caution), and the hill climb is rather short-lived. The reward for completing the hike is one of the best views in central Pennsylvania. I've made this hike on several occasions, in a variety of weather conditions, and degrees of good and bad moods, and have never regretted doing so.

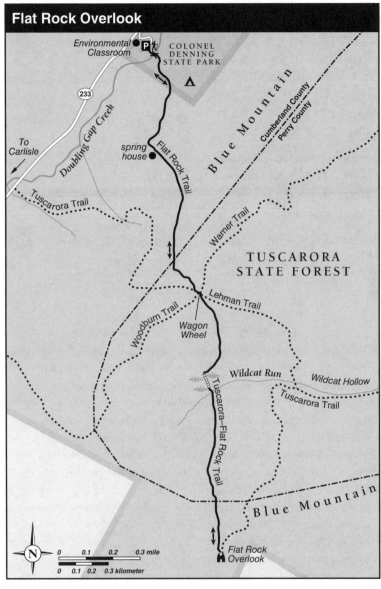

Flat Rock Overlook

Environmental Classroom · P · 🏛

COLONEL DENNING STATE PARK

To Carlisle

Doubling Gap Creek

233

spring house ●

Flat Rock Trail

Tuscarora Trail

Blue Mountain

Cumberland County / Perry County

Warner Trail

TUSCARORA STATE FOREST

Lehman Trail

Woodburn Trail

Wagon Wheel

Wildcat Run

Wildcat Hollow

Tuscarora Trail

Tuscarora–Flat Rock Trail

Blue Mountain

Flat Rock Overlook

N

0   0.1   0.2   0.3 mile
0   0.1   0.2   0.3 kilometer

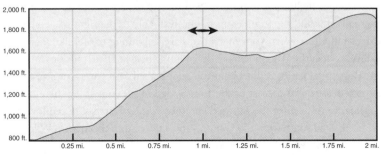

2,000 ft.
1,800 ft.
1,600 ft.
1,400 ft.
1,200 ft.
1,000 ft.
800 ft.

0.25 mi.   0.5 mi.   0.75 mi.   1 mi.   1.25 mi.   1.5 mi.   1.75 mi.   2 mi.

LENGTH 4 miles	**ACCESS** Sunrise–sunset
CONFIGURATION Out-and-back	**MAPS** USGS *Andersonburg;* Colonel Denning State Park map has part of the route; Potomac Appalachian Trail Club *Tuscarora Trail, Map J: Appalachian Trail, PA, to PA Route 641*
DIFFICULTY Strenuous hill climb for 0.5 mile; the rest is moderate.	
SCENERY Outstanding view of the Cumberland Valley	
EXPOSURE Shade	**FACILITIES** Water and restrooms near trailhead
TRAIL TRAFFIC Moderate–somewhat busy on weekends	**WHEELCHAIR TRAVERSABLE** No
TRAIL SURFACE Dirt and rock	**CONTACT** Colonel Denning State Park, 717-776-5272, tinyurl.com/colonel denningsp
HIKING TIME About 1 hour each way	
DRIVING DISTANCE About 25 miles from the junction of I-81 south and PA 114 south of Harrisburg	**SPECIAL COMMENTS** The second half-mile of the hike is a real grind; afterward it is much more pleasant. The area is home to timber rattlesnakes.

You begin this hike from the Environmental Classroom parking area in Colonel Denning State Park. Walk south past the picnic shelter, keeping the amphitheater to your right, and cross the creek at a bridge, where you will see the rattlesnake sign. From the bridge, the trail ascends Blue Mountain by way of a series of wooden steps constructed into the hillside. Blue Mountain in this area makes a Z shape, formed by the uplifting of the Valley and Ridge Province during the Allegheny Orogeny, the formation of these mountains millions of years ago. In effect, this hike begins in the southwestward-tending valley formed by the Z and climbs over the center ridge and across the head of the northeastward-tending valley (Wildcat Hollow) to the Flat Rock Overlook, which is situated at the very bottom of the Z.

From the steps, continue past the tent-camping area on the left, along a gradual incline through a beautiful forest of oak and hickory trees. If you are a fan of oranges and yellows, this place cannot be beat in the fall. I have spotted quite a few deer here early in the morning, and judging by the amount of mast on the ground here during the fall, I wouldn't be surprised if black bears frequent the area.

After 0.25 mile, the trail reaches a prominent dirt road. Turn left on this road and follow it up a steeper incline for another 0.25 mile to the remains of an old spring house. Here, the road ends and the trail begins to climb steeply to the right of a watercourse for the next half-mile. Just when your hamstrings are beginning to feel like piano strings, it abruptly levels out at the Wagon Wheel, the meeting place of five trails on the Blue Mountain ridge. Here, the Flat Rock Trail joins the blue-blazed Tuscarora Trail, a 252-mile-long path that extends from the crest of the Blue Ridge Mountains in Shenandoah National Park, Virginia, to just shy of the Susquehanna River near Harrisburg. Follow the Tuscarora–Flat Rock Trail south from the Wagon Wheel down into the head of Wildcat Hollow, passing by a trail shelter and outhouse on the left after 0.2 mile.

Soon the trail levels out in a swampy area and crosses several wooden boardwalks and a couple of areas where stones have been positioned as treads. The hickory trees here are tall and provide habitat for many birds. When I last passed through this area, I spotted an owl in the early morning flying silently just above the forest floor. After passing the swampy section, the trail begins to climb again to the ridge of Blue Mountain, only much more gently this time. The 0.6-mile ascent is rather remarkable as the trail—and indeed the entire forest floor—consists of large plates and boulders of sedimentary rock. The trail levels out gradually as it reaches the ridge, and the overlook is actually beyond the ridge, downhill from its crest about 75 vertical feet or so. The overlook is, as its name implies, a large flat rock wedged into the mountainside and clear of trees to the south and east. The view of the Cumberland Valley is the stuff of calendars and postcards. Remarkable. Beneath you, Blue Mountain drops steeply away into a large open talus field, giving the whole experience a vertiginous feel. Bear in mind that the Cumberland Valley is only part of the Great Valley, a geological formation that extends from New York to Georgia.

As you cross the ridge and approach the overlook, try to be as quiet as possible. The entire ridgeline is a wonderful roost for birds of prey and other large birds, and you'll have a better chance of seeing some if you approach the overlook silently. In addition to the abundant turkey vultures that can often be found soaring on the wind currents along the ridge, I have seen peregrine falcons from the overlook and several species of hawks.

From the overlook, you can continue along the Tuscarora Trail to the east and make a loop back to the Wagon Wheel via the Lehman Trail or the Warner Trail (see next hike), both of which are significant undertakings, as the terrain gets very rugged to the east. Or you can simply retrace your steps, the common excursion. Be sure to watch your footing when descending from the Wagon Wheel to the spring house.

Nearby Activities

Colonel Denning State Park has plenty of things to do. It has a very nice tent-camping area, as well as a lake with a swimming beach and a seasonal concession area. Environmental programs are often scheduled at the nature center. And plenty of space is available for picnicking.

GPS TRAILHEAD COORDINATES AND DIRECTIONS
N40° 16.796' W77° 25.104'

Follow I-81 south from outside of Harrisburg. Take Exit 57 and turn right on PA 114 for a mile. Turn left on PA 944 and follow it 4.5 miles to PA 34. Turn right on PA 34 and follow it another 5 miles to PA 850. Turn left and follow 850 into Landisburg. At Landisburg, proceed straight on PA 233. Follow that over the mountain. Colonel Denning State Park is 7.7 miles from Landisburg on the left. Park near the Environmental Classroom along the creek.

26 Flat Rock Overlook and Warner Trail Loop

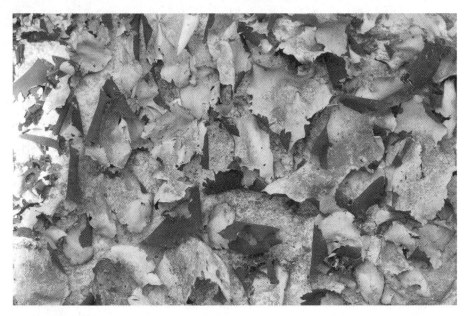

Giant rock tripe

In Brief

Beginning at the Flat Rock Overlook (see previous hike profile), this hike follows the Tuscarora Trail east through Wildcat Hollow. After several miles, it joins the Warner Trail and follows Trout Run to the Wagon Wheel trail junction a mile above the parking area at Colonel Denning State Park.

Description

For the first 2 miles of this hike, follow the directions to the Flat Rock Overlook, provided in the previous profile. After enjoying the view, it's time to grab your pack and take to the Tuscarora Trail. From the overlook, head back uphill a short distance and keep your eyes open for the not-so-obvious blue-blazed trail heading off to the east. If you backtrack as far as the ridgecrest, you've passed it. For the first 0.25 mile or so from the overlook, the route passes over talus in the woods. Nothing suggests a trail except the blazes (which are

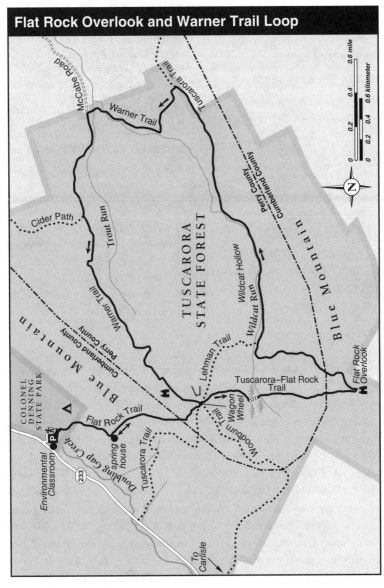

Flat Rock Overlook and Warner Trail Loop

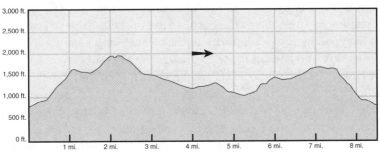

LENGTH 8.5 miles, including the hike to Flat Rock Overlook

CONFIGURATION Balloon

DIFFICULTY Quite strenuous

SCENERY Outstanding view of the Cumberland Valley; the dark and remote Wildcat Hollow

EXPOSURE Shade

TRAIL TRAFFIC Light

TRAIL SURFACE Dirt; some sections are very rugged and rocky.

HIKING TIME 5–6 hours

DRIVING DISTANCE About 25 miles from the junction of I-81 South and PA 114 west of Harrisburg

ACCESS Sunrise–sunset

MAPS USGS *Andersonburg;* Colonel Denning State Park map has part of the route; Potomac Appalachian Trail Club *Tuscarora Trail, Map J: Appalachian Trail, PA, to PA Route 641*

FACILITIES Water and restrooms near Flat Rock Trail trailhead

WHEELCHAIR TRAVERSABLE No

CONTACT Colonel Denning State Park, 717-776-5272, tinyurl.com/colonel denningsp

SPECIAL COMMENTS This is a strenuous hike through a remote section of the Tuscarora State Forest. In spots the trail is very rugged. Use caution and common sense on this route, and allow plenty of time.

prolific), although the path generally follows the ridge of Blue Mountain until it begins to descend into Wildcat Hollow. Although not steep, the descent is rather rocky with uncertain footing in places and would be unpleasant in the rain. If you pay attention, you'll find some wonderful patches of giant rock tripe, a leathery brown-and-green lichen growing on the rocks in the woods. This distinctive lichen grows in large flakes over many years.

As the trail descends into Wildcat Hollow, it gets a little steeper, though a little less rocky. After a rather long 0.85 mile, the terrain levels out and the trail joins an old logging road at the junction with the Lehman Trail. Have a look down the Tuscarora Trail, which follows the logging road next to the creek. Rugged, dark, and rocky, with several fallen trees across it, the trail appears rather forbidding. If the passage looks undesirable, turn left on the Lehman Trail and follow that for a half-mile uphill to the Wagon Wheel. If you decide to continue, you'll traverse some wild and remote terrain. As it descends farther along the creek, the Tuscarora Trail passes through dark stands of hemlock trees. If you are lucky, you may spot signs of the wildlife for which the hollow is named. On my most recent excursion into the hollow, I came across a tree on the trail that was obviously used as a scratching post by a bobcat. Its bark was streaked with long, thin claw marks, too narrow to be those of a bear, which also will mark trees with its claws.

The farther you travel into the hollow, the better the trail gets. Around a mile from the junction with the Lehman Trail, the Tuscarora Trail begins to climb away from the creek, which makes a bend to the north around the end of Wildcat Ridge toward Buck Ridge. The forest in this area is populated by some mature maple and oak trees towering above. The forest floor is matted with ferns and filled with carcasses of large trees in

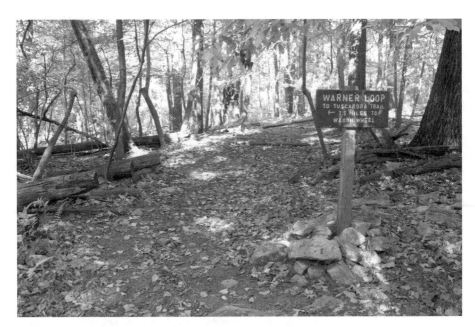

Warner Trail trailhead in Wildcat Hollow

various stages of decay. At about 2.1 miles from the Flat Rock Overlook, the trail passes onto private property identified by two prominent NO TRESPASSING signs nailed to trees astride the path. Just about 0.1 mile beyond those signs, you'll reach the junction with the red-blazed Warner Trail marked by a sign. Turn left onto the Warner Trail, an old roadbed, and follow that through more tall oak and hickory trees back to the creek in Wildcat Hollow. You may notice a significant change in geology in this area. Whereas this hike passed over large boulders of coarse gray sandstone along the top of Blue Mountain, now it passes through an area characterized by plates of dark-maroon Tuscarora sandstone. Soon the forest becomes more populated with hemlock trees, and the creek below is surrounded by large areas of willows.

At 0.7 mile from the Tuscarora Trail, the Warner Trail crosses the creek and immediately heads to the right through the willows (if you continue straight uphill along an obvious path from the creek, you'll soon reach a cabin and private property). Continue along the trail for a short distance and cross McCabe Road, accessible in this area only by four-wheel-drive vehicle. You should spot a sign for the Warner Trail at the road. If you don't, look uphill, as the trail gets braided in the willows and several paths come out to the road a little farther downhill. Cross the road and begin the 2-mile climb up Trout Run back to the Wagon Wheel.

After a half-mile, you'll reach a woven wire fence surrounding a forest-management area, which you will enter by a hanging gate constructed of rebar. You'll eventually leave the area by the same type of gate. These gates can only be lifted outward from the forest-management area and are designed to allow wildlife, deer in particular, to escape but not enter the area. Within the fence are many oak and hickory saplings and young-growth trees, the bark of which is a favorite for deer to browse on. The fence and gates keep the deer away, and hunting is encouraged within these fenced areas.

After exiting the management area, the trail soon joins a very old roadbed and comes out to a significant logging road about 1.7 miles from the creek crossing below. Follow the logging road uphill for a short distance and around a bend to the right. Before it bends back to the left, look for a sign for the Warner Trail on the right conveniently hidden behind a tree. The Warner Trail departs from the road and traverses beneath the crest of Blue Mountain on an old coach road above Colonel Denning State Park. In the fall and winter, this section of trail offers great views across the valley toward Doubling Gap to the north. Soon you reach the Wagon Wheel, completing the 6.5-mile loop, very little of which was on flat ground. Take a well-deserved break and then follow the Flat Rock Trail back to the car.

Nearby Activities

Colonel Denning State Park has plenty of things to do. It has a very nice tent-camping area, as well as a lake with a swimming beach and a seasonal concession area. Environmental programs are often scheduled at the nature center. And plenty of space is available for picnicking.

GPS TRAILHEAD COORDINATES AND DIRECTIONS
N40° 16.796' W77° 25.104'

Follow I-81 south from outside of Harrisburg. Take Exit 57 and turn right on PA 114 for a mile. Turn left on PA 944 and follow it 4.5 miles to PA 34. Turn right on PA 34 and follow it another 5 miles to PA 850. Turn left and follow 850 into Landisburg. At Landisburg, proceed straight on PA 233. Follow that over the mountain. Colonel Denning State Park is 7.7 miles from Landisburg on the left. Park near the Environmental Classroom along the creek.

27 Frank E. Masland Jr. Natural Area Trek

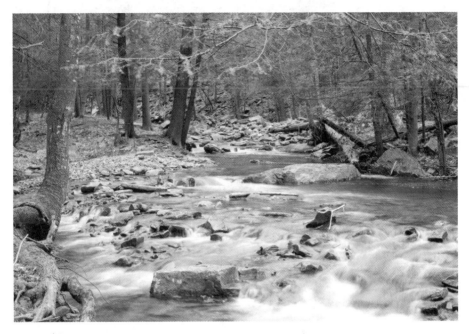

Laurel Run

In Brief

This hike begins with a pretty walk along the North Branch Trail through Laurel Run Hollow, then climbs a hollow to the south of the creek on the Deer Hollow Trail out to Laurel Run Road. After a short walk along the road, it descends back to Laurel Run via the Turbett Trail, goes west, and retraces the first mile to the parking area.

Description

Located in the Tuscarora State Forest in western Perry County, the Frank E. Masland Jr. Natural Area is a 1,270-acre tract of land that encompasses a hemlock-filled section of the north branch of the Laurel Run Valley and a ridge covered with oak and mountain laurel rising to its south.

According to a Bureau of Forestry pamphlet, Frank E. Masland Jr. owned a carpet-manufacturing business in nearby Carlisle during the early 1900s. The naming of this tract

Frank E. Masland Jr. Natural Area Trek

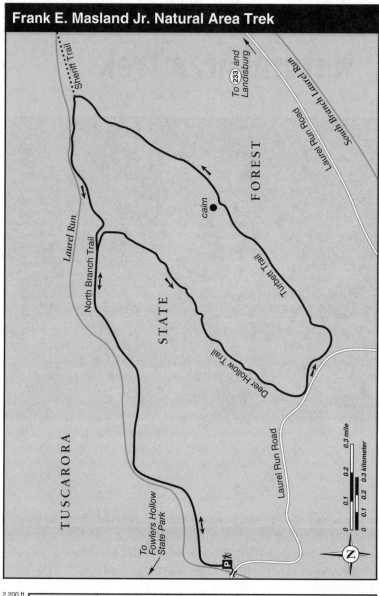

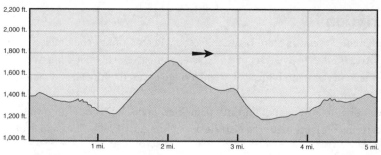

LENGTH 5 miles	**ACCESS** Dawn to Dusk
CONFIGURATION Balloon	**MAPS** USGS *Blain* and *Newburg;* Frank E. Masland Jr. Natural Area pamphlet provided by the Pennsylvania Bureau of Forestry also has a good map, as does the Tuscarora State Forest public-use map available at the forest headquarters in Blain.
DIFFICULTY Moderate	
SCENERY Pretty hollow of Laurel Run; open forest along the ridges	
EXPOSURE Half sun, half shade	
TRAIL TRAFFIC Light	**FACILITIES** None
TRAIL SURFACE Dirt	**WHEELCHAIR TRAVERSABLE** No
HIKING TIME 2.5–3 hours	**CONTACT** Tuscarora State Forest, 717-536-3191, tinyurl.com/tuscarorasf
DRIVING DISTANCE About 15 miles from intersection of PA 233 and PA 850 in Landisburg	**SPECIAL COMMENTS** Bring your fishing rod for Laurel Run.

of land, however, was a result of his commitment to natural-resources conservation around the state and the nation. As the sign at the beginning of the Turbett Trail on Laurel Run Road explains, Masland "dedicated a lifetime to the enrichment of human lives through the conservation of our natural resources." Among the lasting effects that can be attributed to his dedication are the Box Huckleberry Natural Area in Perry County and the Kings Gap Environmental Education Center (see page 241).

The natural area was founded for the protection of a second-growth stand of timber that may be the oldest second-growth stand in the state. The largest trees—the hemlocks, the white and red oak, the red maples, and the poplars—are found in the beautiful valley along Laurel Run. The oaks and pines located on the ridges above tend to be shorter and rather brushy, offering an attractive contrast in scenery. The area is home to a diverse population of woodland birds and a variety of reptiles, and is a habitat for many of the common woodland mammals of Pennsylvania.

Begin this hike from the small parking area on Laurel Run, where the red-blazed North Branch Trail begins. Follow the trail downstream through the valley not far from the south bank of the creek. Laurel Run has many large pools that provide habitat for native brook trout. The fish are often visible from the shore, and you may wish to bring some tackle along with you to test the waters.

At 0.6 mile, the trail climbs above the creek a couple of hundred feet to bypass a cliff along its south bank. Initially the climb is quite steep, but it eases off quickly. The trail walking is pleasant with good footing, but the hillside that the trail traverses is quite steep and thus probably not a good place for children. After passing through the high section, descend into a marshy area where the path becomes less distinct. Follow the red blazes through it, and shortly thereafter (1.2 miles), you'll cross a small creek. Just beyond it is the sign for the Deer Hollow Trail, onto which you will turn right to make a loop over the ridgetop before descending back to the creek. The junction with the Deer Hollow Trail marks the end of the North Branch Trail proper, although the trail continues down the Laurel Run Valley. The name of it changes here to the Sheriff Trail, and you'll pick that up in a couple of miles at the end of the loop and use it to return to this spot.

From the junction, follow the Deer Hollow Trail uphill along the bed of an intermittent creek. The trail gets a bit indistinct in places and the red blazes are not as prolific as they are in the valley. If you stick to the creek bed at places of uncertainty you should have no problems. The creek passes through pretty upland populated by small oak, pine, and much mountain laurel—great habitat for deer and very pleasant in late May and June when the mountain laurel is in bloom.

After 0.75 mile, the trail ends at Laurel Run Road (2 miles), which forms the boundary of the natural area. Turn left on the road and follow it south for 0.15 mile to the trailhead for the Turbett Trail. The trailhead is obviously marked with a large sign, and there is some room for parking. Turn left onto the Turbett Trail and follow it across a ridge in an ecosystem similar in character to that encountered along Deer Hollow.

At about 2.5 miles, you'll pass an enormous, well-constructed cairn in the middle of the Turbett Trail. Continue down the obvious path along rather flat terrain for what feels like a long way, and then begin the descent back to Laurel Run. The descent gets rather steep before reaching the level of creek. If you are thinking about doing the Deer Hollow–Turbett loop in the opposite direction, take the topography into consideration. The loop walks better counterclockwise.

At 3.3 miles, you'll reach the end of the Turbett Trail at the Sheriff Trail by the creek. A large log located at the junction makes a fine place to rest your feet after the descent. Turn left onto the Sheriff Trail and follow it west. After about 0.7 mile, you'll cross a significant wooden footbridge; just beyond that is the junction with the Deer Hollow and North Branch Trails. Follow the North Branch Trail back to the car.

Nearby Activities

The natural area has a certain middle-of-nowhere quality to it. However, **Laurel Run** and **South Branch Laurel Run** (accessible from Laurel Run Road) are both excellent fishing streams. **Fowlers Hollow State Park,** not far to the north, has picnic facilities. **Colonel Denning State Park,** not far to the east on PA 233, has picnic and recreational facilities.

GPS TRAILHEAD COORDINATES AND DIRECTIONS
N40° 15.063' W77° 31.773'

From Landisburg, follow PA 233 west 3.75 miles to Laurel Run Road on your right. Turn right on Laurel Run Road and follow it for another 11 miles to a bridge over Laurel Run in a hemlock-filled hollow. Parking is available on the right at the trailhead before crossing the creek.

28 Hemlocks Natural Area Loop

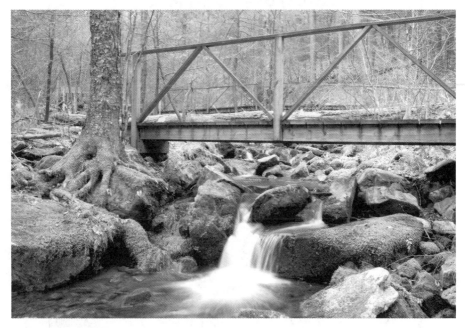

Patterson Run

In Brief

From the north trailhead for the Hemlocks Natural Area, this hike follows the Patterson Run and Rim Trails along the east side of the Patterson Run. About halfway through the natural area, the hike crosses the creek and follows the Hemlock Trail along the west side of the ravine to the south end of the natural area. From there, the hike returns via the Rim and Patterson Run Trails along the east side of the ravine.

Description

Located in western Perry County, the Hemlocks Natural Area is a 120-acre tract of land that is home to a stand of virgin eastern hemlock trees. The extent of the natural area is located in the steep-sided ravine through which Patterson Run flows, and in all likelihood this stand of trees was saved from the bite of the saw by the topography. According to the information brochure provided by the Tuscarora State Forest, the oldest trees date back

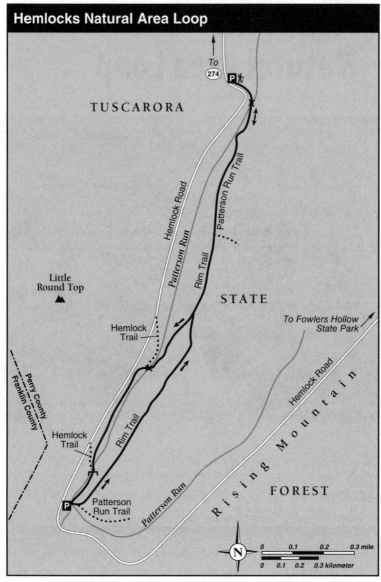

Hemlocks Natural Area Loop

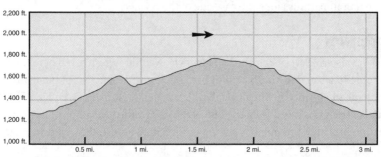

LENGTH 3.1 miles

CONFIGURATION Balloon

DIFFICULTY Mostly easy with some rocky sections

SCENERY Old-growth-hemlock forest

EXPOSURE Shaded

TRAIL TRAFFIC Light

TRAIL SURFACE Mostly dirt

HIKING TIME 1.5–2 hours

DRIVING DISTANCE About 31.5 miles from intersection of PA 34 and PA 274 in New Bloomfield

ACCESS Sunrise–sunset

MAPS USGS *Doylesburg;* map of natural area is available at the Tuscarora State Forest office on PA 274 in Blain.

FACILITIES Pit toilet near south trailhead, seasonal water and restrooms at nearby Big Spring State Park

WHEELCHAIR TRAVERSABLE No

CONTACT Tuscarora State Forest, 717-536-3191, tinyurl.com/tuscarorasf

SPECIAL COMMENTS Although it's a long drive from Harrisburg for a short hike, the scenery here is outstanding. The outing can easily be combined with a hike on the nearby Tunnel Trail (see page 150) and a picnic at Big Spring State Park for a wonderful day rich in natural and cultural history.

280 years. Many of them measure more than 2 feet in diameter and more than 100 feet tall. Some of the trees are absolutely huge, and few places exist in the east where you can see trees with the stature of these hemlocks.

The Pennsylvania state tree, the eastern hemlock, was all but eradicated during the lumber boom in the 19th century. Interestingly, the timber provided by the tree is not considered especially valuable for lumber purposes. It was cut instead for its bark to use for tanning leather. In 1973, the natural area was designated as a National Natural Landmark by the National Park Service. In addition to the hemlock, you will also find here white pine, several varieties of birch, maple, and oak trees, and a healthy understory of mountain laurel, Pennsylvania's state flower. Visiting the natural area in late May and early June will give you the opportunity to see the mountain laurel in bloom.

From the north parking area, follow the orange-blazed Patterson Run Trail down to the creek and across a small footbridge. After crossing the bridge, be sure to veer left on the Patterson Run Trail heading uphill away from the creek. After about 0.3 mile, you'll reach the junction of the Patterson Run Trail and the yellow-blazed Rim Trail. The prior turns left, heading uphill, while the latter continues straight traversing the hillside. Continue straight on the Rim Trail. As you begin this trail, you'll notice the hemlocks getting large, and some of them have a very rough alligator-like bark.

Follow the Rim Trail to a fork in the trail at 0.8 mile. At the fork, turn right and drop down to a footbridge over Patterson Run. On the west side of the creek, you are following the red-blazed Hemlock Trail. From the bridge a spur of that trail heads uphill to the right to Hemlock Road. Turn left and follow the Hemlock Trail to the south along Patterson Run. The terrain is rather rocky for the next half-mile, and in the summer the trail can be a bit overgrown. But from the bottom of the ravine you'll have an excellent view of some of the tallest trees on the steep east slope. Although Patterson Run is not very large, the pools all along it are home to small native brook trout that are easy to spot from the trail. During spawning season they have beautiful colors, speckled on top and bright red or orange on the bottom. They are small, only about 6 inches or so, but every large pool seems to sport one or two.

At 1.4 miles, the trail passes a bench beside the creek and another spur of the Hemlock Trail heads up to the road. The spur is marked by a sign. From the bench, continue following the trail along the creek, and in a few moments you'll reach a pair of footbridges over the creek and a small tributary. Cross the two bridges and you'll see some yellow blazes and a sign indicating the path of the Rim Trail traversing the east slope of the ravine back down the valley. As you follow the Rim Trail above the creek, you'll pass by some of the largest trees in the area, giving you a sense of what Pennsylvania might have been like when it was first settled. In about a half-mile, the trail begins to descend and shortly thereafter meets the fork above the Hemlock Trail and footbridge you passed earlier. Continue straight and follow the Rim Trail and then the Patterson Run Trail back to the car.

Nearby Activities

Camping and picnicking facilities are located at **Fowlers Hollow State Park,** 7 miles to the southeast just beyond the end of Hemlock Road. Picnic facilities are located at **Big Spring State Park.** The **Tuscarora State Forest** has many unpaved forest roads that make for good bike riding. The forest headquarters, on PA 274 in Blain, has maps and information on historical and natural landmarks.

GPS TRAILHEAD COORDINATES AND DIRECTIONS
N40° 15.337' W77° 38.036'

From PA 34 in New Bloomfield, follow PA 274 west approximately 29 miles to Big Spring State Park. Turn left onto Hemlock Road at the park sign. The trailhead and parking are 2.5 miles along on the left at a sign.

---

29 Little Buffalo State Park

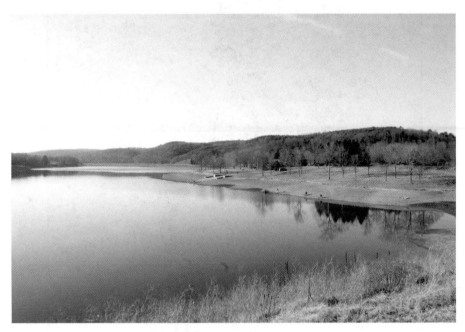

Holman Lake

In Brief

Beginning at the visitor center, this hike makes a circuit of Holman Lake by following trails on ridges to the north and south of the lake.

Description

Little Buffalo State Park is rich with natural and cultural history. The land in the valley along Little Buffalo Creek was purchased from the Iroquois League of Nations around the time of the Revolutionary War, and farming settlements began to be established in the early years of the 1800s. During the 19th century, the land around the present-day park was the site of a large charcoal furnace, a forge (the Juniata Iron Works), a gristmill (Shoaff's Mill), and the Newport and Sherman's Valley Railroad. These businesses contributed to the development of the valley, as well as to the clearing of its forest. As the timber industry declined, the industries and railroad closed down, leaving farming as the area's primary industry. The park was opened in 1972 and, in addition to providing recreational opportunities, has served to preserve some of the cultural history. This hike, which makes a circuit

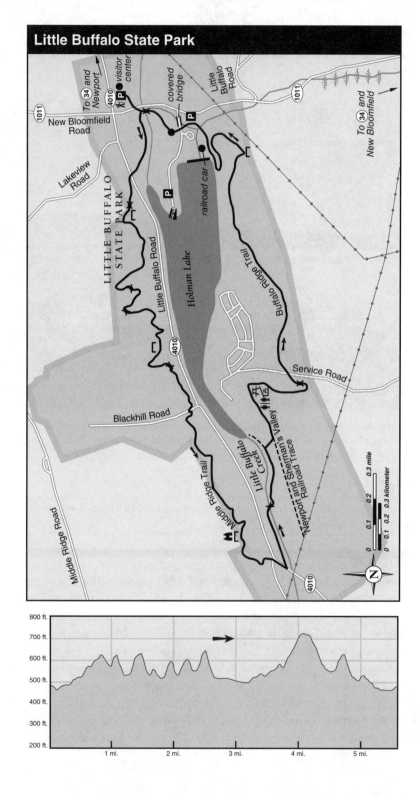

Little Buffalo State Park

LENGTH 5.6 miles	**ACCESS** Sunrise–sunset
CONFIGURATION Loop	**MAPS** USGS *Newport;* a map of the park is available online at tinyurl.com/little buffalospmap.
DIFFICULTY Moderately strenuous	
SCENERY Nice views of Little Buffalo State Park environs and Little Buffalo Creek	**FACILITIES** Restrooms and water at visitor center; a seasonal concession area
EXPOSURE More shade than sun	**WHEELCHAIR TRAVERSABLE** No
TRAIL TRAFFIC Light	**CONTACT** Little Buffalo State Park, 717-567-9255, tinyurl.com/littlebufsp
TRAIL SURFACE Dirt, with short sections of grass and pavement	
HIKING TIME 3–4 hours	**SPECIAL COMMENTS** This hike generally follows the 6.2-mile Volksmarch route through the park, though it's a little shorter and stays more to trails than roads.
DRIVING DISTANCE 5.75 miles from US 22/322 and PA 34 near Newport, west of Harrisburg	

of the park around its 88-acre Holman Lake, passes by several of the historic sites and provides access to some of the park's charming backcountry.

Beginning from the visitor center, walk west across the park road toward the Blue Ball Tavern. Originally opened in 1811 by John Koch, a farmer, the tavern served as a resting place for messengers traveling between Carlisle and Sunbury during the War of 1812. A farmhouse built in 1865 now stands on the site. Pass the farmhouse (now a museum) and a bridge over the creek—don't cross the bridge!—and hike west along the Exercise Trail, keeping the creek to your left. This grassy, mown path passes through a pretty meadow with many nesting boxes for eastern bluebirds, a common resident of the park. As you approach the dam's spillway, the path heads over to Little Buffalo Road and crosses it at some wooden steps. Cross the road, and pick up the trail continuing west as it enters the woods at a little creek. Lots of thicket in the area makes this a good place for spotting some of the many songbirds that visit the park. You are now on the Middle Ridge Trail (as denoted by the park map), although as soon as you enter the woods you'll cross a footbridge by a sign that refers to it as the North Side Hiking Trail. Nonetheless, it is well marked with red blazes—a good thing if you are hiking during the fall, as the abundance of oak and hickory leaves on the ground can make the path virtually invisible.

For the next 2.5 miles, the trail follows the direction of Middle Ridge to the west, climbing out of and back into hollows that divide the ridge toward Holman Lake. The walk is very pretty, through a forest of oaks and hickories with tall white pine trees on the ridges and hemlocks in the hollows, but it does have quite a bit of up and down to it. At about 1.5 miles, the trail descends an uncharacteristically steep hill on a nice path in the pines. Near the bottom, the trail turns sharp right into the hollow and across a footbridge, though a path continues straight out to the road. Keep your eyes open for the junction marked by blazes, and then turn right.

Cross Blackhill Road at 1.8 miles and climb a short hill. At the top of this hill, the path joins a wide-open track through the woods. With loads of thicket on either side of the trail, this is a great area for bird-watching. At one point in a more open area, an infrequently used path heads off to the right to the top of the ridge, a couple of hundred feet away. If you are looking for wildlife, it may be worth the effort to drop your pack and take a peek up there. It seems prime territory for turkey and grouse as well as fox. At about 2 miles, you'll come to a large open meadow on your left that you walk beside for 0.2 mile. The path drops into another hollow, crosses a footbridge, and climbs a short hill. At the top of the hill, you'll find two benches and a nice view back to the east over Holman Lake and the park.

From the benches, the trail continues a short distance to a very large oak tree. The trail makes a right turn into the woods here, while the track continues straight and downhill. The trail winds through the woods for 0.1 mile before crossing back over the track and descending to Little Buffalo Road by a gate and private road. Cross Little Buffalo Road, turn right, and walk west along its shoulder until you cross the bridge over Little Buffalo Creek. Just beyond the creek, step over the guardrail and walk down some steps to a wide track on the south side of the creek. The passage over the guardrail is marked by a sign with a white arrow and is directly beneath some large power lines. Follow the track along the creek, passing a large meadow on your right where you may spot a few deer browsing. In a couple of places the track will fork. Just follow the left forks staying near the creek. The walk along the creek features quite a bit of thicket and some impressive sycamore trees.

After about 0.5 mile along the creek, you'll come to a trail junction with a wide, grassy path heading up to the right. Turn right and follow that path a short distance to the Newport and Sherman's Valley Railroad Grade marked by a white arrow. The white arrows indicate the path of a Volksmarch route around the park. Turn left and walk through a lovely pine forest for a short distance until you reach a junction of several trails heading off to the right at the base of a hillside covered with dense stands of thicket. A white arrow points up along one of the trails. Don't follow it. The trails that head off into the thicket are rather confused and mostly seem to loop back to this spot. That said, the trails are worth exploring for a little while to see what you might see. As I was walking around the area trying to make sense of it, I happened to see a weasel chasing a squirrel out of its den, in addition to a multitude of birds.

From the hillside, continue along the railroad grade (now more of a service road), and follow it until you see some picnic tables and restrooms. The trailhead for the Buffalo Ridge Trail will be on the right, although the sign faces the opposite direction from which you are walking, so keep your eyes open. (If you cross a bridge over a small creek, you've gone too far.) Turn right on the white-blazed Buffalo Ridge Trail and follow it up a beautiful dark hollow, populated by tall pine, hickory, and hemlock trees. At the back of the hollow, cross a footbridge and climb to a service road. Cross the road and follow the trail as it traverses just below the crest of Buffalo Ridge for 0.6 mile, at which point you'll pass a trail heading back west with a sign that says shortcut to main area, about 100 yards east of a water tank.

As the trail descends from here, the walking gets rather rocky for 0.25 mile. Then it improves, climbs back up to the ridge among large pine trees, and reaches a bench near the rocky ridgecrest. This is a peaceful spot and worth planning as a rest spot on your hike. From the bench, follow the path along a ridge in a northeasterly direction, make a couple of switchbacks near its bottom, and descend a set of steps into the east picnic area at the base of the dam. The steps end at the railroad grade at an old railroad car. Turn right and follow the grade to the covered bridge, Clay's Bridge. Built in 1890, it originally crossed Buffalo Creek a mile west of its present location, providing a link to New Bloom-field for residents of the Sherman's Valley. Exemplifying Burr Arch construction, each interior side of the bridge features a wooden structural arch that spans the river. Once through the bridge, turn right onto a paved path and follow it for 0.25 mile back to the Blue Ball Tavern.

Nearby Activities

The obvious activities are at the state park, where you can explore some of the historical sites, picnic, swim, and fish. I highly recommend a walk from the east picnic area up the steps to the crest of the dam for a great view to the west. The park does a fine job with environmental programs and special events. During the Christmas season, the park decorates the east picnic area with lights and ornaments. During the fall, the park hosts the Old Fashioned Apple Festival and activities on Halloween night.

GPS TRAILHEAD COORDINATES AND DIRECTIONS
N40° 27.518' W77° 10.109'

From US 22/322 at Newport, follow PA 34 south 4 miles to Little Buffalo Road/SR 4010. Turn right and follow this road 1.75 miles to New Bloomfield Road. Turn left and the Little Buffalo State Park Visitor Center is on the left.

30 Tunnel Trail and Iron Horse Trail Loop

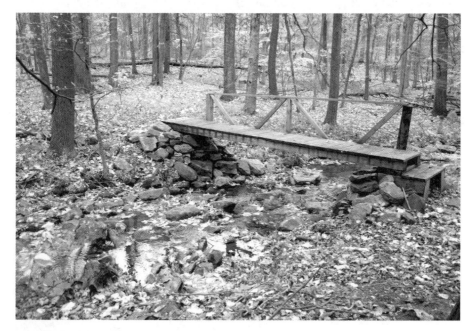

Bridge in vicinity of Big Spring Run

In Brief

From the parking area on Hemlock Road, follow the Tunnel Trail to the abandoned railroad tunnel and descend toward Big Spring Run. Pick up the Iron Horse Trail (IHT) and follow it east, crossing PA 274 and joining the old Path Valley Railroad Grade. Follow the Path Valley grade back to the parking area.

Description

Constructed by the Youth Conservation Corps in the late 1970s, the Iron Horse Trail forms a loop through the Tuscarora State Forest following the paths of two abandoned railroad grades. Although the trail is theoretically a rail-trail, it is considerably more rugged than any rail-trail you'll come across. It's a rocky knee-buster that requires good, sturdy footwear. Linking the IHT with the Tunnel Trail is the common excursion, though

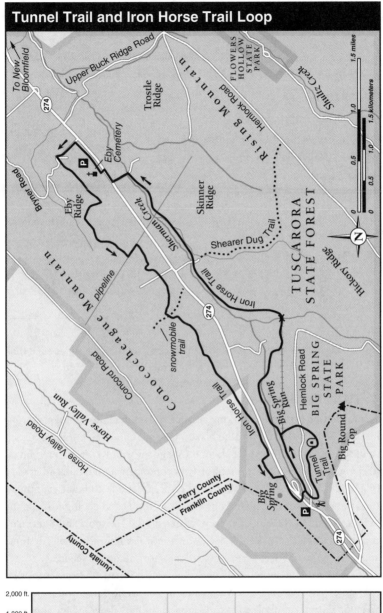

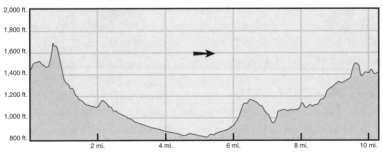

LENGTH The Iron Horse Trail is 9.1 miles and the Tunnel Trail is 1.8 miles. If you join the two (the common excursion) and you don't backtrack, the hike is 10.3 miles long.	from intersection of PA 34 and PA 274 in New Bloomfield
	ACCESS Sunrise–sunset
CONFIGURATION Loop	**MAPS** USGS *Blairs Mills* and *Blain;* Potomac Appalachian Trail Club *Tuscarora Trail, Map J: Appalachian Trail, PA, to PA Route 641*
DIFFICULTY Long and strenuous	
SCENERY Tuscarora State Forest land and much railroad history	**FACILITIES** Seasonal restrooms and water in picnic grounds at Big Spring State Park (parking area)
EXPOSURE Shade	**WHEELCHAIR TRAVERSABLE** No
TRAIL TRAFFIC Iron Horse Trail is light and Tunnel Trail is moderate	**CONTACT** Tuscarora State Forest, 717-536-3191, tinyurl.com/tuscarorasf
TRAIL SURFACE Dirt and rock	
HIKING TIME Allow 5–6 hours for the entire loop. The Tunnel Trail loop takes about an hour.	**SPECIAL COMMENTS** This is not your typical railroad-grade hike, as it's a rather stiff undertaking. The path is often rugged and climbs steep sections around private property.
DRIVING DISTANCE About 28.5 miles	

the latter is a nice, easy outing on its own. When completed as a loop, the Tunnel Trail is 1.85 miles long. The directions here provide information on both of the trails.

PART 1: TUNNEL TRAIL

From the information sign in the parking area, cross Hemlock Road and pick up the Tunnel Trail at a trail sign. Marked by blue blazes, the trail climbs into the woods, curves to the left, and contours the hillside. At about 0.25 mile, descend a set of steps and then turn right and climb a short rocky section. Shortly beyond, gain an old railroad grade and follow it straight up the hillside. After about 100 yards, the grade ends at the entrance to the old railroad tunnel. Never completed due to lack of funds and geological complications, the tunnel was begun in 1803 in an attempt to extend the Newport and Sherman's Valley Railroad from its terminus at New Germantown into Franklin County. The tunnel is an interesting bit of railroad history and is worth the short detour to see it.

From the fence at the tunnel, walk back along the railroad grade and turn right at the first blue blaze on the trail. Walk downhill and, in a short distance, you'll cross Hemlock Road and enter a forest of small saplings. Continue walking downhill for another 0.2 mile and you'll reach the red-blazed IHT. Turn left to return to the parking area (0.3 mile) or right to continue the Iron Horse loop.

PART 2: IRON HORSE TRAIL

If you decide to skip the Tunnel Trail or leave it to the end of the day, hike out of the parking area to the east on a stone-edged gravel path marked by red and blue blazes and an IHT sign. After a short distance, the path bends to the left toward some picnic pavilions.

At the bend, leave the main path and follow the blazes into the woods on a less defined track. As you leave the main day-use area, the trail follows Big Spring Run and soon passes a sign that marks the end of the Perry Lumber Company Railroad Grade, abandoned in 1906. A short distance beyond, you'll pass the junction with the Tunnel Trail. Continue east along the railroad grade for just about a mile, crossing the creek twice over wooden footbridges. Although a wide path, the walking through this section is quite rugged, as the trail surface is formed by broken rock.

Just beyond the second bridge (about 0.8 mile from the Tunnel Trail), the obvious railroad grade continues straight down the valley, but the IHT turns uphill right to circumnavigate private property. The turn is marked by a sign and double red blazes. After a short climb, turn left on an obvious old railroad bed in a stand of maple and birch saplings. Follow the smooth path back down to Big Spring Run, crossing a tributary on the way. You can often hear hawks screeching in this area, and the forest supports a healthy deer population.

About 2 miles from the Tunnel Trail, you'll join the Perry Lumber Company Railroad Grade again. Follow that for a short distance until it crosses the creek onto private property. Continue straight, staying south of the creek. At 2.2 miles, you'll pass a small private cabin and a sign that asks you to respect the owner by staying on the trail. Follow the cabin's access road to a gate and then out to a prominent dirt road at 2.4 miles. This road is the Shearer Dug Trail, and it provides access to some private cabins as well as the Rising Mountain Trail on the ridge to the south. Cross the road, enter the woods, and follow the path over two footbridges and across two pipeline clearings for a mile to another prominent dirt road. An IHT sign is located here. Turn left and follow the road past a stand of pine trees to the highway. Just before the highway, turn right (east) into the woods and parallel the highway for 0.25 mile before crossing to the Eby Cemetery on the north side of the road.

The trail proper reenters the woods through the brush at the southeast corner of the cemetery (right by the road) and parallels the road for 0.5 mile. If you pick up the trail here, you are in for some of the worst hiking imaginable. At this writing, the path near the cemetery was overgrown by thorn bushes fierce enough to destroy my sturdy pair of Carhartt overalls. To avoid such unpleasantness, walk east along the shoulder of the road for 0.4 mile to the eastern trailhead across from a parking area on the south side of the road. From that trailhead, marked by a sign, continue walking east for another 0.25 mile to another dirt road, Bryner Road, by a large clear-cut.

Turn left (north) and pass the clear-cut on your right and a private residence on the left. Beyond both of these, Bryner Road begins to climb slightly and bend to the right. At the point where the road bends back to the left, the IHT enters the woods on the left, heading west now along the grade of the Path Valley Railroad. This is the railroad grade that was supposed to join the Newport and Sherman's Valley line with Franklin County to the west. Although that venture was never realized, the grade did extend as far as the site of the present Big Spring State Park. In the early 1900s, the Perry Lumber Company used it to help move timber out of western Perry County.

The path along the top of the railroad grade for the next 0.6 mile is very pleasant. The woods are thick, making the setting feel remote. At 4.9 miles, the trail makes a sharp right turn and leaves the railroad grade to circumnavigate private property. Follow the red blazes uphill for 0.3 mile to the crest of Eby Ridge by a couple of huge oak trees, where the trail makes a sharp left and drops down to a recent logging road. As you follow the road to the west, Conococheague Mountain will be in view to the north. At the crest of the road, veer left, pick up the red blazes again, and descend a very beautiful ridge along a moss-lined path through stands of pine trees surrounded by tall oaks. It would be difficult to imagine more pleasant walking, and the area is especially beautiful in the fall.

When you reach a clearing at a pipeline, turn left (south) and walk about 0.1 mile to a plastic white-and-yellow pipeline post. The trail enters the woods again at red blazes on the right and follows a railroad spur for 100 yards before it ends abruptly at a small promontory. Continue following blazes through the woods, crossing a footbridge and then a drive for a private camp. Continue up switchbacks to regain the main railroad grade at a good area for spotting woodpeckers. Walk along the pleasant path as it traverses the hillside, avoiding the temptation to veer off on the occasional paths heading downhill. At 6.5 miles, the trail joins a dirt road. Turn right and follow it across another dirt road (marked as a snowmobile trail) and regain the railroad grade just beyond. A short distance beyond, you'll reach a significant fork in the trail and you'll want to stay left.

At about 8 miles, the trail makes a diagonal across an old road right above the highway near the state park. Just when you think it's all over, the trail turns uphill to once again circumnavigate a small plot of private land. Beyond that, follow red blazes through woods back to the highway and into the park. The parking area is just beyond the road.

Nearby Activities

Picnicking facilities are available at **Big Spring State Park,** and camping is available 6.5 miles away at **Fowlers Hollow State Park. Hemlocks Natural Area,** 3.1 miles south along Hemlock Road, is also very much worth a visit (see page 141). Combining the short Tunnel Trail with a hike through the natural area would make for a very pleasant day.

GPS TRAILHEAD COORDINATES AND DIRECTIONS
N40° 15.729' W77° 39.611'

From PA 34 in New Bloomfield, follow PA 274 West approximately 29 miles to Big Spring State Park. Turn left onto Hemlock Road at the park sign and park in the large parking area on the left.

OPPOSITE: *Descending through the pines from Eby Ridge*

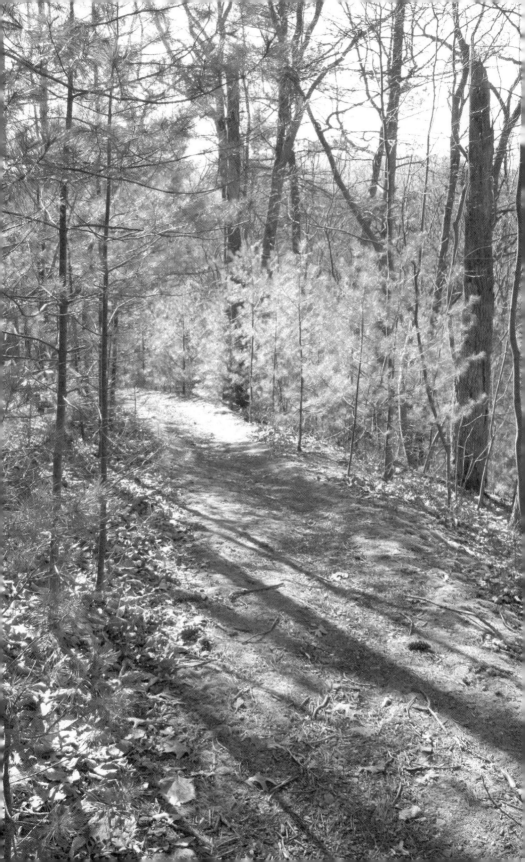

SOUTHEAST

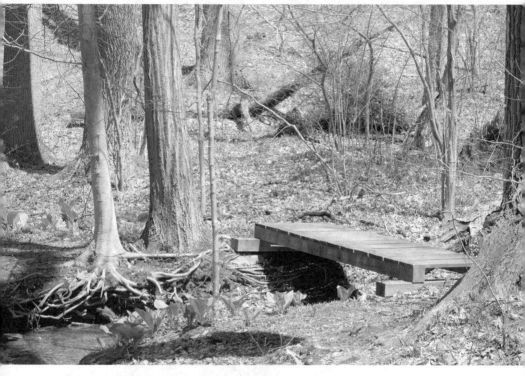

Footbridge along Steinman Run (see Hike 43, page 213)

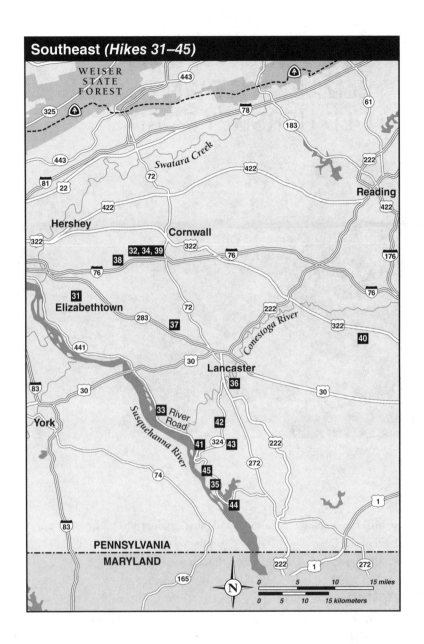

Southeast (Hikes 31–45)

WEISER STATE FOREST

443

325

61

78

183

443

Swatara Creek

81 22

72

422

222

Reading

422

422

Hershey

Cornwall

32, 34, 39

38

322

322

76

176

76

76

31

Elizabethtown

283

72

37

222

Conestoga River

322

40

441

30

Lancaster

36

83 30

30

33 River Road

Susquehanna River

York

42

41 324 43

222

272

74

45

35

44

1

PENNSYLVANIA

MARYLAND

165

222 1 272

N

| 0 | 5 | 10 | 15 miles |
| 0 | 5 | 10 | 15 kilometers |

31 Conewago Trail: ELIZABETHTOWN TO OLD HERSHEY ROAD

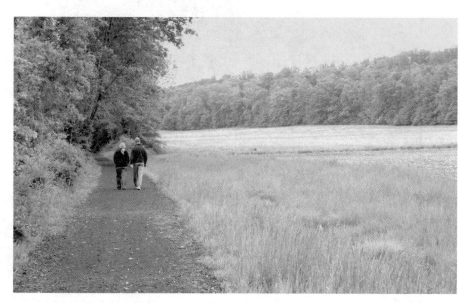

Conewago Trail near Elizabethtown

In Brief

This easy hike traverses an old railroad grade that extends into Lebanon County, following the path of the Conewago Creek and passing by some beautiful corn and farm fields. It is especially pretty late in the day when the sun is low.

Description

Maintained by the Lancaster County Department of Parks and Recreation, the Conewago Recreation Trail is a 5-mile footpath that extends from PA 230 1.75 miles west of Elizabethtown to the Lebanon County line near the town of Lawn. At the 5-mile mark, the trail abruptly becomes the Lebanon Valley Rail-Trail and continues east through Lawn for 12.5 miles (see pages 190 and 194 for hikes on the Lebanon Valley Rail-Trail).

For its length, the Conewago Trail follows the bed of the old Cornwall and Lebanon Railroad line alongside Conewago Creek, which flows just north of the trail. The Cornwall and Lebanon Railroad was built in the 1880s by iron magnate Richard E. Coleman, who

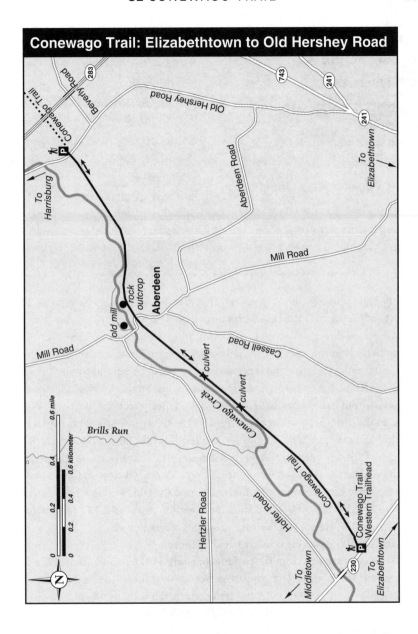

Conewago Trail: Elizabethtown to Old Hershey Road

used it to haul iron ore from his furnaces in Lebanon County to the mills in Steelton on the shore of the Susquehanna River. The rail line was abandoned after the floods from Hurricane Agnes in 1972. In 1979, Lancaster County acquired the land that the railroad line followed, and in 1981 converted the land into a hiking and biking trail.

I discovered the Conewago Trail four years ago after spending two weeks in the hospital battling a serious illness. It was the perfect thing for me during the period of my

LENGTH 4.2 miles	**ACCESS** Sunrise–sunset
CONFIGURATION Out-and-back	**MAPS** USGS *Middletown* and *Elizabethtown*
DIFFICULTY Easy	
SCENERY Conewago Creek, farms, pleasant forest	**WHEELCHAIR TRAVERSABLE** Possibly, when the trail is dry
EXPOSURE More shade than sun	**CONTACT** Lancaster County Parks and Recreation, 717-299-8215, tinyurl.com /conewagotrail
TRAIL TRAFFIC Moderate	
TRAIL SURFACE Gravel and dirt	**SPECIAL COMMENTS** Although it's a nice walk, there have, unfortunately, been some problems with assaults on this trail in the past, so be safe and walk with a partner.
HIKING TIME 1.5 hours round-trip	
DRIVING DISTANCE About 2 miles from central PA 743 and PA 230 in Elizabethtown	

recovery, and I walked it almost every day from September through November. The entire path is nearly level, as is the case with railroad grades, so the hiking is not very difficult. The path passes through sections of shade and sun, so while you are never getting roasted for long periods in the sun, you are also never under a dense canopy of trees for a long period either. Although the trail is popular with hikers, bikers, and runners, it never feels crowded and is an easy place to find some peace and solitude. Additionally, the scenery is lovely as the trail passes cornfields, old farms, and pretty sections of woods. Wildflowers abound in the spring; the colors of the trees and fields are magnificent in the fall.

Although the trail itself extends for 5 miles, this hike covers the first 2-mile stretch out and back from the parking lot on PA 230 near Elizabethtown to the Old Hershey Road at the 2-mile marker. This section of the trail provides easy access, plenty of parking, and avoids having to cross any major highways. Beyond the Old Hershey Road, the trail passes beneath PA 283 (very noisy) and shortly thereafter crosses PA 743 (a heavily traveled road). East of PA 743 are smaller road crossings where you can pick up nice sections of the trail, though the parking is limited at all of those.

This hike heads east from the parking lot along a cinder and gravel surface, immediately entering the woods. Here, you are surrounded by lovely hickory, beech, sycamore, and red-cedar trees. At 0.15 mile, the trail departs the woods and enters a clearing that serves as a crop field to the south of the trail. The field is often planted with corn, though some years it lies fallow. Several small oak trees dot the landscape to the right. The large field extends for a half-mile to the east, is bounded by a forested hillside to the south, and provides for wonderful scenery at all times of the year. I highly recommend a walk near dawn or dusk when the sun is low because the light on this meadow can be quite picturesque. This is also a good place to spot white-tailed deer and wild turkeys en masse, as well as a variety of songbirds, including bluebirds and meadowlarks.

At 0.2 mile, the trail crosses a dirt farm road used to access the field to your right and the wild meadowland to the north of the trail. The trail continues bordered by a narrow

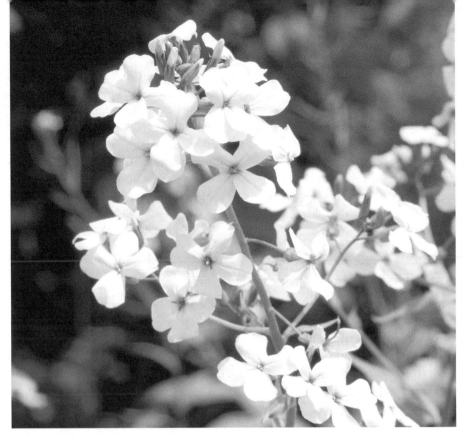

Dame's violet, a common Pennsylvania wildflower

stand of trees on the left and reenters the woods just past the 0.5-mile marker along the trail. Here, you'll be walking under a beautiful canopy of tall trees for the next 0.5 mile until the Mill Road crossing. The sunlight as it plays through these trees creates beautiful shadows on the path and on humid days creates hazy shafts that shine through the leaves. Along the way to Mill Road, the trail passes over two small side streams. In the woods alongside the trail are piles of the old railroad timbers, which are now home to chipmunks, spiders, ants, and other small critters.

At the Mill Road crossing, the trail runs close to a particularly rocky section of the Conewago Creek. It is worth walking over to the creek and the bridge on Mill Road (just to the north of the trail crossing) to have a look at the creek and the old mill building with its characteristic Pennsylvania Dutch architecture. Parking used to be available along the creek here, and the rocky stretch just upstream from the bridge used to draw plenty of people who came to wade and sun themselves on some of the large boulders clogging the creek. In recent years, however, the whole area along this section of the creek has been posted as private property and parking is no longer allowed. Please don't stray from the path except where it crosses roads.

From the Mill Road crossing, the trail climbs briefly and within 0.1 mile enters a cut through a rocky outcrop that obviously had to be blasted to run the railroad line through. Just beyond the outcrop, the trail crosses another small tributary to Cone-wago Creek and then follows the Conewago quite closely for another 0.25 mile before the creek meanders north. On the south side of the trail lies a large farm, the openness of which provides some nice views. The north side of the trail is wooded, much of the land owned by the Hershey Trust.

Within a quarter-mile of the turnaround, two houses are set back in the woods. Shortly thereafter, you arrive at the 2-mile marker and the crossing with the Old Hershey Road. On the east side of the road, you'll find a small parking area with room enough for three cars, and it can provide an alternate starting point for the hike. In the spring, some lovely wildflowers grow in the area of the parking lot, the colors of which are worth the walk itself.

Nearby Activities

Elizabethtown has several restaurants and all of the amenities that you might need. **Twin Kiss** (901 N. Hanover St.; 717-367-1694), between the two traffic lights on PA 743, has good hot dogs, and **Lucky Ducks Bar and Grille** (45 N. Market St.; 717-366-4041, lucky ducksbarandgrille.com), on the main drag through town, has nice outdoor seating by a small creek. On Saturday mornings, there is a large market on the right a couple of miles farther down PA 230 toward Middletown.

GPS TRAILHEAD COORDINATES AND DIRECTIONS
N40° 09.868' W76° 38.528'

From PA 283, follow PA 743 south into Elizabethtown. Turn right at the second traffic light (PA 230). Follow PA 230 for 1.75 miles. The parking area for the trailhead is on your right.

---

32 Clarence Schock Memorial Park

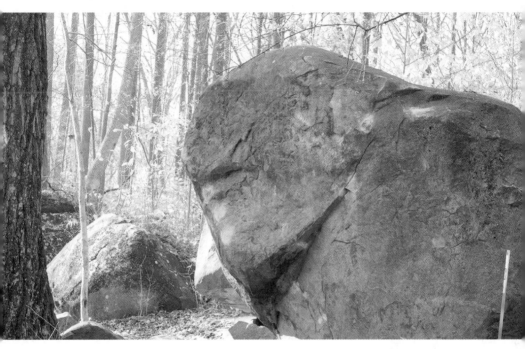

One of the climbing boulders

In Brief

This hike follows the main trail from Clarence Schock Memorial Park's Environmental Center on Pinch Road to the observation tower atop Governor Dick Hill. From there it follows several of the secondary trails into the hollow at the headwaters of Chickies Creek. From the hollow, it traverses below the ridge of Governor Dick Hill and then loops back to the Environmental Center.

Description

The beginning of this hike, to the observation tower on top of Governor Dick Hill, is deservedly popular: The view from the top of the 66-foot-tall observation tower on its summit offers a wonderful panorama of the surrounding countryside. On a clear day, you can see parts of Lancaster, Lebanon, Dauphin, York, and Berks Counties. After the tower,

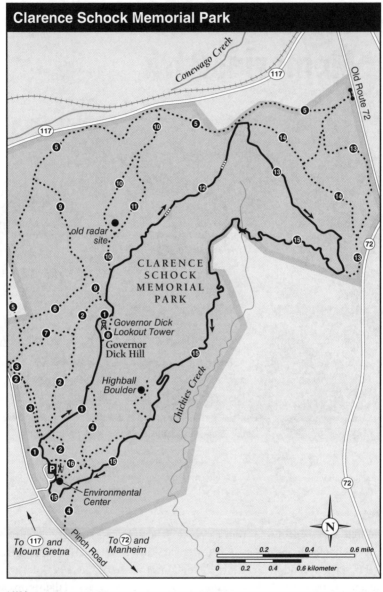

Clarence Schock Memorial Park

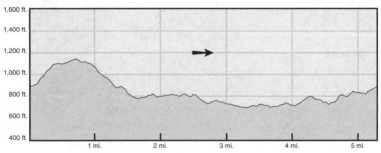

LENGTH 5.3 miles

CONFIGURATION Loop

DIFFICULTY Moderately strenuous

SCENERY Excellent views of Lancaster, Lebanon, and Dauphin Counties

EXPOSURE Shaded

TRAIL TRAFFIC Moderate

TRAIL SURFACE Dirt and rock

HIKING TIME 2.5–3 hours

DRIVING DISTANCE About 13 miles from PA 283 and PA 743 in Elizabethtown

ACCESS Sunrise–sunset

MAPS USGS *Manheim* and *Lebanon;* a park map is available at the visitor center and online at tinyurl.com/schock memorialparkmap.

FACILITIES Portable toilet and vending machine at parking area; picnic tables on top of Governor Dick Hill

WHEELCHAIR TRAVERSABLE No

CONTACT Clarence Schock Memorial Park at Governor Dick, 717-964-3808, parkatgovernordick.org

SPECIAL COMMENTS The observation tower atop Governor Dick Hill provides one of the best views in Lancaster County.

though, you'll encounter considerably less trail traffic until the final mile or so where the trail passes by several large boulders and rock outcroppings that are popular with local rock climbers.

First-time visitors invariably wonder about the origin of the name of Governor Dick Hill. It was named in the latter part of the 19th century for an African American woodchopper and charcoal burner who worked exclusively in this area. His name was Dick, and his coworkers referred to him as "Governor." The hill was named for him after he died.

Begin this hike at the parking area for the Governor Dick Environmental Center located on Pinch Road. From your car, head to the back (northeast) corner of the lot where you will find a sign that says TO THE TOWER. Follow the trail past a bench and into the woods, where you will see a white blaze. Very quickly you will come to a fork in the trail with a signpost noting that Trail 16 heads off to the right. Stay to your left here following the sign for the tower. The trail at this point is marked by yellow blazes. At 0.1 mile the footpath meets a prominent dirt service road, which is Trail 1. Turn right (northeast) onto the road and follow it uphill, passing several side trails as you ascend. For a short distance the road gets a little steep, but the walking is never difficult.

At 0.4 mile, you'll reach a junction with Trail 4, which departs to the right. A bench and information plaque are located here, the latter providing some of the history of the park. The 1,105 acres of woodland on which the park is located were purchased in 1934 by Clarence Schock of the Schock Independent Oil Company (SICO), who donated the land to the Mount Joy school district in 1953. The SICO Foundation built the observation tower in 1954. The land has been deeded to be maintained in its natural state and used solely for recreational purposes. The Clarence Schock Foundation (formerly the SICO Foundation) still contributes funds to maintain the area and is a generous contributor of scholarships for students attending local colleges.

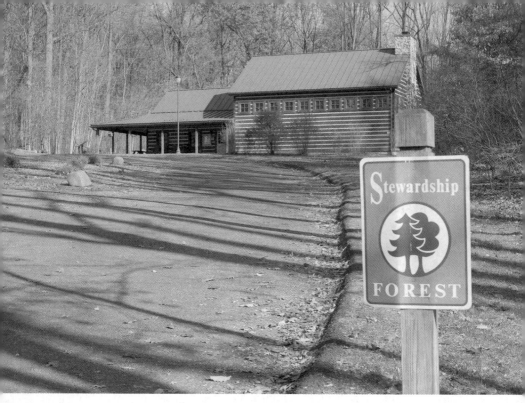

Schock Park's Environmental Center

From the information sign, continue following the road up a gentle incline for another 0.3 mile to the summit of Governor Dick Hill, where you will find the observation tower as well as several picnic benches. The tower can be climbed from the inside via a series of ladders. Take a break here and get ready for the remainder of the hike, which gets significantly more rugged.

From the tower, continue hiking to the north to a sign that reads PINCH ROAD RT 117. That is Trail 2. Follow it a short distance to a prominent trail junction with Trail 10 and a sign that points to Trails 11 and 12. Turn right onto this trail, following red and white blazes, and descend 0.1 mile to the junction of Trails 10 and 12. The hike follows Trail 12, marked with blue blazes, downhill to the right. If you are so inclined, Trail 10 veers uphill to the left and in a short distance reaches a meadow where it joins Trail 11. The meadow is a pleasant spot to stop for a break and to have a look around. After exploring, head back to Trail 12 and follow it downhill for a mile, passing a couple of boardwalks over marshy areas until the trail ends at the junction with Trail 13. Turn right (east) here and after a short distance you come to another junction of Trails 13 and 14. Turn right on 13 (green blazes) and follow that beneath a ridge for nearly a mile until it joins Trail 15.

Turn right (west) onto Trail 15 (white blazed). In this area the hike begins to level out and the trail continues into a hollow with several springs that form, in effect, the headwaters of Chickies Creek (spelled *Chiques* on some maps). As you get closer to the springs, the trail passes over and around boulders and over a couple of creeks. At 3.3 miles, you'll reach a footbridge over a creek, and beyond that the trail begins traversing the hillside beneath Governor Dick. At 4.4 miles the trail makes a sharp S-turn down a steep hillside, and at 4.7 miles comes to a trail spur that leads off to a prominent boulder about 20 feet tall on the right. You are now in the bouldering area that is popular with climbers who travel from as far as New Jersey to test their skills on the rocks. As you continue along Trail 15 you will pass by at least a half-dozen bouldering areas, some right along the trail and others nearby that are accessed by trail spurs.

At 5 miles, Trail 4, which you passed just before reaching the observation tower, enters from the right and joins Trail 15 for a short distance. At 5.1 miles you'll come across a sign that points uphill to the right toward the Environmental Center. Be sure to make this right turn, staying on Trail 15 (Trail 4 continues straight and downhill, eventually out to Pinch Road). After another quarter-mile, Trail 15 ends at the parking area for the Environmental Center.

Nearby Activities

Mount Gretna is a charming little community that's worth exploring. During the summer, be sure to finish up your hike with a trip to **The Jigger Shop** (202 Gettysburg Ave.; 717-964-9686, thejiggershop.com) for ice cream or a hamburger.

GPS TRAILHEAD COORDINATES AND DIRECTIONS
N40° 14.280' W76° 27.550'

From PA 283, follow PA 743 south toward Elizabethtown. At the first traffic light, make a sharp left turn—you'll be going in almost the opposite direction—onto PA 241. Follow 241 for 7.75 miles until it ends in the town of Colebrook. Turn right onto PA 117. After 100 yards, PA 117 turns left toward Mount Gretna. Take this left and follow 3 miles to the intersection with Pinch Road. Turn right on Pinch Road and follow it 0.7 mile to the entrance to Schock Park's Environmental Center, on your left.

33 Enola Low Grade Trail

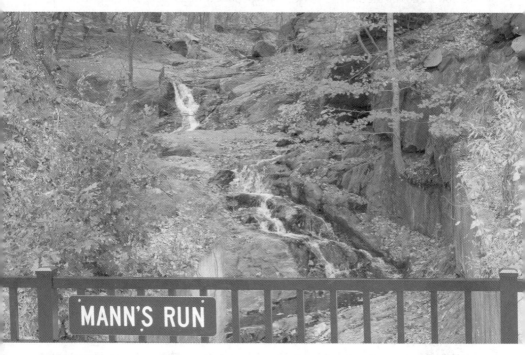

Manns Run

In Brief

This long, flat hike shares the parking area with the trailhead for the Turkey Hill Trail. This hike follows the shore of Lake Clarke on the Susquehanna River south from the trailhead to the Safe Harbor Dam, crossing several creeks along the way. The hike can be shortened to fit one's abilities and desires as necessary.

Description

I first discovered that the Enola Low Grade Trail in Manor Township had been completed while kayaking on Lake Clarke, the still-water section of the Susquehanna River formed by the Safe Harbor dam, during the spring of 2014. I was surprised to see people bicycling and hiking along the banks of the lake as far south as the Safe Harbor Dam. I thought that it would provide readers of this book with a nice complement to the Turkey Hill Trail, which begins from the same parking area. I have recently discovered that sections of the Turkey Hill Trail are, at the time of this writing, closed due to construction in the area.

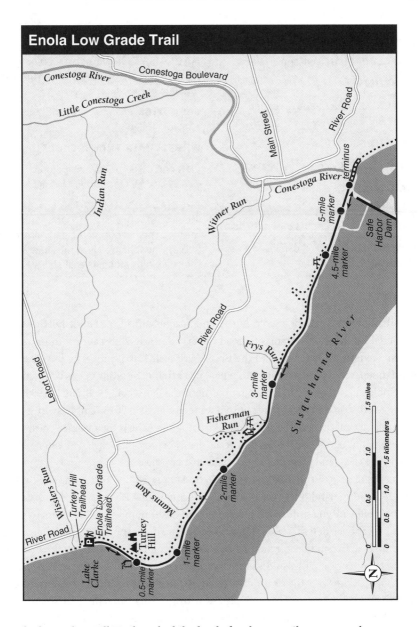

Presently the Turkey Hill Trail can be hiked only for about a mile to a recently constructed lookout near the windmills atop Turkey Hill. Although only a mile long, the hike is fairly steep at points and is moderately difficult. The view from the lookout is superb and is certainly worth planning into a visit to the area.

You'll begin this hike along the Enola Low Grade Trail by the large information sign at the spacious parking area. The rail-trail is 12 feet wide and constructed of cinders and crushed gravel, making it suitable for hikers and bicyclists, and it's traversable by wheelchair.

LENGTH 10.5 miles round-trip	**ACCESS** Sunrise–sunset
CONFIGURATION Out-and-back	**MAPS** USGS *Safe Harbor;* a map of the rail-trail is available online at tinyurl.com/enolalowgrademap.
DIFFICULTY Easy	
SCENERY Susquehanna River and Turkey Hill	**FACILITIES** Picnic shelter and portable toilets
EXPOSURE Sun	**WHEELCHAIR TRAVERSABLE** Yes
TRAIL TRAFFIC Moderate–heavy	**CONTACT** Manor Township Parks, 717-397-4769, manortownship.net/parks
TRAIL SURFACE Cinders and crushed gravel	
HIKING TIME 3–4 hours for entire hike	**SPECIAL COMMENTS** This hike offers little in the way of shade. During summer, it's coolest during the early-morning hours, when the trail is in the shadow of the steep hills along its east side.
DRIVING DISTANCE 5.6 miles from Columbia	

The trail follows the path of the old Atglen and Susquehanna Low Grade rail line that was constructed by the Pennsylvania Railroad during the early 20th century to move freight between Trenton, New Jersey, and the Enola Yard near Harrisburg. The line allowed the railroad to separate its freight traffic from passenger traffic, resulting in less congestion at its Philadelphia yards. The last freight shipment along the line was in 1988, and in 1990 the rails were removed. Construction of the rail-trail was completed in 2013. This is a very good hike for spotting several species of birds that make a riparian habitat their home. These include, most commonly, egrets and herons and occasionally osprey. Bald eagles are often seen soaring above the river, and there are several pairs that nest nearby.

The beginning of the hike passes beneath Turkey Hill, which is capped by several power-generating windmills overlooking the Susquehanna River basin. A short distance from the trailhead you will reach a restored caboose, number 23832, painted red and black. This caboose dates to 1947 and was used as the rear car on the freight line in which the rear brakeman and the conductor worked as the train made its way to the Enola Yard. Near the caboose you will also find the first of several overlook platforms that allow you to get a view of the river that is unobstructed by the chain-link fence that runs along the trail. The fence is there to keep people from trespassing onto the still active rail line below. The setting here is quite striking. With the wide river valley banked by steep cliffs to your right and Turkey Hill rising steeply on your left, you have a real sense of the expanse of the valley and the effect of the river on the landscape over the years. This stretch of the Susquehanna River basin is known as the Conejohela Valley.

As you continue along the trail, you will reach a covered picnic table near mile marker 1. From here you can see as far as the Safe Harbor Dam, 4 miles downstream near the end of the trail. At 1.8 miles the trail crosses Manns Run, one of three small tributaries of the Susquehanna River that pass beneath this stretch of trail. (A sign on the bridge says

MANN'S RUN, with an apostrophe; however, I've gone with the USGS here and omitted it,) The view up each of these small streams is quite beautiful in the fall when the leaves are changing. At 2.4 miles into the hike, you will come to another covered picnic table. This one is accompanied by a wheelchair-accessible portable toilet. Just beyond the picnic table is another viewing platform that offers a nice panorama of the river and the escarpment above its western shore. Another 0.1 mile along the trail brings you around a large bend in the river to the bridge over Fisherman Run, which runs out into a sluice that channels it over the tracks below and deposits its flow into the river.

Just beyond mile marker 3.0, the trail passes over Frys Run. A blue-blazed trail begins here on the south side of the stream. According to a trail worker with whom I spoke, that trail climbs the hillside above the river and parallels the rail-trail several hundred feet above to a point upstream from the dam where it descends back down to the rail-trail. As you progress down the trail about another mile, the hillside to your left (east) gets increasingly steep, eventually turning into cliff faces which, by virtue of the rust color staining along them, are iron rich. This stretch of cliffs is a popular rock climbing area. If you look closely at some of the most sheer and improbable-to-climb sections of cliff you should be able to spot bolts and hangers the climbers use for protection while ascending the faces. On a fall or spring weekend you are likely to see some climbers in action here as well.

About 0.3 mile beyond those cliffs you will reach the Safe Harbor Hydroelectric Dam, which was constructed during the 1930s along with two other dams to the south as part of a large public hydroelectric project along the Susquehanna River. The construction of the Safe Harbor Dam created Lake Clarke on the Susquehanna River. The dam flooded an area of the river basin that once sported several rapids and small waterfalls. Downstream from the dam, the river is characterized by many small rocky islands with rapids running among them. While the dam with its concrete and power wires is really nothing much to look at, the river downstream is quite beautiful and a little imagination can help you to picture what the valley must have been like before construction of the dam. Just beyond the dam, the trail ends at a small concrete rail house located just above Conestoga Creek, one of the major Lancaster County watersheds. From the end of the trail, turn and follow the path back to the beginning.

GPS TRAILHEAD COORDINATES AND DIRECTIONS
N39° 58.013' W76° 27.381'

From US 30 east of York, take the first exit east of the Susquehanna River at signs for PA 441 and 462. Follow PA 441 south 4 miles into Washington Boro, where it ends at the intersection with PA 999 and turns into River Road. Check your odometer here. Follow River Road south 1.9 miles from the intersection with PA 999. The parking area is accessed by a paved entrance on the right and is identified by a large brown LANCASTER COUNTY CONSERVANCY sign.

34 Governor Dick

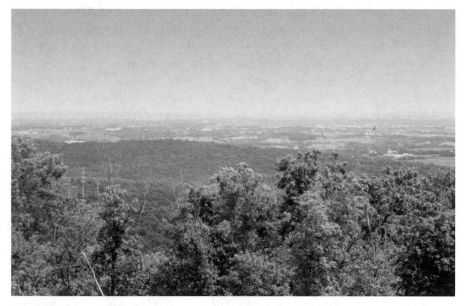

The view of Lancaster County to the southeast from the observation tower

In Brief

This wonderful hike follows the path of an old railroad grade through the woods and then heads uphill to the observation tower via a dirt road. After stopping to take in the great views from the tower, you descend along a gentle path that traverses the hill until a short steep section drops down to the original trail.

Description

Governor Dick Hill is a popular hiking destination for people who live in the small townships around the southern Lebanon County hamlet of Mount Gretna. And for good reason: The 66-foot-tall observation tower on its summit offers a wonderful panoramic view of the surrounding countryside. On a clear day, you can see parts of Lancaster, Lebanon, Dauphin, York, and Berks Counties.

First-time visitors invariably wonder about the origin of the name of the hill. It was named in the latter part of the 19th century for an African American woodchopper and charcoal burner who worked exclusively in this area. His name was Dick, and his co-workers referred to him as "Governor." The hill was named for him after he died.

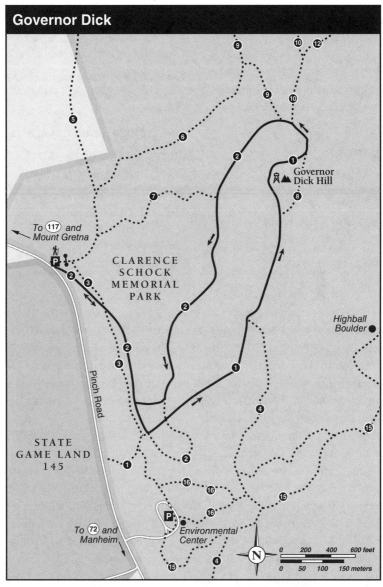

Governor Dick

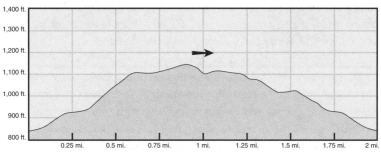

LENGTH About 2 miles	**MAPS** USGS *Manheim;* a park map is available at the visitor center and online at tinyurl.com/schockmemorialparkmap.
CONFIGURATION Loop	
DIFFICULTY Moderately strenuous	
SCENERY Excellent views of Lancaster, Lebanon, and Dauphin Counties	**FACILITIES** Portable toilet at parking area; picnic tables on top of Governor Dick Hill
EXPOSURE Shaded	**WHEELCHAIR TRAVERSABLE** No
TRAIL TRAFFIC Moderate–heavy	**CONTACT** Clarence Schock Memorial Park at Governor Dick, 717-964-3808, parkatgovernordick.org
TRAIL SURFACE Dirt and rock	
HIKING TIME 1–1.5 hours	
DRIVING DISTANCE About 13 miles from PA 283 and PA 743 in Elizabethtown	**SPECIAL COMMENTS** The lookout tower on top of Governor Dick Hill provides one of the best views in Lancaster County.
ACCESS Sunrise–sunset	

The 1,105 acres of woodland on which the hill lies were purchased in 1934 by Clarence Schock of the Schock Independent Oil Company (SICO), who donated the land to the Mount Joy school district in 1953. The SICO Foundation built the observation tower in 1954. The land has been deeded to be maintained in its natural state and used solely for recreational purposes. The Clarence Schock Foundation (formerly the SICO Foundation) still contributes funds to maintain the area and is a generous contributor of scholarships for students attending local colleges.

The popularity of the area for recreational purposes, though, predates Schock's acquisition of the land. In 1889, the Cornwall and Lebanon Railroad completed the construction of the Mount Gretna Narrow Gauge Railway. The narrow gauge shuttled visitors between the station that the C&L Railroad had established at the present site of Mount Gretna and the summit of Governor Dick Hill, a 4-mile ride. The current trailhead and parking area on Pinch Road, in fact, lie at a site where the old railroad passed. With the area's pretty woodlands and lake, the Pennsylvania Chautauqua Society founded the town of Mount Gretna around 1890. It has been a popular summer resort for travelers since.

Many of the hikers on Governor Dick Hill tend to follow the same 1-mile path from the parking lot to the summit and back again. For the sake of variety, I tend to be inclined more toward the loop hike configuration, so the hike described here offers a slight variation from the standard, with just a few hundred feet added distance.

The main trail begins at the parking lot, where you will find trash cans and a portable toilet. Two yellow gates block old roadbeds that extend from the lot. Begin this hike by passing by the right-hand gate. The hike climbs gently on a wide but somewhat rocky track through a lovely forest of oak and hickory trees. Keep your eyes open for birds along this hike. In one day during the spring, I spotted three pileated woodpeckers. As you climb, you'll notice many rough trails that take off into the woods. Most of these are the effects of mountain bikers and hikers who have cut between switchbacks. For the sake of the preservation of the area, I encourage you to stay to the main numbered trails.

At 0.3 mile, you will reach a trail junction with numbered trail signs and a rough and rocky path heading uphill to your left. That path is Trail 2 and is the common route up. You will return via that path. For the purposes of this hike, though, continue straight past that junction along Trail 3 for another 150 feet until you come to the junction with an old dirt road. Another trail marker with the number 3 on it is located here, and at this point turn left and follow the road. The road climbs rather steeply for approximately 0.25 mile before it levels out for the remainder of the hike to the top of Governor Dick Hill, easily recognizable by the large observation tower. Do not neglect to climb to the top of the tower via a series of ladders inside it! The view is worth the bit of effort. Several picnic tables are available for having a snack in the meadow around the base of the tower.

For the descent, follow Trail 2 down the hill. Several trails take off in various directions from the top of the hill, so be sure that you get the right one. Trail 2 leaves the meadow below the tower to the north and is identified by a sign that says PINCH AND RT. 117. The trail proceeds on nice level ground curving to the right (northeast). After 0.1 mile, you will pass a small trail that enters from the right. Trail 2 bends sharply to the left, and in another 0.05 mile reaches a junction with a significant trail descending to the right. Continue straight on Trail 2 (turning right will take you to Route 117). This broad, easy-to-follow path traverses the side of Governor Dick Hill descending steadily but gently.

At 1.7 miles into the hike, you'll come to an unnumbered trail junction giving you the choice of continuing straight across the hillside or turning to the right and descending steeply along a rather rough section of trail. Take the right-hand path. The steep and rocky section is only a couple of hundred feet long and ends at the junction with the main trail that you passed an hour or so ago on your ascent. Turn right here and in ten minutes you are back at the car.

Nearby Activities

Mount Gretna is a charming little community that's worth exploring. During the summer, be sure to finish up your hike with a trip to **The Jigger Shop** (202 Gettysburg Ave.; 717-964-9686, thejiggershop.com) for ice cream or a hamburger.

GPS TRAILHEAD COORDINATES AND DIRECTIONS
N40° 14.650' W76° 27.777'

From PA 283, follow PA 743 south toward Elizabethtown. At the first traffic light, make a sharp left turn (you will be going almost in the opposite direction) onto PA 241. Follow 241 for 7.75 miles until it ends in the town of Colebrook. Turn right onto PA 117. After 100 yards, PA 117 turns left toward Mount Gretna. Take this left and follow it 3 miles to the intersection with Pinch Road. Turn right on Pinch Road and follow it 0.5 mile to the parking area on your left.

35 Kellys Run and Pinnacle Overlook Loop

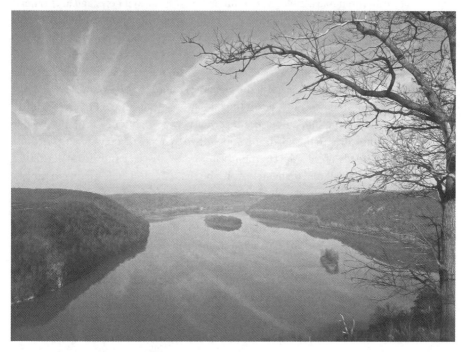

View of the Susquehanna from the Pinnacle Overlook

In Brief

This hike follows the Conestoga Trail from the Pinnacle Overlook above the Susquehanna River southbound into Kellys Run. The route then follows the Kellys Run Trail upstream to the Pinnacle Trail and back out to the overlook.

Description

Kellys Run Natural Area, through which this hike passes, is part of the 5,000-acre Holtwood Environmental Preserve. The preserve was established for recreation purposes by Pennsylvania Power and Light, which used to operate the hydroelectric dam at Holtwood.

In April 2016, the current landowner, Talen Energy, abruptly and unexpectedly closed part of the preserve to public use—including sections of the Kellys Run Trail, which used to be easily accessed from the Holtwood Recreation Area. This is an unfortunate turn of

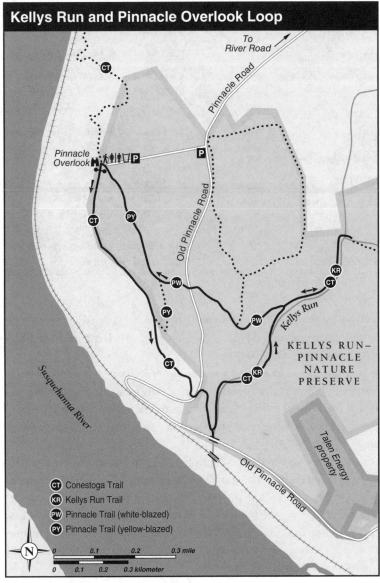

Kellys Run and Pinnacle Overlook Loop

To
River Road

Pinnacle Road

CT

Pinnacle
Overlook P

P

Old Pinnacle Road

CT

PY

PW

PY

KR
CT

Kellys Run

PW

KELLYS RUN–
PINNACLE
NATURE
PRESERVE

CT

CT KR

Susquehanna River

Old Pinnacle Road

Talen Energy property

CT Conestoga Trail
KR Kellys Run Trail
PW Pinnacle Trail (white-blazed)
PY Pinnacle Trail (yellow-blazed)

N

0   0.1   0.2   0.3 mile

0   0.1   0.2   0.3 kilometer

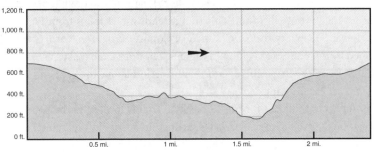

1,200 ft.

1,000 ft.

800 ft.

600 ft.

400 ft.

200 ft.

0 ft.

0.5 mi.   1 mi.   1.5 mi.   2 mi.

LENGTH 2.4 miles	**FACILITIES** Seasonal toilets and water at Pinnacle Overlook
CONFIGURATION Balloon	
DIFFICULTY Moderate	**WHEELCHAIR TRAVERSABLE** No
SCENERY Kellys Run natural area, Pinnacle Overlook, Susquehanna River	**CONTACT** Lancaster County Conservancy, 717-392-7891, lancaster conservancy.org/preserves
EXPOSURE More shade than sun	
TRAIL TRAFFIC Light	**SPECIAL COMMENTS** Recent land closures have made the remarkable Kellys Run Natural Area harder to access— at press time, Kellys Run can be accessed only from the Pinnacle Overlook. This hike provides offers a trek into the heart of the natural area, from the overlook into the most remote and beautiful reaches of Kellys Run.
TRAIL SURFACE Dirt	
HIKING TIME 2–3 hours	
DRIVING DISTANCE 8.1 miles from the intersection of PA 372 and PA 272 in Buck	
ACCESS 8 a.m.–sunset	
MAPS USGS *Holtwood*	

events, as the natural area has been designated by Audubon Pennsylvania as a featured site on the Susquehanna Birding and Wildlife Trail and by the US Department of the Interior as a National Recreation Trail.

The land closure and associated access issues may change in the future, but until that actually happens, Kellys Run can now be accessed only from the Pinnacle Overlook, north of the natural area. *Do not attempt to enter the restricted section*—Talen has zero tolerance for trespassing. The route described provides a nice loop hike into this remote and beautiful terrain.

Start at the Pinnacle Overlook, which offers an impressive panorama of the Susquehanna River to the north and the west. Directly beneath the overlook are several islands and the deepest part of Lake Aldred, formed by the Holtwood Hydroelectric Dam a few miles to the south. During the summer and fall, you can drive to the overlook, where in addition to the gorgeous view you'll find several benches, plus seasonal restrooms and water. During the winter, you will need to park by the gate on West Pinnacle Road and walk the final quarter-mile to the overlook.

The first section of the hike follows a short length of the orange-blazed Conestoga Trail for 0.7 mile into Kellys Run. This trail extends for 61 miles from Pumping Station Road in Lebanon County to Lock 12 in York County across the Norman Wood Bridge. Maintained by the Lancaster Hiking Club, the Conestoga Trail makes use of roads, trails, and rights of way for its path. For more information about the trail and the club, visit tinyurl.com/lancasterhiking.

The Pinnacle trailhead for the Conestoga Trail is located at the south edge of the overlook—look for the orange blazes. Departing the overlook, the trail traverses the hillside southbound above the Susquehanna River, trending out along a ridge that slopes

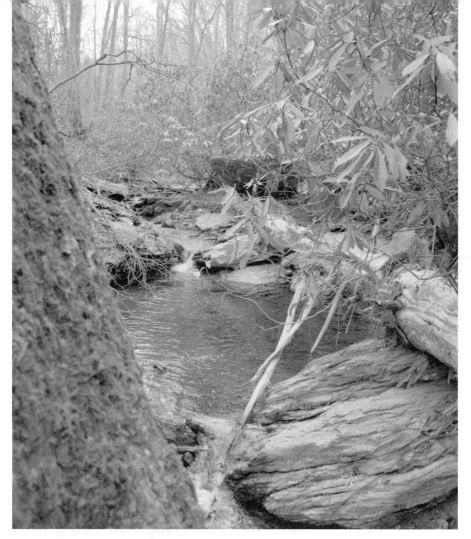

Deep in the heart of Kellys Run

towards the mouth of Kellys Run. You'll enjoy several nice views of the river as you make your way along the trail, descending gradually as you progress. At 0.4 mile, the trail passes a junction where the yellow-blazed Pinnacle Trail enters from the left; this is one of several trails in the Pinnacle area identified by the color of their blazes. The yellow trail will take you back to the parking area if you choose to do so, though you'll miss the best part of the hike.

About 0.1 mile beyond the yellow trail, the Conestoga Trail crosses the track of Old Pinnacle Road. From the road, the trail descends much more steeply and ultimately drops into Kellys Run via a set of steps in the hillside and joins the blue-blazed Kellys Run Trail. The Conestoga Trail now turns left and shares the path with the Kellys Run Trail upstream. A short walk downstream from the trail junction takes you to again to Old Pinnacle Road and the absolutely decrepit and disused bridge over Kellys Run. *The land south of the bridge is closed to the public—you trespass at your own risk.*

Although you could fight your way through the brush down to the Susquehanna River, there are better hikes for gaining access to it. The real attraction of this hike is the secluded Kellys Run. From the junction of the two trails follow them both upstream through the lovely hemlock- and rhododendron-filled glen. For the next 0.3 mile, the scenery is outstanding. The creek tumbles down toward the Susquehanna River, past tall rock outcrops, into pools, and over boulders and ledges. In late May and June, the rhododendrons are in bloom, adding even more to the spectacular scenery.

After crossing the creek twice, first to the south side and then back to the north, you'll come to the junction with the white-blazed Pinnacle Trail, which ascends 0.7 mile back out to the overlook. This is your path back to your car. Before you set off along it, the Kellys Run and Conestoga Trails continue east along the creek another 0.4 mile to a small tributary entering from the left (north) before they begin to climb out of the drainage. Walking out and back to the tributary is well worth the effort because it takes you through even more of this beautiful natural area.

To return to the overlook, head west on the Pinnacle Trail to follow it uphill. Although a little steep at first, the walk out of Kellys Run is quite lovely and offers some excellent opportunities for birding and wildlife viewing. Along this path, I've seen many songbirds common to Pennsylvania, as well as owls and many hawks; I've also seen a fox resting on the trail near the overlook.

At 0.15 mile, the trail meets an unmarked path heading right—keep left and follow the trail across two old roadbeds, the first of which, Old Pinnacle Road, is identified by a NO HORSES sign. At a third road of grass and dirt, turn right and follow the white blazes about 0.3 mile farther to the Pinnacle Overlook. The path here follows the edge of a pretty field on the right, with the Susquehanna River Valley through the trees to the left.

Nearby Activities

A few miles north, you'll find **Shenks Ferry Wildflower Preserve** (see page 203) and **Tucquan Glen Nature Preserve** (see 221). Both are Lancaster County Conservancy preserves, and each has a nice hike that can easily be done in a day along with the Kellys Run hike.

GPS TRAILHEAD COORDINATES AND DIRECTIONS
N39° 50.725' W76° 20.634'

From Buck, travel west on PA 372 4.9 miles. Turn right on River Road and follow it 1.8 miles. Turn left onto West Pinnacle Road. The overlook is 1.25 mile ahead on the right; West Pinnacle Road ends just beyond the overlook.

36 Lancaster Central Park

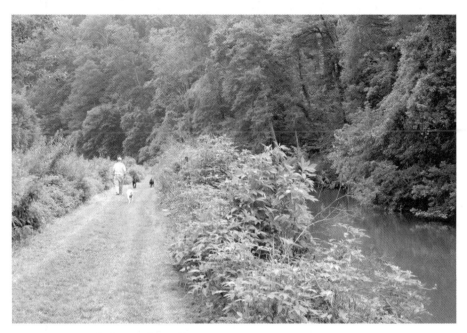

Conestoga Trail along Mill Creek

In Brief

This pretty hike initially follows Mill Creek as it meanders throughout the park before it joins the Equestrian Trail and passes some of the recreation areas in the park.

Description

Located 6 miles south of the city of Lancaster, Central Park is named for its location in the center of Lancaster County. Like many relatively urban parks, Central Park boasts quite a number of recreational facilities, making it a popular destination for people all around the county. The 544-acre park has ballfields, playgrounds, tennis courts, a pool, a fitness trail, equestrian trails, gardens, picnic pavilions, an environmental center, and, with five sites, the smallest public campground in the state.

The park is also rich in local history. In 1979, an ancient Indian burial ground was uncovered north of Golf Road near the microwave tower that this hike passes by. Robert Fulton conducted his first tests of the paddle-wheel boat on the Conestoga River, which composes the northwestern boundary of the park. And one of the park byways, General Hand Lane, is named for Edward Hand, George Washington's adjutant general, whose

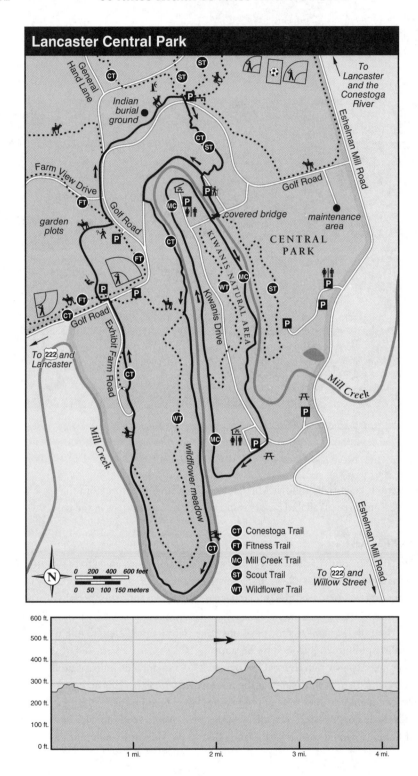

Lancaster Central Park

LENGTH 4.2 miles (1.5 miles on Mill Creek Trail loop and 2.7 miles on Conestoga/Equestrian Trails loop)

CONFIGURATION Figure-eight

DIFFICULTY Moderate

SCENERY Mill Creek, Central Park environs

EXPOSURE Slightly more sun than shade

TRAIL TRAFFIC Light

TRAIL SURFACE Mixed gravel, dirt, and grass with a short section of pavement

HIKING TIME 45 minutes for Mill Creek Trail loop; 1.5 hours for Conestoga/Equestrian Trails loop

DRIVING DISTANCE Approximately 7 miles south of PA 283 and PA 222 in Lancaster

ACCESS Daily, sunrise–sunset

MAPS USGS *Lancaster;* a park map is available online at tinyurl.com /centralparklancastermap.

FACILITIES None at parking area; water, restrooms, and picnic areas available en route

WHEELCHAIR TRAVERSABLE No

CONTACT Lancaster County Parks and Recreation, 717-299-8215, tinyurl.com /lancastercentralpark

SPECIAL COMMENTS This hike combines 3 trails throughout the park. Although each is easy to follow, care needs to be taken at some key junctions indicated in the text.

home is preserved in the park at the site of Rock Ford Plantation near the intersection of General Hand Lane and Williamson Road.

Central Park is home to 10 trails that are open to hiking, including a section of the Conestoga Trail system, which extends from northern Lancaster County south to the Mason-Dixon Trail in York County. This hike follows four trails throughout the park and creates two loops, both of which are focused around Mill Creek, the small stream that forms the southern boundary of the park.

This hike begins at the center point of the two trail loops, at the covered-bridge parking area off of Kiwanis Road. The first loop, along the Mill Creek Trail through the Kiwanis Natural Area, is 1.5 miles long and takes about 45 minutes to complete. The second loop follows the Conestoga and Equestrian Trails for most of their length and is approximately 2.7 miles long, taking about one hour and 20 minutes to complete. Putting both loops together is worth the effort, though if time doesn't permit, each offers a pleasant hike of its own.

PART 1: MILL CREEK TRAIL LOOP

Begin this section of the hike by walking over the covered bridge next to the parking lot. At 25 feet or so beyond the bridge, the trail drops down to river level via a steep but brief hillside to the left. The trail follows Mill Creek upstream in an open grassy area for 0.15 mile before passing power lines and entering the woods. Upon entering the woods, the trail is well marked with yellow blazes on the trees. The trail follows the level of the creek for a short distance before climbing to the top of the peninsula that is home to the Kiwanis Natural Area. At 0.5 mile, the trail exits the woods at an intersection with Kiwanis Drive at a large picnic area with tables, a pavilion, restrooms, and water. The only route-finding difficulty you might have on this loop is here, trying to figure out where the trail reenters the woods.

To find the trail, cross Kiwanis Drive where it comes to a T-intersection just after you leave the woods. A large parking lot will be on your right, and you should walk along the grass next to the lot keeping it to your right. When you reach the corner of the lot, look downhill toward the woods, and you will spot the trail entering the woods marked by a yellow blaze. Once in the trees, the trail descends steeply, curving to the right (north), past the foundation of what appears to have been an old pump house, and down to the level of the creek. You have just passed over the top of the peninsula. When you reach the creek, pause to admire the large sycamore trees that line the banks. Cardinals and the occasional goldfinch add a splash of contrast to the lush green forest in the summer.

The trail now follows the creek (still upstream) around the peninsula's tip. At 1 mile, you will pass the junction with the Wildflower Trail. It climbs back over the peninsula and provides a slightly shorter excursion back to the covered bridge. Continue along the level of the creek around the peninsula and, at 1.5 miles, the trail will pass beneath the covered bridge. Hike back up to the road, walk through the bridge, and into the parking area.

PART 2: CONESTOGA LOOP

Leave the parking lot heading north, following white blazes on trees through a small grassy area beside the creek. You are now following the Scout Trail. In 0.1 mile, however, the trail comes to a junction with the Conestoga Trail System, which enters from the woods on the right. The Scout Trail turns right here and shares the path with the Conestoga Trail for 0.5 mile. Remember this spot, as it will be the end of the loop that you make.

Instead of turning right, continue straight ahead, staying at the level of the river along the Conestoga Trail, marked by salmon-colored blazes. The trail soon enters the woods and bends to the left following the direction of the creek. At 0.15 mile, the trail begins to show signs of being paved. Then it clearly turns into a former paved road and begins to climb. Be wary for the next bit of route finding: At 0.3 mile, the trail drops very steeply off the road to the left back to the level of the river. The sharp left turn is marked by salmon-colored arrows painted on the surface of the road and is easily missed.

Once you regain the level of the river, the trail is very obvious and becomes less precipitous. At 0.6 mile, the Conestoga Trail joins the Equestrian Trail, which comes in from the right. Veer to the left here and enjoy the walk along the wide-open track, often grassy, as it passes through the Muhlenberg Native Plant and Wildflower Meadow, arguably the most beautiful spot in the park. For the next mile, the trail follows Mill Creek as it makes a long bend through the park. The far side of the creek rises up a steep forested hillside, while the side where the trail passes is open and gentle.

At approximately 1.6 miles, the trail leaves the creek and meets up with Exhibit Farm Road in an open grassy area flanked to the right by a large cornfield. A large rock with a salmon blaze marks the junction with Exhibit Farm Road. Follow the grass along the cornfield (there are trail signs) for another 0.2 mile until you reach the intersection of Exhibit Farm Road and Golf Road. Cross Exhibit Farm Road and then cross Golf Road. At this point, the Conestoga Trail turns left, paralleling Golf Road. Our hike continues straight (generally north) along the Equestrian Trail, passing a parking area to your right and then a playground on your left before entering a large grassy area with several large pine trees. Follow the line of pine trees to the end of the grassy area, turn right at another trail post in the northwest corner of the field, and follow the trail through a passage between some tall shrubs and trees next to the tennis courts.

At the end of this passage, the trail meets Golf Road, turns left, and follows the wide grassy shoulder of Golf Road for approximately 0.5 mile. Shortly, it crosses Farm View Drive and then General Hand Lane. At 0.1 mile past General Hand Lane, the shoulder gets very narrow and the trail climbs through a small, steep, wooded area approximately 100 feet back from the road. The trail emerges from the woods into a meadow with several trees and a large microwave tower on top. Head toward the tower following trail signs passing it on the right. Just beyond the tower (mile 2.4), you'll find a water fountain. From the fountain, the trail proceeds 0.1 mile over to a bench and a small parking area along Golf Road.

Here, the Equestrian Trail crosses the path of the Scout and Conestoga Trails. The Equestrian Trail continues to follow the shoulder of Golf Road, while the Scout and Conestoga Trails cross Golf Road and enter the woods at a tree marked with salmon and white blazes. Follow the path of these two trails into the woods, where they wind downhill for 0.2 mile to the grassy area where the loop began. The short passage through the woods is an ideal place to spot white-tailed deer.

Nearby Activities

Central Park provides all sorts of recreational activities, including a swimming pool, ballfields, a garden, and a campground. Downtown Lancaster is home to a host of shops, markets, and restaurants that are worth a visit. If you are hiking on Saturday, stop by the **Central Market** in town to pick up some snacks and drinks for a picnic in the park.

GPS TRAILHEAD COORDINATES AND DIRECTIONS
N40° 00.931' W76° 16.937'

From US 30 just north of Lancaster, follow US 222 South approximately 6 miles to Golf Road on the left. There is a sign for Lancaster Central Park. Turn left and follow Golf Road 1.5 miles to the intersection with Kiwanis Road. Turn right and, just before the covered bridge, bear right into the parking area along Mill Creek.

37 Lancaster Junction Recreation Trail

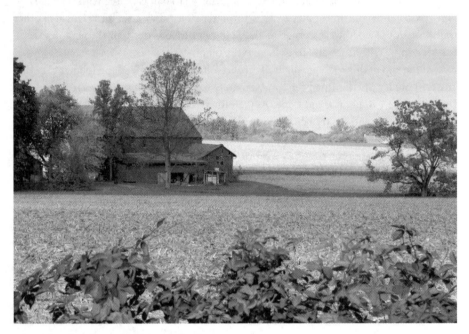

Farmland to the west of the trail

In Brief

The trailhead for this hike is about 50 feet from the highway, but heading north it quickly quiets down, joins Chickies Creek, and follows the railroad grade for 2.4 miles to Auction Road. Return via the railroad grade.

Description

Extending for 2.4 miles from PA 283 outside of Salunga north to Auction Road, the Lancaster Junction Trail follows the grade of the old Reading–Columbia Railroad line. The trail is popular with hikers, bikers, and horseback riders, and it offers a nice outing for the kids. Hiking the trail provides you with some classic Lancaster County farmland scenery and lovely views of the upper stretch of Chickies Creek. The creek eventually drains into the Susquehanna River near Chickies Rocks, a large quartzite outcrop that overlooks the river about 7 miles directly southwest. The trail scenery is particularly attractive in the

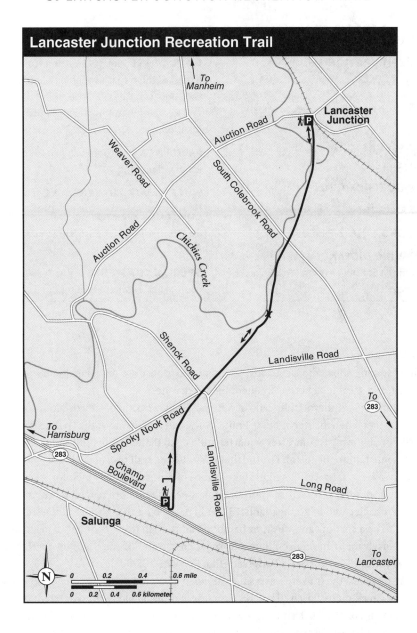

Lancaster Junction Recreation Trail

morning and late day when the sun is low and the shadows are long. Bordered by trees and brush, the trail is generally sheltered and makes for a good hike on a windy day. Common wild mammals that you may encounter are red foxes, groundhogs, and gray and ground squirrels. Bird activity is abundant in the thickets and woods lining the trail. Cardinals, bluebirds, warblers, chickadees, and catbirds are common. Hawks can often be

LENGTH 4.8 miles

CONFIGURATION Out-and-back

DIFFICULTY Easy

SCENERY Upper Chickies Creek and Lancaster County farmlands

EXPOSURE About half shade and half sun

TRAIL TRAFFIC Moderate–heavy

TRAIL SURFACE Cinders

HIKING TIME 2–3 hours

DRIVING DISTANCE Less than a mile from the Salunga exit on PA 283 west of Lancaster

ACCESS Sunrise–sunset

MAPS USGS *Columbia East* and *Manheim*; a map of the trail is available online from the Lancaster County Department of Parks and Recreation at tinyurl.com/lancaster junctionmap.

FACILITIES Restrooms and water at trailhead parking

WHEELCHAIR TRAVERSABLE If dry

CONTACT Lancaster County Parks and Recreation, 717-299-8215, tinyurl.com /lancasterjunctiontr

SPECIAL COMMENTS A good hike with young kids. Excellent birding.

sighted soaring above the farmlands, pheasant and grouse are occasionally spotted along the trail, and great blue herons frequent the creek waters.

From the southern trailhead on Champ Boulevard, head north along the trail, passing a metal bench after about 0.1 mile. Although the setting at the trailhead is rather noisy from highway traffic, after a quarter-mile or so that is left behind and the environment is much more peaceful. For the first 0.5 mile, the trail proceeds directly north and then, by a large farm on the right, takes more of a northeasterly tack for the next 0.7 mile. At 0.65 mile, you'll cross Spooky Nook Road. Just before reaching the road, note the interesting stand of grassy plants 15 feet high or so on the left side of the trail. They appear to be a sort of cane, rush, or bamboo and though they seem out of place in central Pennsylvania I have also come across a dense stand of the same on the Lakeside Trail at Gifford Pinchot State Park (see Hike 52, page 255).

At 1.2 miles, the trail crosses a small stream over an old concrete bridge and parallels Chickies Creek quite closely. The creek is clear and placid along this stretch of trail as it winds among some tall oak and impressive sycamore trees. Signs of woodpeckers are obvious on the old trees. Just past the 1.5 mile mark, the trail crosses South Colebrook Road. I walked for a distance in this area with a gentleman who lived nearby and who told me that occasionally the fish and game department releases ring-necked pheasants in the area. He had seen quite few, though he explained that the foxes tend to get them pretty quickly.

At 1.8 miles or so, you'll pass a grassy area to the left with some tall trees scattered about it and goats wandering around. Hawks often perch in the tall trees surrounding it. Soon after, the trail crosses a private farm road and a large produce farm on the right. Please keep to the trail as the road on either side is posted as private.

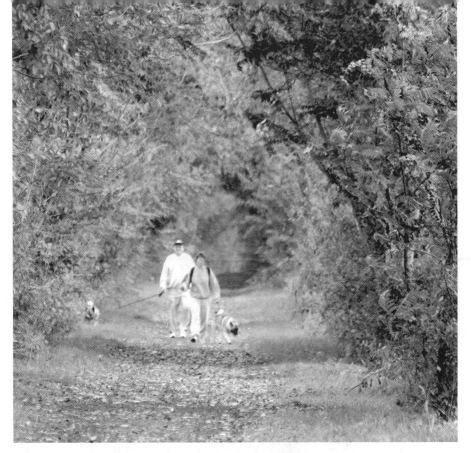

Hikers on the rail-trail

At 2.2 miles, you'll pass a second bench on the side of the trail, and just ahead, the gate at the parking area on Auction Road at the settlement of Lancaster Junction. A rail line enters from the southeast by a scenic old warehouse.

GPS TRAILHEAD COORDINATES AND DIRECTIONS

N40° 06.078' W76° 25.002'

Take the Salunga exit off PA 283 west of Lancaster. Make the first right north of the bridge over PA 283 onto Champ Boulevard. Park at the end of Champ Boulevard.

38 Lebanon Valley Rail-Trail:
LAWN TO COLEBROOK

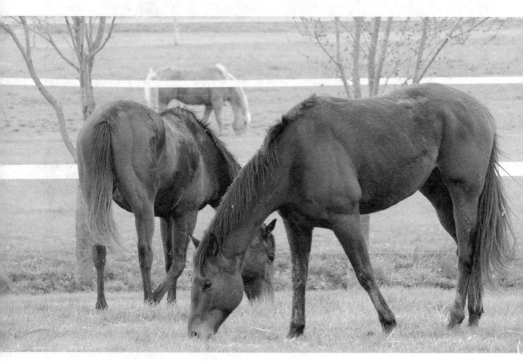

Horses at one of the stables

In Brief

This pretty hike follows the Lebanon Valley Rail-Trail from the trailhead at Lawn to the trailhead at Colebrook. Along the way it passes a couple of horse farms, the Horse-Shoe Trail, and an attractive section of woodlands.

Description

One of a number of central Pennsylvania rail-trails, the Lebanon Valley Rail-Trail (LVRT) is certainly one of the most varied and attractive. I tend to hike this trail and its Lancaster County extension, the Conewago Trail (see page 158), more than any trails in the area, in part because it is on my way home from work but also because it's so peaceful and scenic. Along its 15-mile length between the city of Lebanon and the Lancaster County line, the trail passes through farmland, wooded lots and hollows, historic towns, past ponds, and

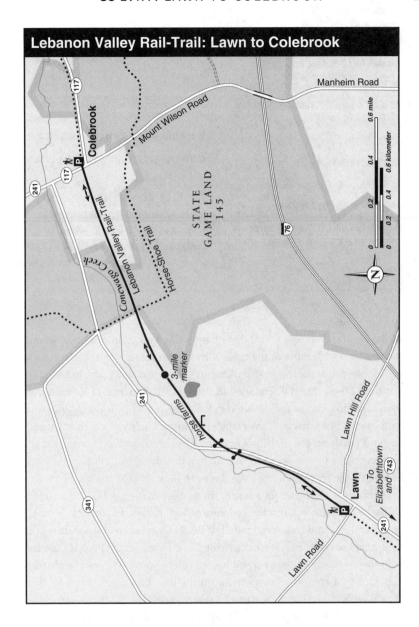

along Conewago Creek. Aside from the abundance of serenity the trail offers, it also offers opportunities for seeing wildlife, especially some of the birdlife that is so abundant and varied in this region of Pennsylvania.

One thing I especially like about the LVRT is the frequency of access points that allow one to select from one of a half-dozen or more hikes to do along it. The hike described here covers the section from the towns of Lawn to Colebrook. I selected this section because it

LENGTH 4.2 miles

CONFIGURATION Out-and-back

DIFFICULTY Easy

SCENERY Farmland and Conewago Creek

EXPOSURE Mixed sun and shade

TRAIL TRAFFIC Moderate–heavy

TRAIL SURFACE Cinders

HIKING TIME About 2 hours

DRIVING DISTANCE 5.7 miles from the junction of PA 743 and PA 241 in Elizabethtown

ACCESS Sunrise–sunset

MAPS USGS *Elizabethtown*; a map of the entire Lebanon Valley Rail-Trail is available online at lvrailtrail.com/trail.pdf.

FACILITIES Benches, portable toilet at trailheads

WHEELCHAIR TRAVERSABLE Yes

CONTACT Lebanon Valley Rails to Trails, lvrailtrail.com

SPECIAL COMMENTS Although hunting is not permitted along the trail, this hike does pass by areas where hunting is allowed. I recommend wearing blaze orange during hunting season, from late October until late December.

doesn't join any of the other sections that I have written about in this book, because of its particular beauty, and because of the availability of refreshments near the Colebrook trailhead. The hike begins at the trailhead parking area and community park in Lawn, which are located at mile 2.0 on the trail. Founded in 1888 under the name of Roseland, the town changed its name to Lawn in 1889. It is a very small town, and quite pretty with several scenic old residences. The town park has a ballfield, a picnic shelter, portable toilet and several benches. Head northeast out of the town, passing by private yards on your right as the trail eventually becomes a wooded path separated from the surrounding farmland by a couple of hundred feet. At the transition area from the open park into the woods, you'll see several birdhouses that provide shelter for some of the numerous songbirds, which include cardinals, goldfinches, nuthatches, titmice, cedar waxwings, robins, and others.

For the first half-mile, the trail parallels PA 241, and then at 0.6 mile it comes to a gate and a road crossing. Be careful crossing here. Once across PA 241, the trail veers away from the road, and highway noise becomes less obtrusive. For the next half-mile, the trail passes by a couple of horse farms on the left. The meadows, with their white split rail fences, not to mention the horses that wander around them, are quite beautiful. In the fall the landscape is lit up with color. In the spring, you will find wildflowers and blossoming plants along the trail. Several tall willows line the meadows, and they hold a wonderful light green during the spring when the leaves are just coming out. About 0.2 mile beyond the road crossing, there is a bench on the right side of the trail that offers a nice place to sit.

Not far beyond the bench, the trail crosses over a seasonal creek that flows in from the south and passes through another horse farm. Three birdhouses are stacked in an unusual arrangement atop a post at the stream crossing. This is a good spot for taking some photographs of the landscape. Continue past the creek and in a short time you will pass mile marker 3.0 on the right. At this point the trail passes through mostly wooded terrain, though the forest is not very dense and at places you can still see out to the surrounding fields to the north. At 1.4 miles into the hike, the trail crosses the Horse-Shoe Trail, which extends 140 miles from the Appalachian Trail to the west to Valley Forge National Park outside of Philadelphia to the east. I have made a loop out of this hike by following the Horse-Shoe Trail uphill to the south and then east through a large meadow atop the hillside on your right. If you choose to do that, consider that doing so entails hiking along the shoulder of Mount Wilson Road back into Colebrook for 0.25 mile. It is not a bad walk along the road, and the upper meadow is very pretty, but Mount Wilson Road can be busy.

After the junction with the Horse-Shoe Trail, the rail-trail runs fairly close to the Conewago Creek before that veers off to the north. After another 0.5 mile of walking in the woods you will reach Mount Wilson Road and the trailhead at Colebrook. Retrace the route back to the parking area.

Nearby Activities

Near the Colebrook trailhead on PA 117 are **Twin Kiss** restaurant (901 N. Hanover St.; 717-367-1694), which has hamburgers and hot dogs, and the **Colebrook Tavern** (1510 Mt. Wilson Road; 717-964-3551). Mount Gretna, about 6 miles from Lawn, has a couple of restaurants, more hiking, a swimming pond, as well as concerts and events during the summer. A good portal for information about Mount Gretna events is located online at mtgretna.com.

GPS TRAILHEAD COORDINATES AND DIRECTIONS

N40° 13.296' W76° 32.367'

From PA 283, follow PA 743 south toward Elizabethtown. At the first traffic light, make a sharp left turn (you will be going almost in the opposite direction) onto PA 241 and follow it 6.7 miles until the town of Lawn. Turn left onto Lawn Road and right into the parking area for the Lawn Community Park.

39 Lebanon Valley Rail-Trail:
MOUNT GRETNA TO CORNWALL

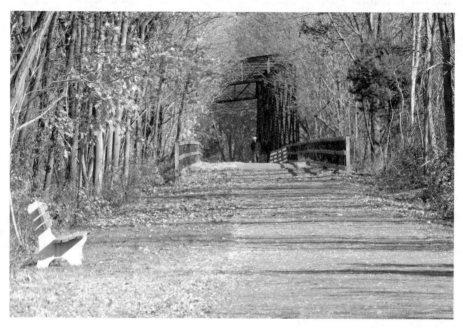

Rail-trail near Cornwall

In Brief

This hike follows the Lebanon Valley Rail-Trail (LVRT) 3.8 miles from the trailhead in Mount Gretna to the town of Cornwall. Along the way, it passes environs that are ideal for viewing wildlife. Just before reaching Cornwall, the trail crosses a scenic old railroad bridge.

Description

This hike follows the LVRT for 3.8 miles from the Mount Gretna Spur to the village of Cornwall. The rail-trail currently extends for 15 miles from the Lebanon–Lancaster County line 6.4 miles to the west of Mount Gretna to the city of Lebanon. At the western terminus, the trail becomes the Conewago Trail and continues for another 5 miles into Elizabethtown (see page 158).

You can begin this hike in either Mount Gretna or Cornwall. I usually go from Mount Gretna simply because it is closer to where I live. I suspect that on a summer weekend, though, parking might be easier to find in Cornwall than in Mount Gretna,

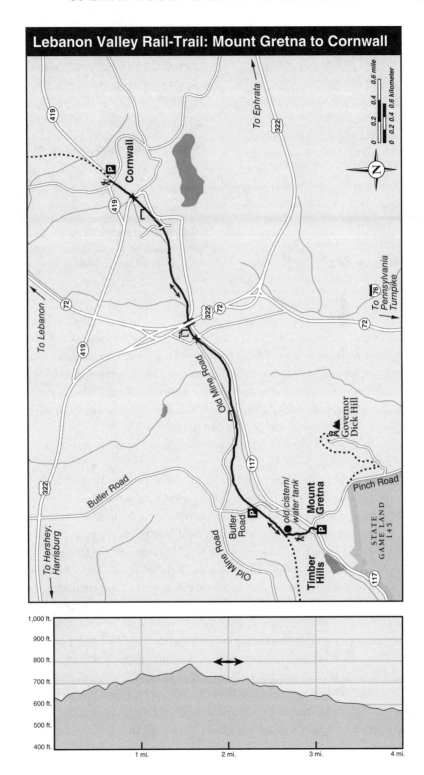

LENGTH 8 miles

CONFIGURATION Out-and-back

DIFFICULTY Moderate

SCENERY Oak-and-hickory forest, some spots of railroad history

EXPOSURE More shade than sun for the first 2 miles, and then it is mostly in the sun

TRAIL TRAFFIC Light during the week, moderately heavy on weekends

TRAIL SURFACE Cinder and dirt

HIKING TIME 3–4 hours

DRIVING DISTANCE 12 miles from PA 283 and PA 743 north of Elizabethtown

ACCESS Sunrise–sunset

MAPS USGS *Manheim* and *Lebanon* quads; a map of the trail is available online at lvrailtrail.com/maps.htm.

FACILITIES None

WHEELCHAIR TRAVERSABLE When the trail is dry

CONTACT Lebanon Valley Rails to Trails, lvrailtrail.com

SPECIAL COMMENTS The trail has been designated by Audubon Pennsylvania as a Susquehanna River Birding and Wildlife Trail.

which gets rather crowded. Mount Gretna was established in 1892 as the site of the Pennsylvania Chautauqua, one of more than 200 Chautauqua communities established in the late 19th and early 20th centuries. Founded at Lake Chautauqua in New York in 1874, the Chautauqua communities were dedicated to the self-education of people from all walks of American life. Each community held its own programs in the arts, sciences, and religion for guests and residents. The current town of Mount Gretna still bears that heritage, as its theater puts on performances during the summer and offers a highly regarded music series.

I begin this hike at the main parking area in Mount Gretna rather than at the trailhead proper because I am uncertain about the parking at the trailhead. Although there are no signs that prohibit parking, many private residences are located around the trailhead and parking nearby might infringe on the rights and privacy of property owners.

From the main lot in town, walk across PA 117 heading east and turn left onto Timber Road. Mount Gretna Pizzeria provides a good landmark for the turn, as well as a good slice of pie on your return. Follow Timber Road across a creek and continue a short distance to where it bends left. The trailhead for the Mount Gretna Spur of the rail-trail is on the right at the bend. The trail is paved initially and soon passes by what appears to be an old stone cistern on the right and a water tank on the left.

At 0.2 mile from the parking area, you come to the junction with the LVRT. Turn right and follow its level cinder track all the way to Cornwall. The rail-trail follows the path of the old Cornwall and Lebanon Railroad line that ran between Lebanon to the northeast and Conewago to the west. It was completed in 1883 by iron magnate Robert Coleman, and a bench acknowledging his historical significance is located on the Mount Gretna Spur.

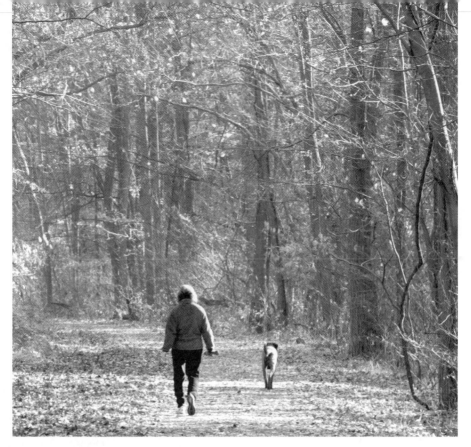

Along the trail near Mount Gretna

The trail has been designated by Audubon Pennsylvania as a Susquehanna River Birding and Wildlife Trail, part of a network of trails in the Susquehanna basin that are acknowledged for bird and wildlife viewing. On the way into Cornwall, you'll find occasional benches on the side of the trail that provide wonderful locations for resting and watching, the next of which is just a tenth of a mile along the trail.

At 0.6 mile, the trail crosses Butler Road outside of Mount Gretna, and just beyond the crossing you'll find the first trail-mileage marker (7) and another bench on the left. The trail is quite wide beyond Butler Road, because it has a mulch shoulder to the left that horseback riders are supposed to use. As you continue generally east, you will see many private residences through the woods.

At 1.75 miles, just past the crest of the railroad grade, you'll find a pair of benches. Old railroad ties that were discarded when the trail was developed lie in piles to either side of the path. Just beyond, a hollow drops off rather steeply to the north by a private residence. This is a wonderful section for spotting birds. In particular, the woodpeckers and flickers seem to be abundant throughout this section of the trail.

At 2.5 miles, pass a bench and then cross over Old Mine Road on a bridge. Between this bridge and the underpass at US 322 0.2 mile beyond, a dense thicket lines the trail to the north, and just beyond that is an open field. This is a superb stretch for bird sightings as several species of songbirds make their homes in this area, including cedar waxwings, nuthatches, warblers, chickadees, and juncos. After you pass beneath US 322, thicket lines both sides of the trail, and the bird-watching remains good. A decent pair of binoculars and a fair bit of patience can be helpful, as the birds tend to be small and very quick.

As you approach Cornwall, signs of development become more abundant. At 3.2 miles, the trail passes a large sump pond on the right. At 3.4 miles, it passes beneath a bridge and then by a private development on the north just outside the town of Cornwall.

Soon you'll pass by mile marker 10 and a bench; then walk across the old iron truss railroad bridge, which has been recently renovated. Just to the north of the bridge is the Cornwall Elementary School, with a couple of historic buildings on its property. Just beyond the bridge, the trail is paved and about 0.2 mile beyond that is the trailhead at PA 419 in Cornwall, the turnaround. Across the road, a large parking area is located just to the right of the trail. The parking area was the site of the old Cornwall and Lebanon Railroad Cornwall station, which burned in 1933.

In the 1800s, Cornwall was the source of a large deposit of high-grade iron ore, which accounted for the development of the railroad in this area. The original line, the North Lebanon Railroad, was completed in 1855. Industrialist Robert Coleman came in some years later and developed the Cornwall and Lebanon line, which provided competition to the North Lebanon Railroad. In 1972 the C and L was abandoned as a result of damage to the tracks from Hurricane Agnes, which also flooded the ore mines in Cornwall.

Nearby Activities

Mount Gretna is a summer resort with plenty of activities going on and recreational opportunities, including a beach and canoe rentals. The historic village is worth driving around to admire some of the quaint and unusual architecture. For food, try **The Jigger Shop** (202 Gettysburg Ave.; 717-964-9686, thejiggershop.com) during the summer. The **Mount Gretna Hide-A-Way** (40 Boulevard St.; 717-675-7987, mtgretnahideaway.com) is just beyond the town center, heading east; turn right onto Boulevard Street and it's on the left. It's open year-round and has an outdoor deck during the summer.

GPS TRAILHEAD COORDINATES AND DIRECTIONS

N40° 14.879' W76° 28.264'

From PA 283, follow PA 743 south toward Elizabethtown. At the first traffic light, make a sharp left turn (you will be going almost in the opposite direction) onto PA 241 and follow it 7.75 miles until the town of Colebrook. Turn right onto PA 117. After 100 yards, PA 117 turns left toward Mount Gretna. Take this left and follow 3 miles to the town of Mount Gretna. Park in the large public parking area on the right at the town center.

40 Money Rocks County Park

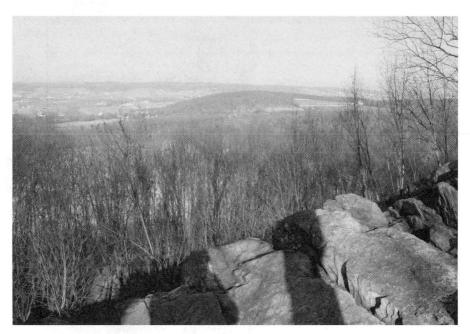

The Welsh Mountains from the overlook

In Brief

This hike begins with a short walk from the parking area out to the Money Rocks Overlook and then heads west on the Cockscomb Trail. From the Cockscomb area, it heads north and west along the hillside. At a T-intersection, it descends north to the Iron Horse Trail (IHT). After completing the IHT loop, this hike returns to the Cockscomb Trail, and completes that loop by climbing out of a hollow and along the ridge back to the Cockscomb outcrop.

Description

Located in eastern Lancaster County, the little-known Money Rocks County Park spans more than 300 acres in the Welsh Mountains of Pennsylvania, the second largest tract of forested land remaining in the county, the largest being the Furnace Hills along US 322 to the west (see page 73). This pleasant hike covers most of the trails in the park. It offers views of the surrounding countryside as well as opportunities to see ruffed grouse, wild turkey, and white-tailed deer, all of which are common to the park.

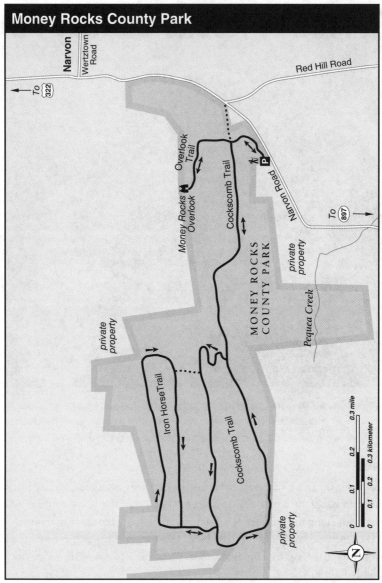

Money Rocks County Park

Narvon

Wertztown Road

Red Hill Road

To 322

Overlook Trail

Money Rocks Overlook

Cockscomb Trail

P

Narvon Road

To 897

private property

Pequea Creek

MONEY ROCKS COUNTY PARK

private property

Iron Horse Trail

Cockscomb Trail

private property

0.3 mile
0.1 0.2
0.3 kilometer
0 0.1 0.2

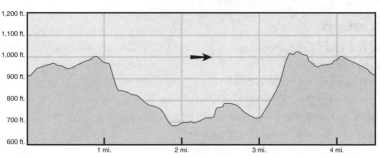

1,200 ft.
1,100 ft.
1,000 ft.
900 ft.
800 ft.
700 ft.
600 ft.

1 mi.   2 mi.   3 mi.   4 mi.

LENGTH 4.5 miles	**ACCESS** Sunrise–sunset
CONFIGURATION Figure-eight with a section of out-and-back	**MAPS** USGS *New Holland, Honey Brook;* a trail map is available online at tinyurl .com/moneyrocksparkmap.
DIFFICULTY Moderate	
SCENERY Welsh Hills and nice views to the north from Money Rocks	**FACILITIES** None
	WHEELCHAIR TRAVERSABLE No
EXPOSURE Shaded	**CONTACT** Lancaster County Parks and Recreation, 717-299-8215, tinyurl.com /moneyrockscp
TRAIL TRAFFIC Generally light	
TRAIL SURFACE Dirt and rock	
HIKING TIME 2.5–3 hours	**SPECIAL COMMENTS** Use caution when hiking during hunting season. Muzzle loading and archery seasons extend well into January.
DRIVING DISTANCE 5.1 miles from US 322 and PA 23 in Blue Ball	

The trailhead for the white-blazed Overlook Trail, the first section of this hike, is located at the east edge of the parking area near a large wooden information sign. Begin by following the white blazes from the trailhead north along an old roadbed for 0.3 mile to the Money Rocks Overlook, crossing the Cockscomb Trail (a roadbed marked by a prominent sign) en route. The overlook offers the best views on this hike of farms, towns, and distant wooded hills to the north. According to the Lancaster County Department of Parks and Recreation, legend has it that the rocks were so named because farmers from the Pequea Valley to the south hid their money among the rocks. Consisting mostly of a Chickies Formation white-and-pink quartzite formed by erosion of the softer rock surrounding it, the overlook sits atop cliffs and outcroppings ranging from 15 to 50 feet high. A metal railing safeguards one section of the cliffs, though care should be taken at all places when scrambling about the area. The best view and resting spots are located among the square boulders about 100 feet past the railing. Take note of the large rectangular boulder on the crest with names carved into it; some of them date back to the mid-1800s.

After enjoying the view, make your way back through the forest of white oak, black birch, and mountain laurel to the red-blazed Cockscomb Trail and turn right (west). This trail follows the flat ridge for 0.3 mile to a junction with a dirt road that is posted with private property signs. Bear right and follow the red blazes over to the edge of the ridge where the Cockscomb Trail begins a gentle descent along the north-facing hillside. A short distance along the descent, you'll be able to spot the Cockscomb on the ridgecrest to the left (south). Another smaller quartzite outcrop, the Cockscomb provides views mostly from late fall to early spring when the leaves are off the trees. In this area, about 1.1 miles into the hike, the Cockscomb Trail forks at a tree marked with multiple red blazes. Turn right (north) and follow the trail down the steep, rocky hillside for a short distance to an old roadbed at the next level. Turn left (west) and follow the road as it traverses the hillside. According to the park map, several small trails connect this section of the trail with the IHT several hundred feet downhill. Those trails are unmarked and much of the area surrounding the park is private land belonging to mining companies.

To be safe, follow the roadbed (the lower stretch of the Cockscomb Trail) for 0.6 mile to a major T-intersection identified by a tall oak tree with double red blazes. The Cockscomb Trail, red-blazed and distinct, turns left uphill. To pick up the Iron Horse Trail, turn right and head downhill on an unmarked track that is more distinct in the spring and summer than fall and winter. Follow it for 200 yards, staying right of a small watercourse. Soon you will reach a sign marking the IHT, marked by blue blazes. Continue past that sign on the now more prominent trail to a second sign at an old railroad grade. Turn right (east) and follow the grade for 0.5 mile of very pleasant walking to a third IHT sign pointing uphill. Beyond the third sign, the grade passes onto private property barricaded by two large concrete blocks. Leave the grade and follow the trail uphill into the woods, crossing an old carriage road and then reaching a second former road with a trail sign onto which you'll turn right. This takes you back to the first IHT sign and the end of the 1.4-mile lower loop.

Trace your steps back up to the Cockscomb Trail, and follow it uphill into a pretty and dark hollow. Cross a creek and then continue about halfway up the hollow until you reach a fork in the trail. Continuing straight along the main track takes you into private property. Turn left (east) and cut back across the hollow and gain the Cockscomb Ridge by climbing a short steep section with timbers that serve more to retard erosion than to facilitate walking. Once upon the ridge, just below its crest to the south, about a mile of easy walking returns you to the car.

GPS TRAILHEAD COORDINATES AND DIRECTIONS
N40° 05.718' W75° 58.932'

Follow US 322 east from the intersection with PA 23 in Blue Ball 3.9 miles. Turn right onto Narvon Road (poorly marked). The parking area is 1.2 miles south on the right at a high point of the road.

41 Shenks Ferry Wildflower Preserve

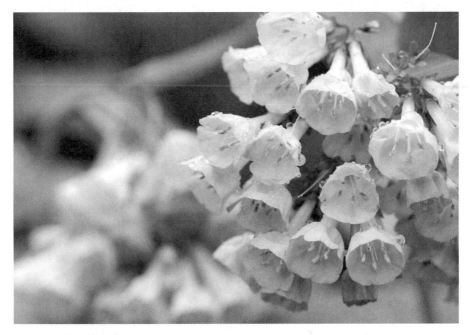

Virginia bluebells

In Brief

This hike covers all the trails in the Shenks Ferry Wildflower Preserve. It follows the main trail to the end of the hollow, and on the return it crosses the creek and follows an old path through the woods above Grubb Run Hollow.

Description

I had repeatedly seen signs for the Shenks Ferry Wildflower Preserve as I was exploring the glens and trails along the lower Susquehanna River in Lancaster County during the fall of 2006. A visit to the area was quite inviting, though I decided to put it off until the spring, figuring that would be the best time to visit. I spent the whole winter thinking of the place, conjuring images of blue skies, open meadows filled with grasses and flowers. I picked a weekday in mid-April, got up early on a rainy morning and drove down to the preserve. What I found was remarkable, though not at all what I expected.

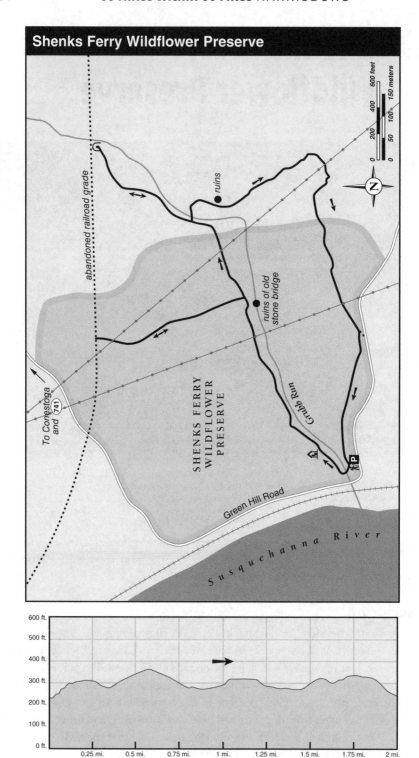

Shenks Ferry Wildflower Preserve

LENGTH About 2 miles

CONFIGURATION Loop or out-and-back (the most popular option)

DIFFICULTY Easy if you hike out-and-back, moderate if you do the loop

SCENERY Beautiful hollow filled with wildflowers

EXPOSURE Shade

TRAIL TRAFFIC Can get very busy

TRAIL SURFACE Dirt

HIKING TIME 1–3 hours or more, depending on how much time you spend looking at the wildflowers

DRIVING DISTANCE 12 miles from PA 72 and US 222 in Lancaster

ACCESS Sunrise–sunset

MAPS USGS *Safe Harbor;* a map of the preserve is available at the trailhead.

FACILITIES Portable toilet along the trail

WHEELCHAIR TRAVERSABLE Possibly, if the trail is dry

CONTACT Lancaster County Conservancy, 717-392-7891, lancaster conservancy.org/preserves

SPECIAL COMMENTS The main trail along Grubb Run would be good for kids and is probably wheelchair accessible. If doing the loop, which involves crossing Grubb Run, the trail is a bit more rugged and not well maintained.

The wildflower preserve is located in something of a dark forested glen along a creek (Grubb Run) just before it flows beneath the railroad tracks and into the Susquehanna River. Your first indication of approaching something special comes when you reach the level of the river and begin driving south next to the railroad tracks. When I first visited in April, the hillside on the left was completely covered (no exaggeration) in bluebells—more than I had even seen in one place before. After parking the car at Grubb Run, I was pretty amazed at the variety of plants and flowers I saw as I walked along the trail: jack-in-the-pulpits, fiddlehead ferns, trillium, Dutchman's-breeches, columbines, more bluebells. The flowers were everywhere.

The wildflower preserve is part of the Holtwood Environmental Preserve in southern Lancaster County, which also, incidentally, is home to the Kellys Run Trail and Nature Preserve a few miles farther south (see page 176). Shenks Ferry Wildflower Preserve is a small tract of land, only about 50 acres according to the life list and trail map you can pick up at the trailhead. But the area provides habitat for more than 70 species of spring wildflowers and another 60 species that bloom throughout the summer months.

This hike covers most of the trails in the sanctuary. Begin hiking at the trailhead on Green Hill Road, identified by a sign with a map and photographs of some of the indigenous wildflowers. Follow the wide dirt path back into the hollow. As you walk above Grubb Run, a hillside rises to your left and descends to the creek on your right. In late April, the hillside to your left is covered with Virginia bluebells and white trillium.

After about 0.1 mile or so, you pass beneath a power line and at about 0.25 mile, you'll reach the ruins of an old stone bridge and a culvert that passes beneath the path. A side trail departs to the left and follows a small tributary for 0.2 mile up a small hollow to a power line

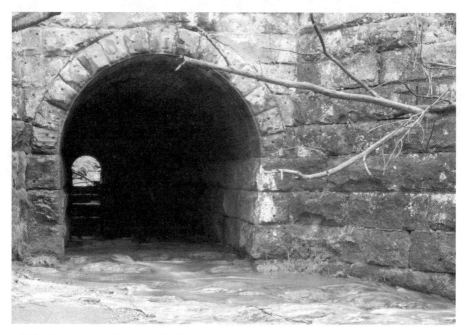

Old railroad tunnel over Grubb Run

and old railroad grade. In early spring, the hollow is filled with Dutchman's-breeches (a common and beautiful white-and-yellow early-spring flower) and a variety of yellow composites. I also found it to be a good place to see a wild turkey.

After the side trip, return to the main trail, turn left, and continue walking in an upstream direction. You'll pass some power lines quite soon that cross over the main creek at the confluence of Grubb Run and a significant tributary entering from the southeast. Beyond those power lines, Grubb Run flows over long bedrock shelves, giving the stream a distinctive character. Follow the main trail for 0.35 mile to its end at an old stone tunnel through which Grubb Run flows beneath an old railroad grade (1.1 miles including side trip).

From the tunnel, you can either backtrack along the path to the trailhead or you can make a loop of the hike. To do the latter, follow the trail back to the power lines that cross the confluence of the creek and its tributary. The trail map indicates that a side trail crosses Grubb Run just downstream from the confluence. I was unable to locate that path and found the following to be a good alternative: Just before reaching the power lines, several trails descend to the level of the creek upstream from the confluence. This is probably the easiest place to cross Grubb Run, though it is necessary to walk in the water. Cross the creek at its shallowest point and follow the obvious trail around the tip of the peninsula formed by the two streams. As you round its end, you'll come to the ruins of an old homestead against the hillside of the hollow from which the tributary runs. This small hollow is extremely beautiful, as it is carpeted with a variety of wildflowers.

From the ruins, cross the tributary near the end of the peninsula to a gain an obvious trail ascending the hillside along a small steep creek parallel to the power-line cut. Many unusual wildflowers can be found along that little steep creek. It is the only place that I have found the small white miterwort, with its geometrically unique and complex petals. Follow the trail uphill for a short distance, crossing to the right side of the creek. At the top of the climb, the trail makes a sharp right turn beneath the power line at several signs posting private property. At the power line, the path becomes less distinct and somewhat overgrown. Cross the power-line cut, and when you enter the woods again, turn right following a faint path back down toward Grubb Run. After a short distance, you'll reach a wide path onto which you will turn left. Although the path is quite obvious here, it is frequently obstructed by deadfall.

Soon the trail reaches another power line in the vicinity of a private residence. The trail becomes quite indistinct here. Pass beneath the power line and as you enter the woods again, follow the path (s) of least resistance out to Green Hill Road, just 100 feet or so to your left. Alternately, you can walk beneath the power line over to Green Hill Road, though the terrain is quite swampy. Turn right on Green Hill Road and follow it a short distance downhill to your car.

Nearby Activities

The two towns closest to the preserve are **Conestoga** and **Safe Harbor.** Conestoga, the home of the Conestoga wagon, has a museum and historical society. **The Conestoga Wagon Restaurant** (717-872-4811, theconestogawagon.com), on Main Street, serves great food. The staff is also very friendly.

Just north of the hydroelectric plant on River Road in Safe Harbor, you'll find **Conestoga River Park.** It has picnic areas and a playground. From there, the drive east along the shore of the Conestoga River is quite lovely.

GPS TRAILHEAD COORDINATES AND DIRECTIONS
N39° 54.139' W76° 21.994'

From Lancaster, follow PA 324 south to New Danville. When PA 324 turns, continue straight onto New Danville Pike into Conestoga, where it becomes Main Street. Pass through the town and at an obvious fork in the road, bear left onto River Corner Road. Cross River Road and pick up Shenks Ferry Road. At Green Hill Road, turn left and follow it downhill beneath a stone tunnel to the railroad tracks at the river. Turn left at the tracks and follow Green Hill Road south. The trailhead is about 0.5 mile on the left. Park along the road.

42 Silver Mine Park

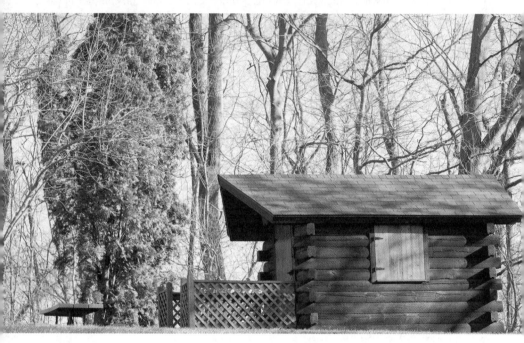

Cabin along the upper Hike and Bike Trail

In Brief

This pleasant hike takes in most of the varied environments of both the north and south sections of Silver Mine Park in Pequea Township. It begins near the site of the old mine shaft and kiln on the north side of Silver Mine Road and heads back along an old carriage road to one of the park's two catch-and-release ponds. The hike makes a wide counter-clockwise loop around the pond before heading over some more uplands and then out to the Hike and Bike Trail trailhead on Silver Mine Road. The hike follows the Hike and Bike Trail along Pequea Creek to the playing fields on the south side of the park, makes a loop around the southernmost picnic pavilion, and departs from the Hike and Bike Trail near the south catch-and-release pond, where it crosses Silver Mine Road and returns to the car.

Description

Named for the old silver-and-quartz mine in the area, Silver Mine Park is the only community park in Pequea Township, located on the eastern side of the lower Susquehanna River in Lancaster County. Although at 151 acres it is a small park, the scenery and

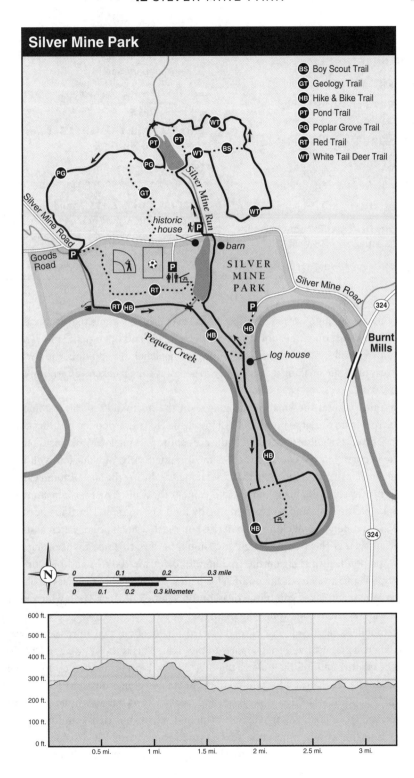

Silver Mine Park

BS Boy Scout Trail
GT Geology Trail
HB Hike & Bike Trail
PT Pond Trail
PG Poplar Grove Trail
RT Red Trail
WT White Tail Deer Trail

Silver Mine Run

historic house

barn

SILVER MINE PARK

Goods Road

Silver Mine Road

Pequea Creek

log house

Silver Mine Road

324

Burnt Mills

324

N

| 0 | 0.1 | 0.2 | 0.3 mile |

| 0 | 0.1 | 0.2 | 0.3 kilometer |

600 ft.
500 ft.
400 ft.
300 ft.
200 ft.
100 ft.
0 ft.

0.5 mi.   1 mi.   1.5 mi.   2 mi.   2.5 mi.   3 mi.

LENGTH 3.3 miles

CONFIGURATION Loop

DIFFICULTY Easy

SCENERY Pond, park fields, Pequea Creek

EXPOSURE Mix of sun and shade

TRAIL TRAFFIC Medium

TRAIL SURFACE Dirt and paved

HIKING TIME 1.5–2 hours

DRIVING DISTANCE About 7.5 miles from downtown Lancaster

ACCESS Sunrise–sunset

MAPS USGS *Conestoga;* a map of the park is available online at tinyurl.com /silvermineparkmap.

FACILITIES Picnic pavilions, portable toilets

WHEELCHAIR TRAVERSABLE Yes for the Hike and Bike Trail

CONTACT Pequea Township, 717-464-2322, pequeatwp.org/park-info

SPECIAL COMMENTS A guide to the history of mining and geology of the park, written by Don Wise of Franklin and Marshall College, is available online at tinyurl .com/silverminegeologyguide.

environs are surprisingly varied. The park has several hiking trails that traverse creeksides, ponds, forest, open meadows, as well as ballfields and open park land. The main Hike and Bike Trail is paved and is accessible by wheelchair. In addition, the park offers several areas to picnic, making it a nice place to get away for a weekend afternoon of walking and relaxing.

Begin this hike at the small parking area on the north side of Silver Mine Road, directly across from the large pond south of the road. There is a wooden box that contains trail maps as well as a guide to geology of the area at the parking lot. Walk north out of the lot past a gate onto an old carriage road. Almost immediately, on your left, you will see the stone remains of an old lime kiln that operated here during the late 19th and early 20th centuries that was used to make mortar and cement for walls. The two-kiln stone structure is quite picturesque and worth stopping by for a photograph. Continue beyond the kiln and in 0.2 mile you will climb a small rise and reach a small pond. Catch and release fishing is allowed at this pond, though you should be sure to abide by licensing regulations. At the pond, turn right on the trail and follow it for 200 feet and pick up a road heading uphill and away from the pond. This path is not named but is marked dark blue on the park map and takes you to the head of the White Tail Deer Trail, which makes a loop in meadows and woods above the pond to the east.

Hike uphill along the old gravel road toward a field, about two-thirds of the way up the hill, where a green-blazed trail departs to the right. This is the White Tail Deer Trail. Turn right (south) and follow it along the hillside into a pretty hardwood forest past a bench. The trail eventually bends around to the north and comes out to a field at 0.6 mile, where you will see a large farm off to your right (east). Keep your eyes open for a sign for the White Tail Deer Trail, which will point you off toward your right (continuing north) and back into the woods, where the trail descends and bends back to the west. After descending a short distance, you will reach the orange-blazed pond trail near a sign that

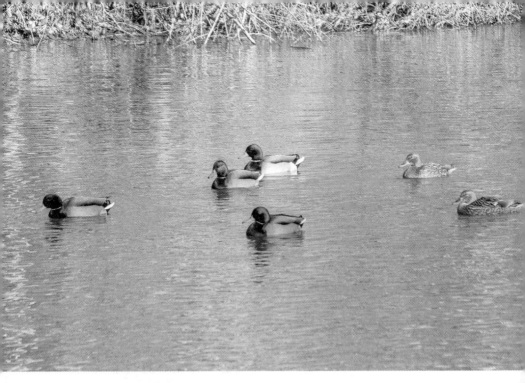

Mallards in the upper pond

indicates horses are not allowed. Turn right and shortly you will be back at the pond. Cross a footbridge over Silver Mine Creek and follow the trail around the pond back to its south end (1 mile). Upon reaching the south end of the pond, locate and turn right on the gray-blazed Poplar Trail on your right. It heads up and west up a short and steep hill away from the pond toward a clearing near some power lines.

Pass underneath the first set of power lines and angle to the southwest to walk beneath a second set of power lines. The trail is a little indistinct in this area as it passes around a cornfield, but as it begins to descend the blazes become more obvious. Soon the trail curves around to the southeast and passes back beneath the power lines, then passes through a short section of woods and emerges at Silver Mine Road. At Silver Mine Road, you will pick up the paved Hike and Bike Trail, which begins at a small parking area down-hill from you about 100 yards to the right (west). You need to cross Silver Mine Road and you should be very cautious about doing so; the road is very winding in this area and approaching cars can have a difficult time seeing you. Make your way to the parking area and follow the Hike and Bike Trail south, first through some woods and then to the banks of Pequea Creek, where you will find a little fishing platform and a bench (1.6 miles).

Upon reaching the creek, the trail heads directly east and departs the shore of the creek. There is a small path that follows the creek more closely, though it might be covered by debris from recent flooding. At 1.8 miles, you will come to a footbridge over Silver Mine Run, which flows out from beneath the dam to your left. A bench near the creek provides a nice rest spot. From this point in the hike you will be walking through the attractive park fields for the rest of the hike. There are trees where you can take some shade if you are walking on a hot, sunny summer day, but the walking will be mostly in the sun. The path curves around to the south and at 1.8 miles you will pass a cutoff trail that heads uphill to your left. Beyond that you walk along a long field with a row of trees toward the southern edge of the park. At 2.3 miles, the trail intersects the loop on the Hike and Bike Trail at the southernmost field in the park. Turn right and follow the loop counterclockwise past some grand sycamore trees growing along the creek for almost a half-mile to where it joins the upper section of the Hike and Bike Trail. Turn right and follow that north. The leg of the Hike and Bike Trail that you followed to the loop is about 50 yards to your left, downhill and beyond a narrow section of forest.

At 3 miles, you will pass a small log house along the trail and just beyond that the upper end of the cutoff trail that you passed on your way out to the loop. Just past the cutoff, leave the Hike and Bike Trail, and follow the faint track (not on park map) through the grass angling left (northeast) so that you stay above the cutoff trail and are heading toward the south pond. When you reach the hillside the track becomes much more obvious and it bends around to the north and joins a dirt path at the southeast corner of the pond. Turn right on the path so that you are heading counterclockwise around the pond and follow it out to Silver Mine Road past an old barn. Turn left on Silver Mine Road and walk down to your car and the parking area, about 200 feet. Alternately, you could turn left when reaching the pond and walk around it in a clockwise direction back to the parking lot and your car.

GPS TRAILHEAD COORDINATES AND DIRECTIONS
N39° 56.670' W76° 18.784'

From downtown Lancaster, follow Prince Street south until the intersection with PA 324, New Danville Pike. Follow New Danville Pike south 4.7 miles to the intersection with Silver Mine Road. Silver Mine Road angles off to the left between Penn Grant Road and New Danville Pike. Follow Silver Mine Road 1.6 miles. The trailhead parking is on the left directly across the road from the pond.

43 Steinman Run Nature Preserve

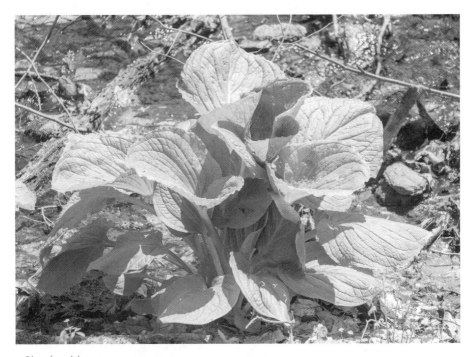

Skunk cabbage

In Brief

This lovely hike follows the blue-blazed trail from the parking area along Trout Run to Clearview Road. After crossing Clearview Road, the trail climbs and descends into Steinman Run, which it follows for half a mile before returning to Clearview Road. Crossing the road, it climbs to a high point before descending 0.5 mile to the parking area.

Description

Steinman Run Nature Preserve is a 245-acre tract of wildland that is protected by the Lancaster County Conservancy. This very beautiful hike provides one of those experiences that make you glad for the conservancy's efforts. In the spring and summer it is rich with birdlife and wildflowers. During autumn the preserve is a great place to take in the

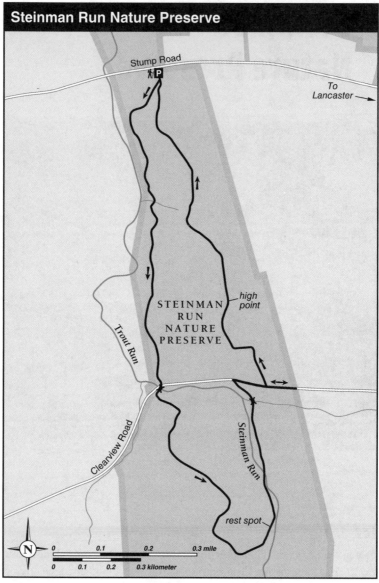

Steinman Run Nature Preserve

Stump Road

P

To Lancaster →

STEINMAN RUN NATURE PRESERVE

high point

Trout Run

Clearview Road

Steinman Run

rest spot

N

| 0 | 0.1 | 0.2 | 0.3 mile |
| 0 | 0.1 | 0.2 | 0.3 kilometer |

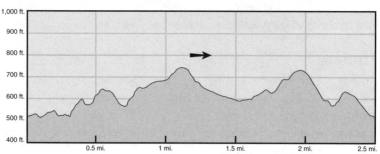

| 1,000 ft. |
| 900 ft. |
| 800 ft. |
| 700 ft. |
| 600 ft. |
| 500 ft. |
| 400 ft. |

| 0.5 mi. | 1 mi. | 1.5 mi. | 2 mi. | 2.5 mi. |

LENGTH 2.5 miles	**ACCESS** Sunrise–sunset
CONFIGURATION Loop	**MAPS** USGS *Conestoga;* a map is some-times available at the parking area or can be accessed online at tinyurl.com /steinmanrunmap.
DIFFICULTY Moderately easy	
SCENERY Wooded hollows of Trout and Steinman Runs	
	FACILITIES None
EXPOSURE Shade	**WHEELCHAIR TRAVERSABLE** No
TRAIL TRAFFIC Light	**CONTACT** Lancaster County Conser-vancy, 717-392-7891, lancaster conservancy.org/preserves
TRAIL SURFACE Dirt	
HIKING TIME 1.5 hours	
	SPECIAL COMMENTS Beware of poison ivy along the creek in the section of the hike past Clearview Road.
DRIVING DISTANCE 14 miles from PA 283 and PA 72 in Lancaster	

fall colors. And if there is enough snow in the winter the trail is suitable for cross-country skiing. Please do your part for helping to keep the experience pleasant for others by stay-ing on the main trail (there are plenty of deer trails), picking up trash, and refraining from crossing onto private land especially in the area of Trout Run.

From the parking area, follow the lower (right) of the two blue-blazed trails to the south to do the hike in a counterclockwise direction (it walks best this way). The dirt path traverses the hillside above the upper reaches of Trout Run, staying above and a couple of hundred feet east of the creek, which flows through private property. The trail in this section passes through a forest of saplings and young oak, ash, hickory, and birch trees. Their youthful appearance is due to the fact that this section of the preserve was logged prior to 1981.

At about 0.3 mile, the path crosses a small seasonal tributary to the creek, which flows over exposed schist bedrock. After crossing the creek, the trail climbs steeply for a short distance to the remains of an old logging path before traversing the hillside again. Continue traversing the hillside for another 0.4 mile until you reach Clearview Road, a prominent dirt road which is now disused. Turn right on Clearview Road and immediately turn left following the blue-blazed trail as it now climbs a small ridge on the west side of Trout Run. The path ascends the ridge and then descends into Stein-man Run in a lovely hollow. This forested area has a wide variety of mature trees includ-ing birch, beech, cherry, poplar, and chestnut. The terrain here is generally flat and is good habitat for deer. At about 0.5 mile from Clearview Road, you reach the level of the creek where you'll find plenty of logs and rocks. This is a nice place for a break. Just downstream from this spot you will cross the creek using some rocks for the crossing. This crossing used to be navigated by a footbridge, but that was destroyed during the heavy rains and flooding in the fall of 2011.

Continue along the creek for another 0.25 mile, where you will reach a footbridge over a small tributary to Steinman Run. The bridge crosses over a small pool in the creek, and if you look you may spot some very small trout in this pool or some frogs in the area. Another 100 yards takes you back to Clearview Road, passing the ruins of what looks to have been a set of steps or aqueduct along the way.

Upon reaching Clearview Road turn right (east). About 200 yards along Clearview Road is a gate at a parking area with a nice view near a large farm and a sign for the nature preserve. About halfway between the spot where you reach Clearview Road and the gate, the trail leaves the road to the left (north). The junction is well marked with blazes. Continue the hike by following this leg of the trail as it climbs gently along a ridge before dropping into a small hollow. After climbing out of the hollow the trail climbs a short distance before flattening out near the high point of the hike at 2 miles. There are no views from the high point, but it is nice to know that the next half-mile descends all the way to the car.

Nearby Activities

The trailhead for the **Trout Run Nature Preserve** is about 200 feet west of the Steinman Run parking area along Stump Road. That trail provides a nice out-and-back hike of about 2 miles that can be added to the Steinman Run Loop. For more information, see the first edition of this book or visit lancasterconservancy.org/preserve/trout-run.

GPS TRAILHEAD COORDINATES AND DIRECTIONS
N39° 54.310' W76° 17.082'

From Lancaster, follow PA 272 south to Smithville. Turn right (west) on Pennsy Road. Turn left on Sigman Road. Sigman Road is a little difficult to identify, as it appears as little more than a driveway. It is about 100 yards beyond the intersection of Rawlinsville Road and Pennsy Road (exercise caution at this intersection) in the midst of several houses. Take Sigman Road to its end. Turn right on Stump Road. Parking is about 0.5 mile down on the left.

---

44 Susquehannock State Park

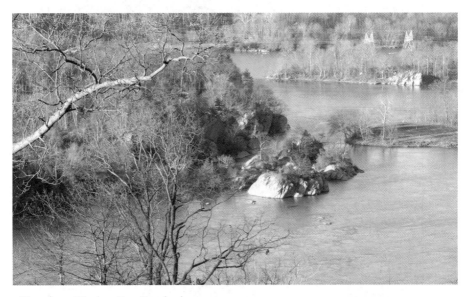
View from Wisslers Run Overlook

In Brief

This hike links several of the park trails to make a pleasant outing. It begins with a stroll out to the Hawk Point Overlook and then follows the Overlook Trail to the Wisslers Run Overlook. From there, it heads north on the Fire Trail for a short distance before descending into a hollow on the appropriately named Rhododendron Trail. It follows this trail out of the hollow and down to Wissler Run. Departing Wissler Run, it follows a small tributary past the Neel Foundation site to the Holly Trail, where it turns left and returns to the Fire Trail near the Wisslers Run Overlook.

Description

Named for the Native American tribe that inhabited the area before the development of the region by English settlers, Susquehannock State Park is another of those remarkable locations in the river hills southeast of Lancaster known for its wonderful scenery and opportunities to see wildlife and wildflowers. The park has been designated by the Audubon Society as part of a global network of places recognized for their outstanding value

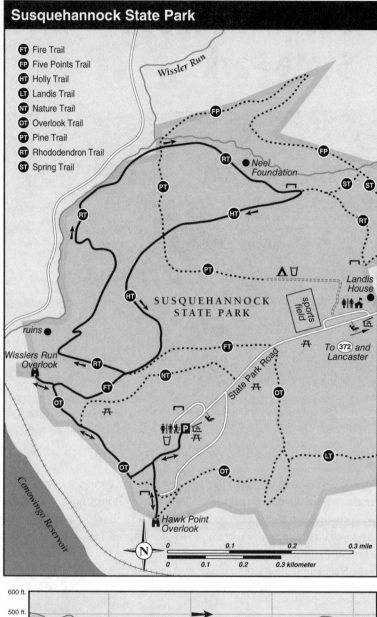

Susquehannock State Park

- **FT** Fire Trail
- **FP** Five Points Trail
- **HT** Holly Trail
- **LT** Landis Trail
- **NT** Nature Trail
- **OT** Overlook Trail
- **PT** Pine Trail
- **RT** Rhododendron Trail
- **ST** Spring Trail

Wissler Run

Neel Foundation

SUSQUEHANNOCK STATE PARK

sports field

Landis House

ruins

Wisslers Run Overlook

State Park Road

To 372 and Lancaster

Conowingo Reservoir

Hawk Point Overlook

N

| 0 | 0.1 | 0.2 | 0.3 mile |

| 0 | 0.1 | 0.2 | 0.3 kilometer |

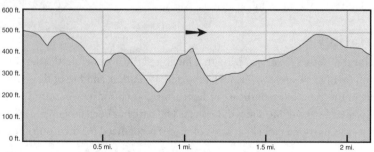

LENGTH 2.15 miles

CONFIGURATION Balloon

DIFFICULTY Easy, with 1 climb

SCENERY Wonderful views of Susquehanna River, rhododendrons, Wissler Run valley, and abandoned homesteads

EXPOSURE Mostly shaded

TRAIL TRAFFIC Light

TRAIL SURFACE Dirt

HIKING TIME 1.5–2 hours

DRIVING DISTANCE About 10.2 miles from intersection of PA 372 and PA 272 in Buck

ACCESS Sunrise–sunset

MAPS USGS *Holtwood;* a park map with all of the trails listed is available online at tinyurl.com/susquehannockspmap.

FACILITIES Seasonal restrooms and water

WHEELCHAIR TRAVERSABLE No, though the first overlook is accessible by wheelchair.

CONTACT Susquehannock State Park, 717-548-3361, tinyurl.com /susquehannocksp

SPECIAL COMMENTS Break-ins have occurred at the parking area. Be sure to take all valuables with you or to store them out of sight.

for bird conservation. Along the edge of the escarpment above the Susquehanna River, you can see bald eagles (many of whom nest in the area), ospreys, black and turkey vultures, a wide variety of hawks, and visiting seabirds. In the woods, you'll encounter many small species such as warblers, woodpeckers, sapsuckers, and bluebirds. If you visit the park at a time when the park office is open, pick up the *Field Guide to the Natural History of Susquehannock State Park* to help you identify its diverse natural features.

Begin this hike at the main parking area and follow the gravel path southwest to the Hawk Point Overlook. The overlook provides a nice start to the hike with an expansive view of the Conowingo Reservoir (the most southern impoundment lake on the Susquehanna River formed by the Conowingo Hydroelectric Plant in Maryland) and Mount Johnson Island to the south. Mount Johnson Island was the first bald eagle sanctuary established in the world, and the birds are common visitors to the environs of Susquehannock State Park. The overlook features a spotting scope and a bird identification chart that will help you to distinguish between the vultures, eagles, and osprey you may see from this point.

After visiting the Hawk Point Overlook, take the gravel path back toward the parking lot and pick up the Overlook Trail as it heads north out of the day-use area along the edge of the river escarpment. The trail follows a wide-open track marked with orange blazes and as it begins to descend among tall trees to Wisslers Run Overlook. This second overlook provides you with a great view upstream to the north toward Lake Aldred and the Holtwood Dam. Beneath you flows Wissler Run as it empties into the river by a storage plant, and several small islands dot the lake immediately west.

From this overlook, walk back to a trail junction just uphill from the overlook and turn left onto the Fire Trail. Traverse the hillside and climb slightly for 0.25 mile to a junction with an old roadbed descending to your left. This is the Rhododendron Trail and you'll turn left on it and follow it into Wissler Run. As you descend, you'll see that the trail is appropriately named. Dense stands of rhododendron line the track on both sides for its entire length. In June, when the rhododendrons are in bloom, the trail is a remarkable sight. After 0.1 mile or so, you'll reach a sharp bend to the right and just beyond that a trail junction at the crossing of a small creek bed. If you turn left on the trail and continue along it for 100 yards or so, you'll come to the ruins of an old homestead on the left, just above the level of Wissler Run. You can walk down to have a look or just continue along this hike following the Rhododendron Trail to the right from the junction toward a rock outcrop on the hillside. The trail traverses just beneath it.

Soon you'll climb out of the hollow at a ridge in the woods. Descend the ridge back toward Wissler Run, following switchbacks down to the creek. On the way, you pass several interesting outcrops of sandstone with occasional layers of white quartzite or limestone slicing through them. Now at the level of the creek, you are once again surrounded by rhododendrons. This is a particularly enchanting spot with the creek tumbling over small ledges as it winds its way to the river. From the creek, follow the Rhododendron Trail upstream and then eventually into a hollow formed by a small tributary. At about 1.35 miles, you'll come to a trail crossing. The Five Points Trail heads off to the left and the Pine Tree Trail turns right. Continue straight on the Rhododendron Trail and in about 0.2 mile you'll reach the Neel Foundation. According to the park brochure, this site was the homestead of a veteran of the Revolutionary War, Thomas Neel. The foundation of the house still remains, though little more. Take note of the enormous hickory tree beside it.

Pass by the homestead site and shortly you'll reach the junction with the Holly Trail. Turn right on the Holly Trail and follow it back to the Wisslers Run Overlook. On the way, you will cross the Pine Tree Trail, where you continue straight, and then join the Fire Trail, onto which you turn right just before reaching the Wisslers Run Overlook.

Nearby Activities

The park has many picnic areas, playgrounds, and several ballfields, as well as four group camping areas. North of the park and north of PA 372 along River Road is **Shenks Ferry Wildflower Preserve** (see page 203), which is definitely worth a visit during the spring and summer.

GPS TRAILHEAD COORDINATES AND DIRECTIONS
N39° 48.211' W76° 17.311'

From PA 272 in Buck, follow PA 372 west 5.7 miles to River Road (a sign for the park is located on the left before River Road). Turn left on River Road, cross the dam, and turn right on Furniss Road. Turn right on Silver Spring Road and right again on State Park Road on a bend. Use caution when leaving the park as the entrance is blind to cars approaching from the south.

45 Tucquan Glen Nature Preserve

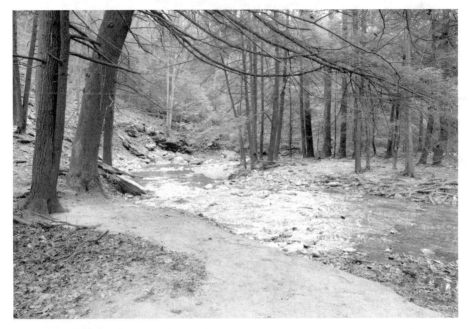

Tucquan Glen Road crosses the creek.

In Brief

This beautiful hike follows the south bank of Tucquan Creek, through its glen filled with hemlock and rhododendron, to the railroad bridge at the Susquehanna River. The route crosses the creek via the bridge, ascends a short steep gulley up the escarpment, and picks up the old Tucquan Glen Road over a promontory and back down to the creek.

Description

Certainly the jewel site of the Lancaster County Conservancy, the 336-acre Tucquan Glen Nature Preserve in Martic Township provides a gem of an excursion. Although not a long hike, you get a lot of great scenery packed into the mile-long gorge of this tributary of the Susquehanna River. The creek has understandably been designated a Pennsylvania Scenic River. The forest along the sides of the glen consist of tall mature poplars, white and pin oaks, and hickory trees. Hemlocks and rhododendrons line the banks of the steep creek as it tumbles over large boulders forming deep pools and steep drops. In late May and June,

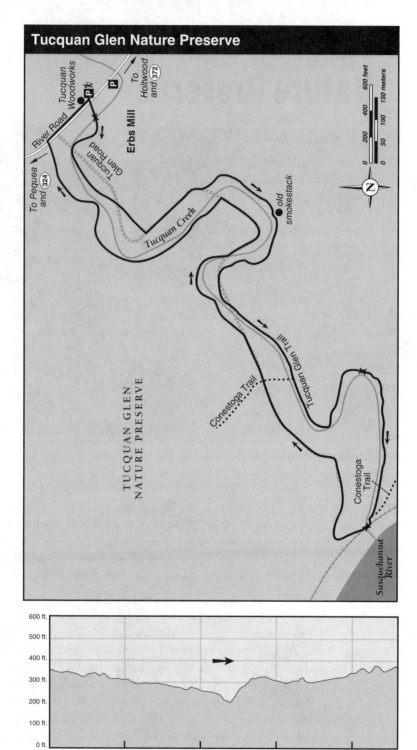

Tucquan Glen Nature Preserve

LENGTH 2.3 miles	**ACCESS** Sunrise–sunset
CONFIGURATION Loop	**MAPS** USGS *Holtwood*; a map of the preserve is available online at tinyurl.com /tucquanglenmap.
DIFFICULTY Moderate	
SCENERY The beautiful gorge of Tucquan Glen	**FACILITIES** None
EXPOSURE Mostly shaded	**WHEELCHAIR TRAVERSABLE** No
TRAIL TRAFFIC Light during the week; can be very busy on summer weekends	**CONTACT** Lancaster County Conservancy, 717-392-7891, lancasterconservancy.org/preserves
TRAIL SURFACE Dirt; rocky in places	
HIKING TIME 1.5–2 hours	**SPECIAL COMMENTS** Several cars have been broken into at the parking area. Be sure to take all valuables with you or secure them in your trunk.
DRIVING DISTANCE About 23 miles from PA 283 and PA 272 in Lancaster	

when everything is in bloom, the place is amazing. According to the *Susquehanna River Birding and Wildlife Trail Guide,* published by Audubon Pennsylvania, Tucquan Glen is home to more than 40 species of wildflowers as well as 21 species of ferns. The glen is also home to great horned owls and is frequented by white-tailed deer.

A couple of notes of caution: First, the rocks can be quite slippery along the trail, so use care to avoid any nasty slips. Although accessible year-round, the rocks can get covered with ice and the route along the south side of the creek may become impassable. The preserve is open to hunting, so be sure to wear blaze orange during hunting season and consider hiking on Sunday.

This hike walks best in a clockwise direction. From the parking area, cross the creek over a small wooden footbridge. The trail is marked for its entire length with blue blazes, and it veers to the right once you cross the bridge. As you enter the preserve, you'll come to the remains of the old Tucquan Glen Road and the trail follows it for a short distance until the road crosses the creek. You'll notice blue blazes over on the north side of the creek. Those mark the path on the other side, but there is no need to cross until you get to the Susquehanna River. Follow the creek through an extraordinary area of hemlock trees. At about 0.5 mile, the gorge narrows and the trail passes through a rock outcrop via some narrow ledges and then crosses a small side creek. Just beyond the creek, the ruin of a large stone chimney stands on the side of the trail.

Continue along the creek and, at approximately 0.8 mile, you'll notice some red blazes enter from the north side of the creek at an unlikely place to cross. This is a section of the 61-mile-long Conestoga Trail, and it shares the path with the Tucquan Glen Trail along the south bank of the creek. From this point to the river, you'll follow red and blue blazes. About 0.9 mile into the hike, the gorge becomes much narrower, and the creek becomes steeper and more choked with boulders. The trail hugs the south hillside, and it crosses a wooden footbridge along a particularly exposed section of rock above a large pool at the base of a cliff. The scenery from the footbridge to the river is outstanding. Beyond the

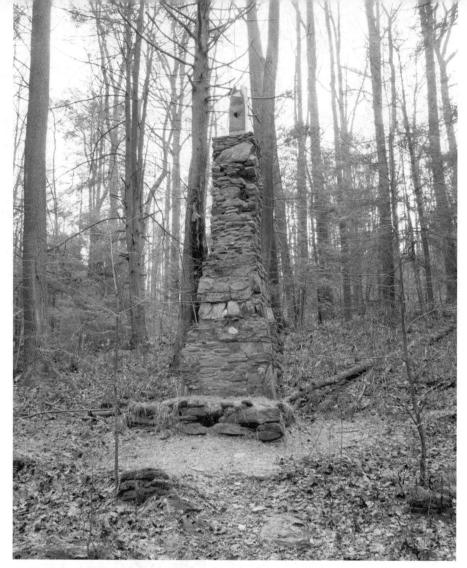

Stone chimney in Tucquan Glen

bridge, the valley gets tighter and tighter and the creek more choked with large sandstone boulders. At 1.2 miles, the gorge opens up and the trail reaches the railroad along the Susquehanna River. From here, the Conestoga Trail continues south, climbing the escarpment above the river.

The second half of this hike is rather different in character from the first, as it generally follows the old roadbed for a good part of the way back to the car. A good portion of the walk stays above the level of the creek providing views into the glen. To complete the loop, cross the creek via the railroad bridge. About 30 feet beyond the bridge, the trail heads directly up a short, steep gulley by a blue blaze. The path improves very quickly, makes a switchback, and joins the old roadbed for a short climb to a promontory above the creek. This is a particularly nice place to sit for a while. If you walk out to the edge of the promontory (use caution!), you'll get a nice view back into the glen at its most rugged point. From the promontory, the road descends pleasantly back down to the level of the creek. At 1.5 miles, it crosses the Conestoga Trail, and at 1.85 miles, the old road crosses the creek. Stay on the north side of the creek and follow the footpath along the bank back to River Road.

Nearby Activities

The **Holtwood Environmental Preserve** to the south is home to the **Kellys Run Natural Area** (see Hike 35, page 176). The nearby **Pinnacle Overlook** offers a place to picnic, plus a fine view of Lake Aldred on the Susquehanna River and the mouth of Tucquan Glen. To get there, head south on River Road a short distance, then turn right onto Pinnacle Road and follow the signs to the overlook. During the spring and summer, **Shenks Ferry Wildflower Preserve** (see Hike 41, page 203), a couple of miles to the north, can't be beat. Take River Road to the north and follow signs.

GPS TRAILHEAD COORDINATES AND DIRECTIONS
N39° 51.831' W76° 20.351'

From Harrisburg and the north, the easiest route is to take PA 283 to Lancaster. Follow PA 272 south to the town of Buck and head west on PA 372 toward Holtwood. Follow 372 for 4.9 miles to River Road/SR 3017. Turn right and follow River Road 2.65 miles. Two small parking areas are located on the west side of the road, directly across from the vacant building for the old Tucquan Woodworks furniture store. If those are full, a larger area is about 100 yards south on the east side of the road, just south of the Tucquan Woodworks building.

SOUTHWEST

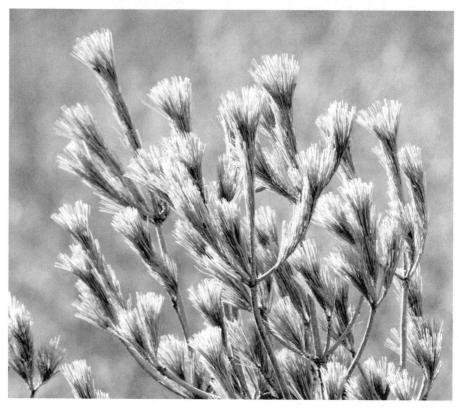

Spring growth on Pole Steeple (see Hike 53, page 260)

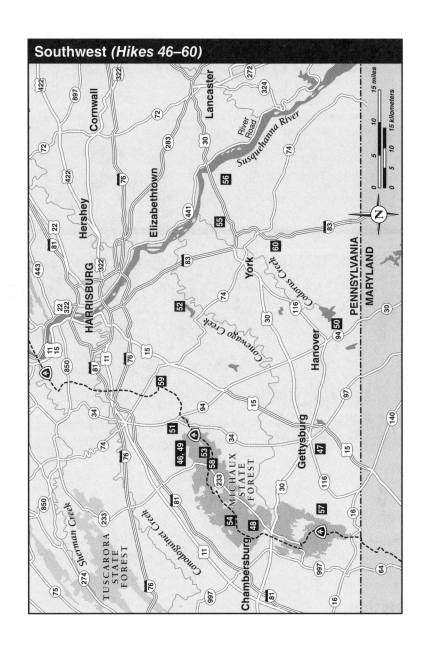

46 Buck Ridge Trail

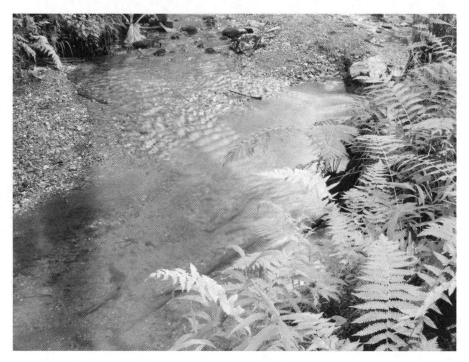

Iron Run

In Brief

Beginning at the Kings Gap Environmental Education Center, follow the Buck Ridge Trail south, along Buck Ridge. The trail descends for most of its length to Pine Grove Furnace State Park.

Description

Stretching between the Kings Gap Environmental Education Center to the north and Pine Grove Furnace State Park to the south, the Buck Ridge Trail offers a wonderful hike through the South Mountain Province of south-central Pennsylvania. The trek follows old logging roads that take you through open fields and dark hollows.

The hike can be done either as a one-way trip or as an out-and-back excursion. If you hike it one-way, you'll want to begin at Kings Gap because the trail walks better from north to south. You'll need to leave a car at the parking area across the street from the visitor center at Pine Grove Furnace State Park.

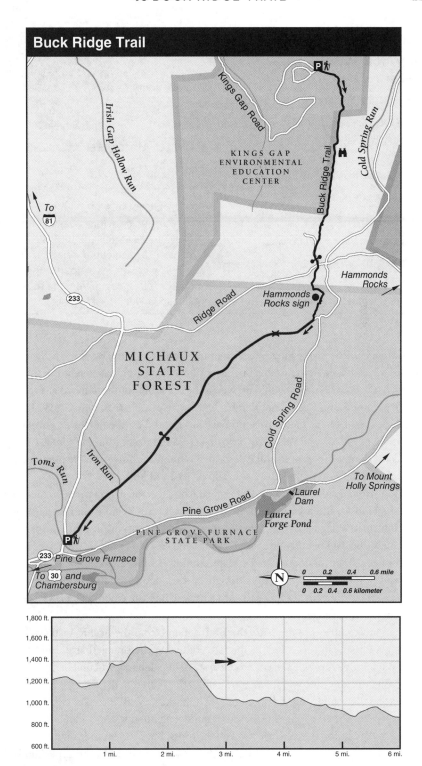

Buck Ridge Trail

LENGTH About 6 miles one-way

CONFIGURATION One-way or out-and-back

DIFFICULTY Moderate

SCENERY Kings Gap and Pine Grove Furnace parks, lovely woods and meadows

EXPOSURE Mostly shade

TRAIL TRAFFIC Light

TRAIL SURFACE Dirt

HIKING TIME 3 hours one-way

DRIVING DISTANCE About 8 miles from I-81 and PA 233 south of Carlisle

ACCESS Sunrise–sunset

MAPS USGS *Dickinson;* Michaux State Forest public-use map; a trail map is available at the Kings Gap and Pine Grove Furnace Visitor Centers.

FACILITIES Water and restrooms available in parks near both trailheads

WHEELCHAIR TRAVERSABLE No

CONTACT Michaux State Forest, 717-352-2211, tinyurl.com/michauxsf

SPECIAL COMMENTS Done as a one-way excursion from Kings Gap to Pine Grove Furnace State Park, this hike requires 2 cars. An out-and-back trip of about 12 miles makes a nice day trip, though it is best begun from the southern trailhead at Pine Grove Furnace.

Although a little on the long side, an out-and-back trip on the Buck Ridge Trail (BRT) provides a reasonable day trip. Personal experience, however, has taught me that for an out-and-back excursion, you would do well to begin at the south trailhead at Pine Grove Furnace because Kings Gap is considerably higher in elevation than Pine Grove. The parking area and trailhead at Pine Grove Furnace are located on the northeast corner of the intersection of PA 233 and Pine Grove Road, across the street from the Pine Grove State Park Visitor Center. Because the hike described is one-way, however, I've provided directions and GPS for both trailheads so you can leave cars at both.

Hiking from Kings Gap to Pine Grove, you'll begin at the parking area on the left, just before the loop for the mansion area begins. Several trails begin from this parking area and an information sign provides a good landmark for identifying it. From the car, follow the Scenic Vista Trail out the old roadbed south and east along the clearing for 200 yards. You'll soon reach the junction with the Maple Hollow Trail, which continues straight, and you'll see a post marked with BRT. Turn right at the junction following the BRT and Scenic Vista Trail as the path descends toward a hollow into the woods. The BRT is marked for its length with orange blazes.

At about 0.5 mile into the hike, the BRT departs from the Scenic Vista Trail to the left along another old road. Stay to the left, following the orange blazes, and begin to ascend Buck Ridge through a pretty understory of huckleberry and blueberry. About 0.5 mile beyond the junction, you'll pass a trail off to the right that descends to the Pond Day Use area and then the 1-mile marker. From that marker, the BRT makes two climbs. The first is steep but not very long, the second is quite long but not very steep.

Just shy of 2 miles, the trail levels out on the top of Buck Ridge, and you'll pass through a forest of mostly oak trees. When I visited the area in June of 2007, the gypsy moths had all but stripped the trees bare of foliage. To look at one of my photographs, you'd swear it was midwinter. Fortunately, the damage to the foliage is only temporary and by later that summer many of the leaves had grown back.

After walking along the ridge for a short distance, you'll pass a marker on the right, indicating that you are at 1,540 feet of elevation. The hike is pretty much downhill for the next 4 miles. Descend from the ridge, pass the 2-mile marker, and then pick up a wide open service road onto which you'll turn left.

Continue along the road for a short distance until you reach a forest-road gate. Pass the gate and cross over a significant forest road, following the orange blazes into woods on the far side. The trail winds downhill for a distance, at times moderately steeply, and it comes to a fork where you will stay right. Just beyond, you'll reach a side trail and a sign pointing the way to Hammonds Rocks. Resist the urge to visit the rocks. Although they afford a nice view, they are much easier to reach by car. Continue downhill for a distance, to where the trail meets an old washed-out logging road. Turn right and continue descending, passing the 3-mile marker in a short distance. Cross a small creek over a footbridge and continue through the woods for another half-mile before entering more of an open clear-cut area for a mile. The area has plenty of thick brush that makes good habitat for a variety of birds.

At about 4.5 miles you'll pass an iron gate with a BRT sign just beyond it. Walk out to the road, cross it, and enter the woods just to the left of a private drive. After circumnavigating the property, you'll come to another old logging road—the Leaf Trail Road—where you'll stay left. Just beyond the junction is the 5-mile marker. Follow this for a mile to a significant dirt road just beyond some private residences. Turn right, walk about 200 feet out to the main road (PA 233) and turn left. About 200 feet along is the parking area for the south trailhead. Across the street, you'll see the ranger station and just beyond that is a general store that sells supplies and refreshments.

Nearby Activities

Pine Grove Furnace State Park has swimming areas, a campground, and places to picnic. **Kings Gap** has several picnic areas and a host of interpretive and educational programs.

GPS INFORMATION AND DIRECTIONS

N40° 05.593' W77° 15.850' (Kings Gap)
N40° 02.014' W77° 18.230' (Pine Grove Furnace State Park)

KINGS GAP: From I-81, take Exit 37 (Newville) and follow PA 233 south 2.3 miles to Pine Road. Turn left onto Pine Road (signs for Kings Gap Environmental Education Center) and follow it another 2.3 miles to Kings Gap Road (sign for Kings Gap). Turn right and follow the winding road up to the mansion area. The parking area, with several trailheads, is on the left, just before the loop at the mansion area begins.

PINE GROVE FURNACE STATE PARK: Follow PA 233 south 7.8 miles from I-81 to the intersection with Pine Grove Road. The parking area for the south trailhead is on your left at the intersection.

47 Gettysburg National Military Park

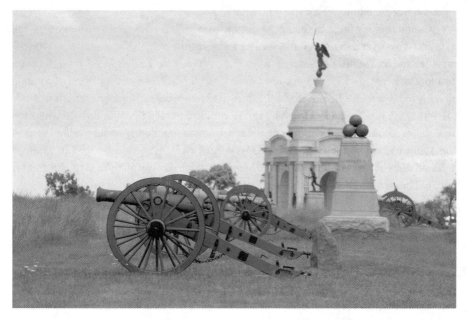

The Pennsylvania Memorial

In Brief

This hike route mostly follows the path of the horse trail through the southern part of the military park. As a result, it tends to see rather little traffic, although it doesn't pass by as many of the heritage sites as the Billy Yank and Johnny Reb Trails (see page 234 for more information).

Description

Although known for its numerous military monuments commemorating the soldiers who fought here for three days in July of 1863, Gettysburg National Military Park is perhaps less well known for its natural history. The park is part of Audubon Pennsylvania's Susquehanna River Birding and Wildlife Trail, and, in addition to the historical setting, the scenery it provides of open farmland and wooded hollows is quite delightful. I have found it to be a wonderful place for wildlife viewing, having seen foxes and a

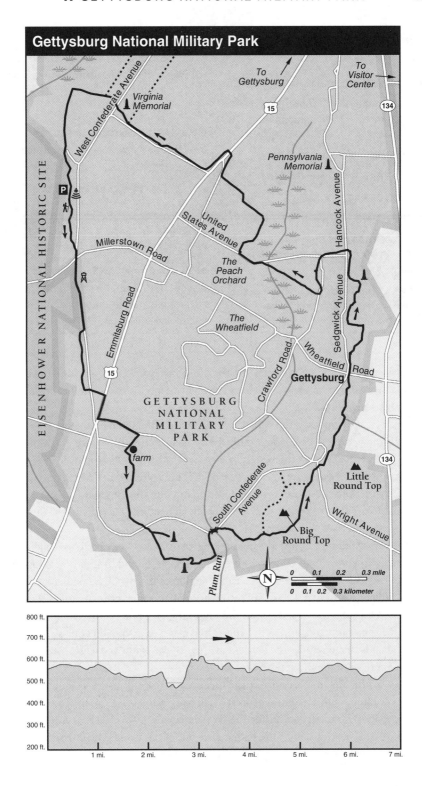

Gettysburg National Military Park

LENGTH 7 miles

CONFIGURATION Loop

DIFFICULTY Moderate

SCENERY Rural farm country, hardwood forests, streams, military monuments and memorials

EXPOSURE More sun than shade

TRAIL TRAFFIC Generally light

TRAIL SURFACE Dirt

HIKING TIME 4 hours

DRIVING DISTANCE 5 miles from intersection of US 15 and US 30 east of Gettysburg

ACCESS Sunrise–sunset; parking at the amphitheater parking area is available during the summer.

MAPS USGS *Fairfield* and *Gettysburg*; a park brochure and map, which includes the hiking trails, is available at the visitor center or online at tinyurl.com /gettbrochure.

FACILITIES Restrooms and refreshments available at the visitor center, portable toilets along trail

WHEELCHAIR TRAVERSABLE Some sections

CONTACT Gettysburg National Military Park, 717-334-1124, nps.gov/gett

SPECIAL COMMENTS This hike is more of a naturalist's excursion through the military park rather than an informative historical hike.

wide variety of birdlife on my visits there. This hike description provides an outing in the park that offers you exposure to its secluded natural areas as well as to the more popular historical sites.

Several useful guides to the park and its historical sites and monuments are available at the visitor center, located on Emmitsburg Road and across from the Gettysburg National Cemetery. Hikers interested in visiting historical sites would do well to purchase a copy of the *Gettysburg Heritage Trail Guide* published by the Boy Scouts of America. It has directions for and interpretive information on the 9-mile Billy Yank Trail and the 3-mile Johnny Reb Trail, as well as other shorter walks. It is available at the visitor-center bookstore.

Begin this hike at the amphitheater parking lot on West Confederate Avenue. Pick up the gravel path about 20 or 30 feet west of the parking lot and turn left, heading south. The hike begins by winding through a short section of hardwood forest before the path reaches Millerstown Road. Cross Millerstown Road and then cross left over West Confederate Avenue and take a walk up to the top of the observation tower for an excellent view of the surrounding countryside. To the north and east, you look out over the farms and woodlands that compose the battlefield area. To the south and west, you can see the peaks of South Mountain 15 miles distant.

After visiting the tower, return to the trail on the west side of West Confederate Avenue and continue south as it enters a forest of tall oak trees. This is a good place in the early morning to look for owls, and during the day you can find woodpeckers and thrushes in the area. After a short distance, the path comes out of the woods and crosses West Confederate Avenue by some of the park's characteristic wooden barricades. Walk across the road, around the small farmhouse, and over toward the corner of Emmitsburg Road (Business 15) and West Confederate Avenue. Cross Emmitsburg Road onto a dirt road heading east and downhill through farm country toward the lowlands around Plum Run and several farms. After about 0.25 mile, you'll come to a gravel track heading off toward a farmhouse to the right and a sign indicating that only authorized vehicles are allowed to continue along the main dirt road beyond that point. Turn right (southwest) onto the gravel track (you'll see a sign indicating that this is the horse and footpath) and follow it around the farmhouse to its drive. Turn left and then pass the barn to its right. Please be respectful of the residents and move through the property quickly and quietly.

Beyond the barn, the trail enters a beautiful lowland area, a good spot for wildlife viewing. If you are a photographer, this is a great place for a long lens and a tripod. Among the reeds and grasses you may spot warblers, cardinals, bluebirds, and perhaps some woodland mammals. Soon the path reaches South Confederate Avenue and a sign indicating that horses should turn left at the shoulder. Instead, cross the road and enter the woods on a footpath. In about 100 feet or so, you'll reach a fork in the trail. The hike continues to the right, but if you turn left, you'll come to a couple of state and regimental memorials and monuments on top of a small rise. Continuing south along the main trail, you'll soon come to another fork. Again the left fork will take you to several memorials and monuments atop a small rise. The right fork (the path of this hike) descends into a beautiful hollow filled with mature poplars, hickories, and catalpas before coming back out to the road next to a stone bridge over Plum Run. Turn right and follow the shoulder over the bridge and then cut back into the woods on the horse path just beyond. The trail gets a little murky for a short distance as it begins traversing around Big Round Top, passing two junctions with a trail that makes a loop over Big Round Top to the left. If you go up to the summit, you'll find several monuments, though the view from the top is not particularly good. You would do well to continue along the trail over to Wright Avenue at the base of Little Round Top.

After crossing Wright Avenue, follow the significant path as it climbs over Little Round Top. This hill was the site of a furious battle beginning on July 2, 1863. Many memorials have been erected near its summit commemorating those who fought and died. From the top, you'll be able to get a good vantage of the extent of the terrain and the battlefield as it stretches out to the north and west.

From Little Round Top, follow the horse path (which passes just east and below the crest of the hill) to the north for a distance until you reach the corner of Wheatfield Road and Sedgwick Avenue. Cross Wheatfield and continue north along the shoulder of Sedgwick and follow the path into the woods again when you reach the Major John Sedgwick Equestrian Monument. Follow the path through the woods for a half-mile to the monument erected for Kearny's New Jersey Brigade atop a hill. From the monument, walk downhill to Sedgwick Avenue and follow it north to the intersection with United States Avenue by the G. Weikert House. Cross Sedgwick and follow the shoulder of United States Avenue to the west. You'll have a wonderful view of the Pennsylvania Memorial and several cannons to the north from here. After a short walk along United States Avenue, the path leaves the road to the left and makes a short circuit through Plum Run. This is a very pretty section of trail that should not be missed. As the trail winds through open fields and then a stand of trees, it passes by a long network of wooden barricades through some low-lands. This is another excellent area for viewing wildlife.

The path returns to the road in the area of the Trostle Farm. Turn left and follow the shoulder around the farm and then turn right onto the gravel path by a sign commemo-rating the site of Bigelow's Last Stand. Follow the path as it winds around through open fields providing lovely rural views and the opportunity to see kestrels, which appear to nest in this area, and red-tailed hawks. The Pennsylvania Memorial stands prominently on the eastern horizon. Soon, the path reaches Emmitsburg Road. Cross the road, and follow the path through open farmland to the left (south), eventually bending back to the west toward a red farmhouse and barn. You'll be able to see the observation tower off to the southwest as you cross this wide-open stretch of farmland.

Follow the trail between the farmhouse and the barn (a roost for hundreds of barn swallows) and continue directly west along the path. As the trail enters the woods again, you will reach a junction, marked by a sign, indicating that you can follow the path straight or make an additional spur to the right (north). If you turn right, you'll add 1.75 miles to the hike by visiting the Virginia Memorial. Our hike, however, contin-ues straight out to West Confederate Avenue. When you reach the road, you can either turn left and follow the shoulder for 0.25 mile to the amphitheater parking area, or you can continue straight across the road and follow the path past a field and to a second junction with the north spur of the trail. At the junction, turn left and walk south to the amphitheater parking area.

Nearby Activities

You should definitely stop by the visitor center to view the exhibits on the history of the battle. There you can get information on an automobile tour of the park (well worth doing) and on visiting **Gettysburg National Cemetery.** The town of Gettysburg, along Business 15, has restaurants and shops galore.

GPS INFORMATION AND DIRECTIONS

N39° 48.336' W77° 15.429'

From US 15 east of Gettysburg, follow US 30 west through the center of town. At the traffic circle, head south on Business 15 to PA 116 West (one block south of the circle). Turn right onto PA 116, then left onto West Confederate Avenue. Begin the hike at the amphitheater parking area, about 2 miles south on the right.

48 Hosack Run

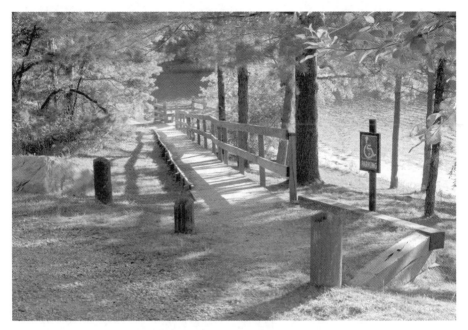

Farm near Emmitsburg Road

In Brief

This hike follows the Greenwood Trail (also known as the Locust Gap Trail) for several miles before joining the Appalachian Trail (AT). It picks up the AT and follows that into Quarry Gap, past the Quarry Gap Shelter, and onto the ridge above. From the ridge, the hike follows the Hosack Run Trail down into a beautiful and remote rhododendron-filled ravine and then rejoins the Greenwood Trail a mile or so from the trailhead.

Description

This hike is without a doubt my favorite hike in the South Mountain Province of central Pennsylvania. The walking is very pleasant; the trails aren't especially crowded; the distance is quite manageable; the scenery is excellent. If you do this hike in June when the rhododendrons are in bloom, you are in for a real treat. In the fall, the colors can't be beat. And even in the summer, the hike tends to stay cool.

Begin this hike at the parking area for the wheelchair-access ramp by the northwest corner of the Long Pine Run Reservoir. The trailhead is across the road, and the trail

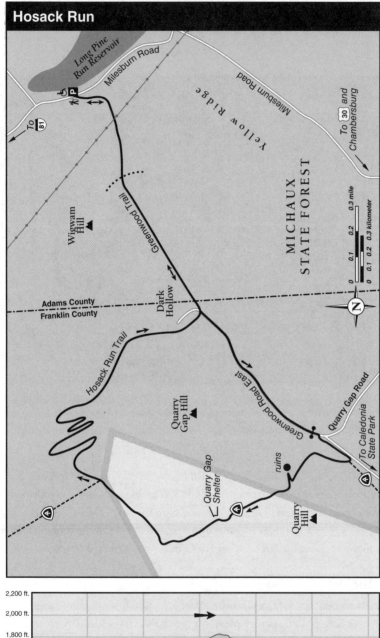

Hosack Run

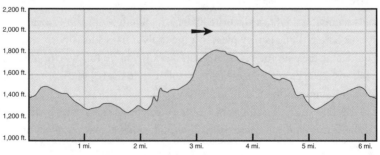

LENGTH 6.2 miles	**ACCESS** Sunrise–sunset
CONFIGURATION Balloon	**MAPS** USGS *Caledonia Park;* Michaux
DIFFICULTY Moderate	State Forest public-use map; Keystone
	Trail Association *Appalachian Trail,*
SCENERY Pretty, open woodlands; steep	*PA Route 94 to US Route 30 (Sections*
and rugged rhododendron-filled ravines	*12 and 13)*
EXPOSURE More shade than sun	**FACILITIES** None
TRAIL TRAFFIC Light	**WHEELCHAIR TRAVERSABLE** No
TRAIL SURFACE Dirt	**CONTACT** Michaux State Forest,
HIKING TIME 3 hours	717-352-2211, tinyurl.com/michauxsf
DRIVING DISTANCE 21.7 miles from	**SPECIAL COMMENTS** My favorite hike
I-81 and PA 233 south of Carlisle	in South Mountain

heads west past a forest gate. The initial trail, the Greenwood Trail, is a biking, hiking, and equestrian trail. It is blazed in blue as far as the AT. Follow the Greenwood Trail, an old haul road, up a hill and around to the right, then out to a power line. The power line clearing is a good place to see wildlife, especially deer and fox, and to watch for birds in the many boxes along its edges.

Pass the power line and follow the path down a gentle grade to the crossing of a path that is unmarked and not on any map. Continue straight downhill. The track is a little rocky in this area for a short distance, but never becomes too unpleasant. At about 1.2 miles, you'll cross a small creek in an area that is thick with rhododendrons, and about 150 feet beyond that is the junction with the Hosack Run Trail, identified by a labeled post. This begins the loop part of the hike.

Continue straight along the Greenwood Trail past a deer exclosure on the left, through some pretty, open pine woods and meadows. This is great habitat for deer, which are abundant, as well as foxes, rabbits, and other woodland wildlife. After about 0.7 mile, you'll cross a second little creek and just beyond that you'll find a forest gate at Quarry Gap Road. Pass the gate and follow the trail across the road and into the woods on the other side. According to the Michaux State Forest map, the trail name at this point changes from the Greenwood Trail to the Locust Gap Trail. According to the AT map, the entire trail from the reservoir is called the Locust Gap Trail. Whatever its proper name, all you have to do is to continue following the blue blazes as the trail climbs gently from the road.

In about 0.25 mile, you'll reach the AT, onto which you will turn right, heading north. After a short distance, the AT is crossed by a forest gate and the ruins of some old buildings are located on the right side of the trail. Follow the AT up into Quarry Gap, a steep and rocky ravine filled with dense rhododendrons. At times the foliage is so thick that the bushes form a tunnel over the trail. Walk another 0.25 mile beyond the gate, and you'll reach the Quarry Gap Shelter.

Continuing beyond the shelter, the AT gets rather rocky for a short distance and then crosses a creek at a log. Beyond the creek, the quality of the trail improves dramatically, but the walking gets quite steep. After a bracing climb of 0.5 mile, the trail levels out and about 200 feet beyond the leveling point the Hosack Run Trail (blue blazes) departs to the right (northeast) at a trail sign (3.3 miles).

Follow the Hosack Run Trail through the woods and into the hollow below via a series of switchbacks down a steep hillside on a good trail. The path is in excellent condition and is well blazed. At just about 4 miles, you'll reach the bottom of the hill and are now in the appropriately named Dark Hollow. The steep-sided gap is filled with hemlock and some of the thickest rhododendron I've ever seen. This is a very beautiful and remote area, filled with the sounds of woodpeckers and thrushes, and much wildlife hiding in the brush. Head down the hollow from here, following the trail as it traverses above the thick bushes around the creek. Soon the trail drops down and crosses the creek in the area of a large boulder field on the left. Soon it crosses back over the creek in an area of some enormous deadfall. Beyond that, you'll soon return to the Greenwood Trail (5.1 miles). Turn left and follow it back to the car.

Nearby Activities

Two state parks are located on PA 233 nearby and both have swimming and picnicking facilities. They are **Pine Grove Furnace State Park,** to the north, and **Caledonia State Park,** just a couple of miles south of Milesburn Road.

GPS INFORMATION AND DIRECTIONS
N39° 56.413' W77° 27.364'

From I-81, take Exit 37 (Newville/PA 233). Follow PA 233 south 20 miles to Milesburn Road. Turn right on Milesburn Road and follow it 1.7 miles to the parking area at the wheelchair-access ramp on the right at Long Pine Run Reservoir. The trail begins at the forest road gate across the street.

49 Kings Gap

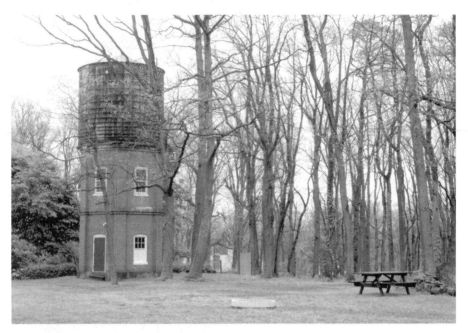

Stone tower near the main gardens

In Brief

Beginning at the trailhead for the Scenic Vista Trail and Buck Ridge Trail, follow the Scenic Vista Trail to the Pond Day Use Area. From there, follow the Watershed and Boundary Trails along the perimeter of the park and ascend back to the trailhead from Kings Gap Hollow via a walk along the Ridge Overlook Trail and Maple Hollow Trail.

Description

Unique among Pennsylvania state parks, the Kings Gap Environmental Education Center is oriented more toward activities and programs that promote a greater understanding of the natural world than toward purely recreational purposes. The center consists of about 2,500 acres of scenic woodlands that are home to several day-use areas, 16 miles of hiking trails, a visitor center, and a majestic 32-room mansion situated on a mountaintop in the South Mountain region of south-central Pennsylvania. The center provides a host of educational opportunities year-round, including environmental-education programs for high school students and teachers, weekend interpretive programs, and backcountry hikes.

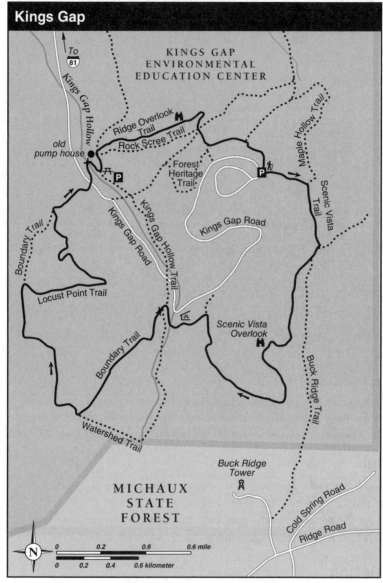

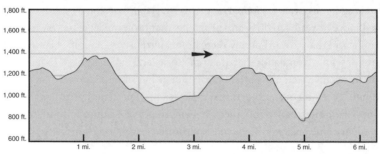

LENGTH 6.3 miles	**ACCESS** 8 a.m.–sunset
CONFIGURATION Loop	**MAPS** USGS *Dickinson;* a trail map is available at the Kings Gap visitor center and online at tinyurl.com/kingsgapmap.
DIFFICULTY Moderate	
SCENERY Kings Gap Environmental Education Center and great views of the Cumberland Valley	**FACILITIES** Water and restrooms available at visitor center
EXPOSURE Mostly shade	**WHEELCHAIR TRAVERSABLE** No
TRAIL TRAFFIC Light	**CONTACT** Kings Gap Environmental Education Center, 717-486-5031, friends ofkingsgap.org
TRAIL SURFACE Dirt	
HIKING TIME 3–3.5 hours	**SPECIAL COMMENTS** The trails on this hike can be quite rocky in places, so a sturdy pair of boots is advisable.
DRIVING DISTANCE About 8 miles from I-81 and PA 233	

The mansion and the views of the surrounding terrain are worth the visit in and of themselves. This hike, though, provides access to some of the more remote regions of the park, offering some wonderful scenery and excellent views.

Begin this hike from the parking area by following the orange-blazed Scenic Vista Trail to the east through a clearing. This trail shares the path with the Maple Hollow and Buck Ridge Trails initially. After about 0.25 mile, follow the orange blazes to the right (south), leaving the Maple Hollow Trail behind. The trail descends toward a hollow into the woods, and after another 0.25 mile the Buck Ridge Trail departs to the left. Continue along the Scenic Vista Trail for a little more than a half-mile to the Scenic Vista Overlook (1.1 miles), where you will find a couple of nice benches and an even nicer view into Kings Gap Hollow to the west.

From the overlook, follow the trail over a ridge and through a splendid, silent forest down into Kings Gap Hollow. At just about 2 miles, the route makes a sharp left turn (northwest), although the obvious path appears to continue straight. Make the left and follow the blazes down the trail to the program pavilion at the Pond Day Use Area (about 2.2 miles). The pavilion is dedicated to the memory of Frank E. Masland, whose family once owned the mansion. You'll find restrooms at the day-use area, and plenty of benches and tables to take a rest and have a snack.

From the pavilion, head downhill and slightly to your right to the obvious information board at the road. Here, you will find a sign that points the way to the Boundary and Watershed Trails along the Kings Gap Trail. Follow the latter downhill for a short distance to the junction with the Boundary and Watershed trails, which follow a common path to the left (southwest). The junction is well marked. Turn left, and just ahead (50 yards) you'll find a sign at a small bridge over the creek that says WATERSHED TRAIL, 1.8 MILES. Cross the bridge, and stay to the right following the Watershed Trail (purple blazes) toward the Boundary Trail.

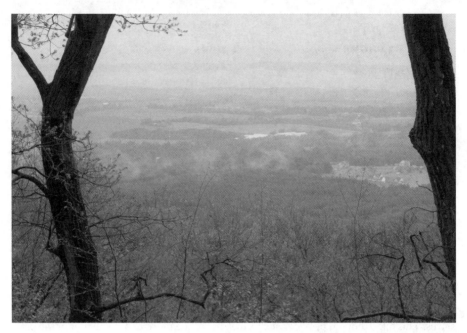

A clearing storm viewed from a point along the Scenic Vista Trail

Continue on the Watershed Trail for 0.75 mile, passing several small side trails, to a T-intersection. The Boundary Trail (green blazes) goes to the right here while the Watershed Trail heads left. Turn right (north) onto the Boundary Trail, so named because it follows the boundary of the park lands. You'll immediately pass a sign facing the opposite direction that says END OF BOUNDARY TRAIL. Follow green blazes uphill and along a straight logging road through pretty, open woods to a forested ridge, where you'll find the junction with the orange-blazed Locust Point Trail (3.7 miles). Turn right and follow that uphill.

The Locust Point Trail makes a side trip of about a mile over a lovely wooded hillside that has a nice viewpoint about 0.6 mile along. Before reaching the viewpoint, the trail makes a sharp left turn and heads downhill. The turn is well blazed, but worth paying attention to, as a side trail there will take you out to a clearing. Follow the Locust Point Trail until it returns you to the Boundary Trail, where you will turn right (northeast) and follow that down to the park road at a picnic bench and parking area (4.9 miles).

From the picnic bench, cross the road angling downhill and follow the sign for the Kings Gap Hollow Trail (slightly to the left) toward the creek below. Shortly you will reach a pretty footbridge. Cross the creek and then turn right onto a wide trail. (If you turn left, you'll come to the remains of an old pump house downstream a hundred feet or so.) After turning right, you will quickly reach the junction with the Ridge Overlook Trail (purple blazes) to your left by some large boulders in the woods. Follow that trail up to the ridge. Just as you attain the ridge and the terrain flattens out, the Ridge Overlook Trail crosses the Rock Scree Trail. Continue straight along the ridge for 0.75 mile to the overlook, identified by a sign. You'll have a wonderful view of the Cumberland Valley to the north and west from here. Looking to the southeast, you should be able to make out the mansion on the hillside above you.

Continue along the ridge to the east for a short distance, where the trail makes a switchback and descends the ridge to the west into a hollow. Soon the Ridge Overlook Trail joins the Rock Scree Trail. Then, just beyond, it crosses the Forest Heritage Trail. Continue straight past a deer exclosure on the left. Just beyond that, you will reach a second crossing of the Forest Heritage Trail (lime green blazes). Turn left (east) here and follow the Forest Heritage Trail for a short distance to the Maple Hollow Trail (yellow blazes). Turn right (south). In a hundred feet or so, the Maple Hollow Trail makes a sharp left and then emerges into a small clearing that offers a view to the north. Follow the trail along a forest cut from the clearing to the right, which will return you in a couple of minutes to the parking area.

Nearby Activities

Kings Gap offers many environmental programs as well as wonderful places to have a picnic. Visit the mansion, the gardens, and the visitor center just uphill from the parking area. **Friends of Kings Gap** maintains the trails in the park and hosts recreational events in and near the park. Consider volunteering to help keep these trails accessible to all users. Information is available at friendsofkingsgap.org.

GPS INFORMATION AND DIRECTIONS
N40° 05.593' W77° 15.850'

From I-81, take Exit 37 (Newville/PA 233) and follow PA 233 south 2.3 miles to Pine Road. Turn left onto Pine Road (signs for Kings Gap Environmental Education Center) and follow it another 2.3 miles to Kings Gap Road (sign for Kings Gap). Turn right and follow the winding road up to the mansion area. The parking area, with several trailheads, is on the left, just before the loop at the mansion area begins.

50 Mary Ann Furnace Trail

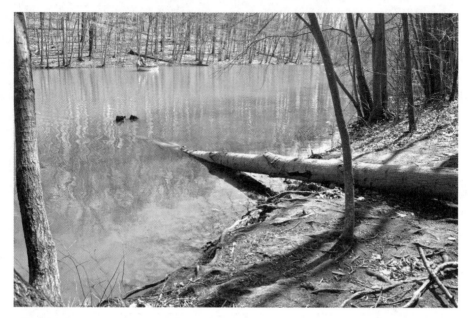

Wonder Cove

In Brief

Following the white-blazed Mary Ann Furnace Trail, this hike makes a loop through the woods along the southwest shore of Lake Marburg.

Description

The Mary Ann Furnace Trail consists of a 3.5-mile network of trails in three loops on the south shore of Lake Marburg at the lake's western end. This 2.5-mile hike follows the white-blazed main loop around the perimeter of the trail network. Lake Marburg is a large (1,275-acre) man-made water impoundment that is popular with fishermen who angle for bass, crappie, perch, muskellunge, and catfish. The lake's construction was a cooperative project between the H. P. Glatfelter Paper Company located in Spring Grove, which needed the water for industrial purposes, and the Commonwealth of Pennsylvania, which administrates the lake for recreational purposes. The lake is home to a large and varied population of waterfowl, and it is quite common to see Canada geese, wood ducks, teal, and herons along its 26 miles of shoreline. The park's woodlands are home to deer, pheasant, rabbits, squirrels, and other small game.

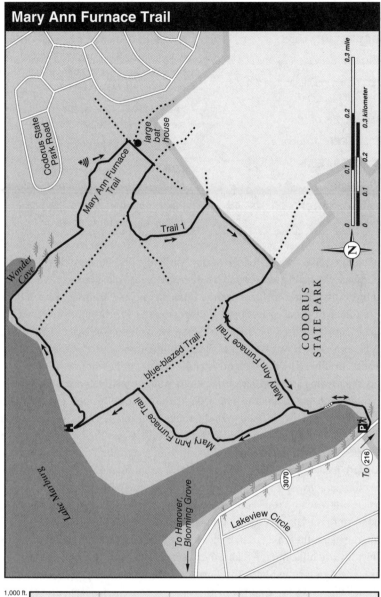

Mary Ann Furnace Trail

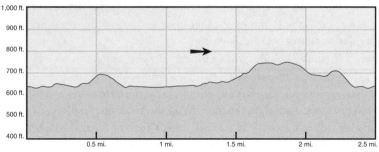

LENGTH 2.5 miles	**ACCESS** Sunrise–sunset
CONFIGURATION Loop	**MAPS** USGS *Hanover;* a map is included in the recreation guide for Codorus State Park, available at the park office and at tinyurl.com/codorusspmap.
DIFFICULTY Easy	
SCENERY Pretty walk in the woods; nice views of Lake Marburg	
EXPOSURE Mix of sun and shade	**FACILITIES** None at the trailhead but plenty in the state park
TRAIL TRAFFIC Moderate	**WHEELCHAIR TRAVERSABLE** No
TRAIL SURFACE Dirt	**CONTACT** Codorus State Park, 717-637-2816, tinyurl.com/codorussp
HIKING TIME 1.5 hours	
DRIVING DISTANCE About 25 miles southwest of York	**SPECIAL COMMENTS** The hike can get a bit buggy in the summer.

The hiking trail is named for the Mary Ann Forge and Furnace that was located on nearby Furnace Creek, the westernmost feeder stream to Lake Marburg. The furnace was founded in 1761 by Mark Bird and George Ross, an attorney from Lancaster, Pennsylvania, and a signer of the Declaration of Independence. The furnace produced cannons, cannonballs, and shot used by the Continental army under George Washington's command. A historic plaque was erected at the site of the Iron Master's house on Black Rock Road near the trailhead by the Daughters of the American Revolution in 1949.

From the parking area on Black Rock Road, walk across the footbridge over Codorus Creek West Branch and follow the path around a small cove through a wetlands area. On a spring morning, this cove is filled with the songs of spring peepers. As you bend around the back of the cove, you'll come to a long boardwalk. Cross the boardwalk and climb a little hill where you will find a fork in the trail with a sign for Trails 1 and 2. Follow the arrow toward Trail 1, heading to the left (north). At about 0.6 mile, the trail comes to a T-intersection at a grassy road. Turn left and follow the path down to the shore of the lake. Just before reaching the shore, the trail makes a 90-degree right turn, though you can walk down to the lake to a pretty vantage point.

From the bend, the trail parallels the shore of the lake through an attractive forest of cedars. Just shy of a mile into the hike, enter a small clearing with a trail approaching from the right and a sign for the Mary Ann Furnace Trail. Continue straight, staying near the shore of the lake. Soon the trail bends to the right and enters a second secluded cove: Wonder Cove. Continue to the back of the cove and follow the small hollow beyond, passing a short section of boardwalk.

Soon you'll climb a hillside, passing beneath the park amphitheater and grassy picnic area—a nice place to stop and hang out for a while. After passing the amphitheater, descend a wide grassy path to a large open meadow at the head of the hollow to a crossing with an old dirt road. Turn right (southwest) on this road, and take note of the large bat box on the left side of the trail just after you turn. Cross the creek through a muddy section of trail and climb a short hill to another trail crossing (1.5 miles).

Turn right (northwest) at the crossing and contour around a hillside past a couple of old wooden posts. In a short distance, you'll reach a field on top of a hill at another MARY ANN FURNACE TRAIL sign. A yellow-blazed trail enters the woods directly ahead, and a white-blazed trail enters the woods about 20 feet to the left of it. Bear left (south) and follow the white blazes into the woods. Wind through the woods until you come to the edge of the hillside field. This spot offers a nice view of the hills in this part of the park.

Follow the trail until it forks and then turn right (southwest), following it along the boundary of private property on your left. When you reach a T-intersection, turn right (northwest) again and descend into a small hollow. At 2.1 miles, a blue-blazed trail heads off straight, and you want to bear left, staying with the white blazes across a small creek. Climb a small hill that seems steep relative to the other grades on this walk. After cresting the hill, descend for a short distance until you reach the trail junction near the boardwalk in the first cove. Turn left, and the parking area is just 5 minutes along.

Nearby Activities

Codorus State Park, through which the trail passes, offers facilities for many kinds of recreational activities, including fishing, swimming, boating, camping, and picnicking.

GPS INFORMATION AND DIRECTIONS

N39° 46.192' W76° 55.793'

From I-83 in York, follow US 30 West 7.5 miles to PA 116 West. Follow PA 116 for 12 miles to PA 216 just before reaching Hanover. Turn left on PA 216 and follow it 3 miles, crossing Lake Marburg. Turn right onto Dubbs Church Road and follow it 1.85 miles to SR 3070, Black Rock Road. Turn right and drive about a mile. The trailhead and parking are on the right, just beyond the bridge over Codorus Creek West Branch at a wetlands area.

51 Mount Holly Marsh Preserve

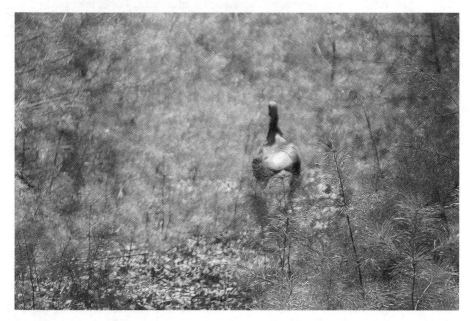

Wild turkey in the pines

In Brief

This lovely and varied hike links most of the trails on the preserve land to make a 5-mile loop of the entire preserve. It begins by climbing to the ridge on Mount Holly via the Lamberton and Ridge Trails, and continues by following the ridge southwest for 1.5 miles to a gate. There it descends into the Mountain Creek Valley via the Briar Trail to the Creek Trail. The hike then follows the Creek Trail south to Mountain Creek and then back north along the creek to the marsh. Near the marsh, the hike picks up the Spring Trail through the open marsh area and eventually to the junction with the Marsh Loop Trail, which it follows back to the parking area.

Description

Although there is a fair bit of climbing at the beginning of this hike, the effort of getting up on the ridge of Mount Holly is worth it. The ridge walk is quite beautiful (especially during the fall), and you will end up seeing an infrequently visited part of the preserve. Begin your hike by crossing Ridge Road from the parking area heading for the signs that

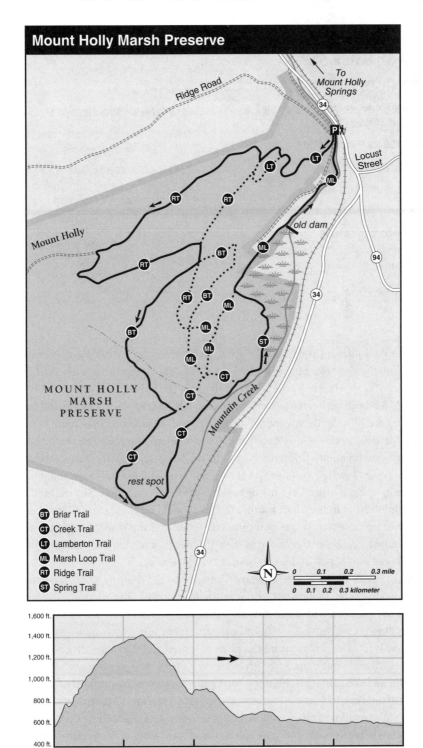

Mount Holly Marsh Preserve

Ridge Road

To
Mount Holly
Springs

34

Locust
Street

Mount Holly

old dam

94

34

MOUNT HOLLY
MARSH
PRESERVE

Mountain Creek

rest spot

34

BT Briar Trail
CT Creek Trail
LT Lamberton Trail
ML Marsh Loop Trail
RT Ridge Trail
ST Spring Trail

N

| 0 | 0.1 | 0.2 | 0.3 mile |

| 0 | 0.1 | 0.2 | 0.3 kilometer |

1,600 ft.
1,400 ft.
1,200 ft.
1,000 ft.
800 ft.
600 ft.
400 ft.

1 mi.   2 mi.   3 mi.   4 mi.   5 mi.

LENGTH 5 miles

CONFIGURATION Loop

DIFFICULTY Moderate

SCENERY Mount Holly Marsh and Mountain Creek

EXPOSURE Mostly shade

TRAIL TRAFFIC Light

TRAIL SURFACE Dirt

HIKING TIME 3 hours

DRIVING DISTANCE About a mile from the intersection of PA 34 and Pine Street in Mount Holly Springs

ACCESS Open

MAPS USGS *Mount Holly Springs;* a map of the preserve is available online at tinyurl.com/mthollymarshmap.

FACILITIES None

WHEELCHAIR TRAVERSABLE No

CONTACT The Nature Conservancy, 800-628-6860, tinyurl.com/mthollymarsh

SPECIAL COMMENTS The preserve is on Pennsylvania Game Commission land, so it is open to hunting; be sure to wear blaze orange during hunting season. The damp area around the marsh and the woodlands is prime habitat for some area snakes, including the copperhead. Be sure to exercise caution should you encounter any snakes.

say Parkside Boulevard and Lakeside Drive. Just beyond those signs you will see an obvious trail on the right climbing the wooded hillside. This is the Lamberton Trail, and it is well marked with white blazes. At first the climb up the hillside is moderately steep, passing a sign for a spring, but it eases off in a short while just before crossing an old haul road traversing the hillside. Follow the white blazes uphill to a second haul road. It is easy to get confused here. If you look uphill and downhill along the road you should see white blazes in both directions. If you turn right, the road, the trail, and the blazes all end after a short distance. Turn left (southwest) on the haul road and follow it downhill for a short distance to where it forks. Take the right fork and follow that uphill. The trail will switchback, climb a little farther, join another old haul road, and come to a trail marker with a number of white blazes, where you turn left (uphill) off the road. In another short distance you will reach yet another road with another trail marker that indicates you have reached the loop section of the Lamberton Trail (0.4 mile).

Make a right turn and follow the road uphill to an old skidway where the Lamberton Trail switchbacks left (southwest). Continue following the blazes and soon you will reach a significant dirt road with a signpost indicating that you have reached the upper section of the yellow-blazed Ridge Trail (0.5 mile). Turn right (northeast) on the road and follow the Ridge Trail as it winds around the ridge of Mount Holly, eventually heading back to the west. The walk through the woods along the ridge is very pleasant and offers views to the north and west through the trees during the winter and beautiful tree cover during the rest of the year. It is very pretty here in the fall. After almost a mile of walking you will reach an intersection of dirt roads. Should you continue straight along the ridge you will encounter a gate after a short distance that indicates the edge of the preserve property. At the intersection, turn left (south) onto the dirt road and begin to descend from the ridge.

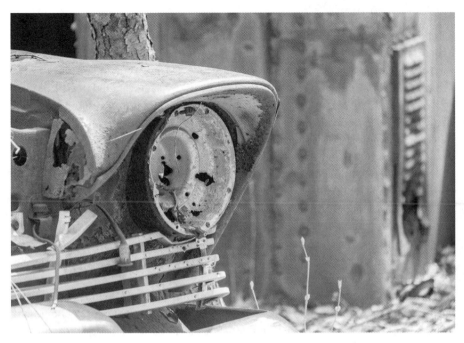

Remains of an old car along Creek Trail

At first the road drops gently, and then it gets steeper at another intersection where an old roadbed heads off to the north and west. Stay to the left here. The road traverses down the hillside through some pine trees until you come to the junction with the Ridge Trail at a clearing (1.9 miles), which in effect marks the end of the loop on that trail. Turn right (south) and in a very short distance the Ridge Trail joins the orange-blazed Briar Trail at an obvious junction.

Turn right (west) onto the Briar Trail and follow that for nearly half a mile to where it crosses over a seasonal creek into a flat clearing. Head to the left (downhill) in the clearing and you will see where the trail enters a beautiful forest of young pine trees. Here I was surprised by a very large wild turkey that ran across the trail right in front of me, and for nearly a mile I could hear turkeys gobbling away in the woods around me. Walking through the pine forest couldn't be more pleasant. The ground is soft, the scenery is lovely, and the light is particularly beautiful in this section of the forest. At 2.7 miles the trail levels out and ends at an old roadbed, which is the red-blazed Creek Trail. Turn right (southwest) and hike along that as it winds its way through the woods for 0.25 mile until it crosses a creek, passes by the rusted carcasses of a half dozen old automobiles, and then loops back to the east. At 3.3 miles you will reach the banks of Mountain Creek, a significant stream that is popular with area fishermen. Right when you reach the creek, you will find a very nice place for a break before heading off onto the last section of the hike through the marsh.

After the break, follow the Creek Trail to the north. It strays away from banks of Mountain Creek and at 3.7 it comes to the junction with the lime-green-blazed Spring Trail. At the junction the Creek Trail turns decidedly to the left. Continue straight (northeast) on the Spring Trail. The terrain gets a little more damp as the trail winds through the woods, and at 4.1 miles it enters a large grassy clearing with scattered trees. This is the area of Mount Holly Marsh proper. Some older maps show this to be the site of an old lake, Mount Holly Spring Lake. I have not been able to locate any history of that body of water, but as you will see a short distance farther along the trail, this area was indeed dammed at one time. Continue along the trail as it hugs the very left edge of the clearing. The walking gets a little spongy and marshy at times—your feet might get a bit wet—and soon the trail leaves the clearing and ends at the Marsh Loop Trail, which follows a wide, open path. Turn right (north) and follow this blue-blazed trail along the perimeter of the marsh on your right. Soon you will pass some private homes constructed on the hillside to your left. Stay on the pleasant dirt path, skirting private property. At 4.6 miles you will reach the remains of the old Upper Mountain Holly Dam along Mountain Creek, another nice place to take a break.

From the dam site the trail continues north for only another 0.25 mile before reaching the trailhead for the Mount Holly Marsh Preserve trail system at Parkway Boulevard, which is marked by a large sign. The trail proper ends. Continue walking north along the road and in 0.2 mile you will reach the parking lot.

Nearby Activities

Pine Grove Furnace State Park, which has swimming ponds, camping, and hiking trails, is 9 miles to the south on PA 34. The nearby town of **Mount Holly Springs** has all of the supplies you might need. And not far away, the town of **Boiling Springs** has a beautiful community park with a pond and is home to the regional Appalachian Trail Conservancy.

GPS INFORMATION AND DIRECTIONS

N40° 06.375' W77° 10.829'

From Carlisle, follow PA 34, Hanover Street, south about 6 miles to Mount Holly Springs. Continue beyond Mount Holly Springs on PA 34 for 0.6 mile to the junction with Lakeside Road, just before PA 34 crosses over Mountain Creek. Lakeside Road is at the end of a large parking area for a restaurant currently under renovation. Turn right on Lakeside Road and follow that to 0.5 mile to the parking area on the left.

52 Pinchot Lake

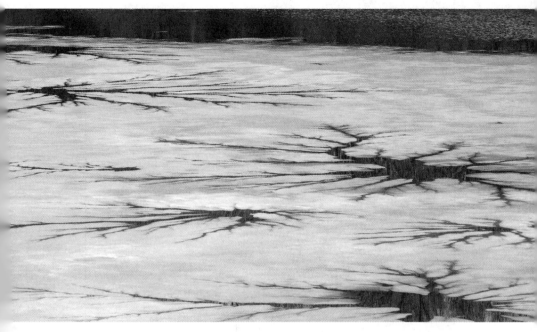

Ice-covered Pinchot Lake

In Brief

This hike generally follows the path of the Lakeside Trail as indicated on park maps around Pinchot Lake.

Description

This hike tends to follow what the Gifford Pinchot State Park brochure refers to as the Lakeside Trail around Pinchot Lake, although this hike incorporates a couple of side trails to circumnavigate the campground area. In places the hike passes through some of the busiest areas of the park, and in other places the most remote. It's a great hike that encompasses some beautiful country and affords some fine opportunities for viewing wildlife.

Begin this hike by exiting the parking area at Boat Mooring Area 2 to the southeast, walking past the handicapped parking space along a paved path toward the restrooms. Just past the restrooms, look to your right and you will see a sign that says LAKESIDE TRAIL. Take this trail, which initially follows the lakeshore through cedar and hickory trees beneath the cabin area.

255

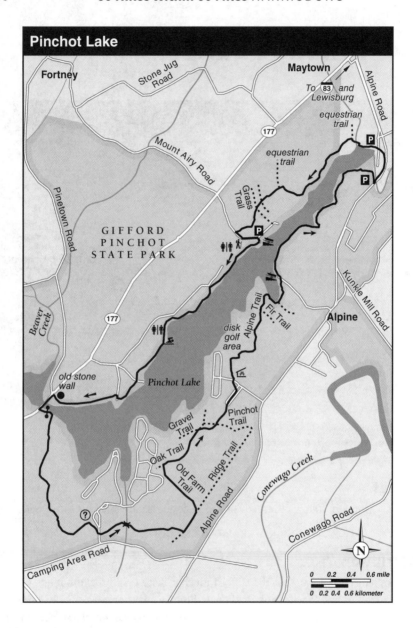

At about 0.5 mile, the trail meets a road and angles to the left through a field of wild-flowers where it splits into two grassy paths. Both take you to the far side of the field, where the trail reenters the woods on dirt. A quarter-mile or so beyond that, you'll reach the Quaker Race Day Use Area, with its picnic pavilions, a swimming beach, and a concession stand that are open during the summer. When you reach the recreation area, hop on the paved path by the first set of restrooms and follow it past the swimming beach to its end at a pavilion. Walk toward the woods between two large sycamore trees and you'll

LENGTH 8.5 miles	**MAPS** USGS *Wellsville* and *Dover;* a map of the park with the trail outlined is available at the park office and online at tinyurl.com/pinchotspmap, though the hike here varies slightly from the Lakeside Trail that is indicated on that map.
CONFIGURATION Loop	
DIFFICULTY Moderately strenuous because of length	
SCENERY Gifford Pinchot State Park environs; wonderful views of the lake and woods	**FACILITIES** Restrooms and water available at various locations along the first 5 miles of the hike
EXPOSURE Mostly shade	
TRAIL TRAFFIC Medium–light	**WHEELCHAIR TRAVERSABLE** No
TRAIL SURFACE Varies from dirt and rocky to paved in places	**CONTACT** Gifford Pinchot State Park, 717-432-5011, tinyurl.com/giffpinchotsp
HIKING TIME 4–5 hours	**SPECIAL COMMENTS** Use discretion about completing this hike following a heavy rain. At about 7 miles, the path crosses a creek that would be impassable with much water in it.
DRIVING DISTANCE About 9 miles from I-83 and PA 177 south of Harrisburg	
ACCESS Sunrise–sunset	

see a LAKESIDE TRAIL sign where it enters the woods. The trail immediately crosses a small footbridge, curves to the left, and climbs gently. As you enter the woods, admire the interesting and beautiful stand of cane to the right.

When you reach a maintenance building, turn right on the dirt road and follow it for a couple of hundred feet until you see a LAKESIDE TRAIL sign on the left near a gate on the road. Turn left on the trail and follow it for 0.4 mile to a spruce tree and a maintenance access gate. The trail veers left and then past an old stone wall onto PA 177 at the intersection with Pinetown Road. Turn left and walk the shoulder across the bridge over the lake.

A prominent blue blaze has been painted on the end of the bridge's guardrail, and there is another LAKESIDE TRAIL sign. For the most part, this hike follows the blue blazes along the south side of the lake. Enter the woods here and follow the lakeshore for a short distance through a forest of maple and oak trees. Soon the trail bends right and climbs from a junction with a trail to the left. As it levels out, the trail widens and appears to be an old bridle path as it heads to the southwest. Eventually the trail passes by a road and large meadow, both of which are on the right.

Just shy of 3 miles, this hike comes to an open area surrounded by pine trees with a small cedar tree with a blue blaze on your left. A grassy path comes in from the right and the trail appears to continue straight. Turn right onto the grassy path and shortly you will come to the campground access road. Cross the road and enter the woods at the LAKE-SIDE TRAIL sign. The campground kiosk will be to your left. It has vending machines and information.

At this point, the park map shows the Lakeside Trail turning immediately to the left and cutting through the campground, whereas continuing straight takes you along the

Ridge Trail. Continue to follow the blazes along the Ridge Trail. At 3.6 miles, the trail reaches a T-junction by a telephone line. Be sure to turn left here. The walking is really lovely along an old roadbed a fair bit above the lake. In another 0.2 mile, you'll reach the junction of the Ridge Trail and the Old Farm Trail.

Here, you have some choices. The blue blazes continue straight along the Ridge Trail, and you can follow them to the junction with the Pinchot Trail that joins the Gravel Trail atop a small hill with a log bench near the lake (about 0.7 mile). At that point, you'll turn right. Or you can turn left on Old Farm Trail (slightly shorter option), which descends to the edge of the campground where it meets the Oak Trail (about 0.25 mile). Neither trail is marked, but a sign on the left says NO PETS ALLOWED IN CAMPING AREA. Turning left brings you to a meadow and small playground. Turn right here and follow the gravel path (which is both the Old Farm Trail and Oak Trail) up a gentle hill, noting the shagbark hickory growing in this area.

Following this latter option, at 4.3 miles you'll reach another trail junction where the Old Farm Trail turns right and heads back uphill and the Oak Trail continues straight to a significant junction 0.2 mile ahead. Here, the Gravel Trail enters from the left and crosses the Oak Trail. Turn right and follow the Gravel Trail by a sign that advises CAUTION: STEEP GRADE. The grade is neither very steep nor very long, though. At the top is a log bench and the junction with the Pinchot Trail.

Take the Gravel Trail as it heads downhill, following the blue blazes. At 4.8 miles, the path enters an open grassy area, and comes to a signpost with a bicycle symbol pointing to the woods on the left. Enter the woods and then cross the access road to the Conewago Recreation Area. The path continues by a disk-golf course to the left and a large pavilion with a restroom to the right. At 5 miles the trail veers left and then forks. A blue blaze on a tree indicates that this hike heads uphill to the right following the Alpine Trail.

Another 0.4 mile and the Midland Trail enters from the left. Turn right onto the Midland Trail and immediately cross a little footbridge. Soon you pass the Fir Trail on the right, and then reach a T-junction with the Boulder Point Trail. Turning left will take you to Balanced Rock, a geological formation along the lakeshore. Turning right keeps you on the Lakeside Trail as it circumnavigates a secluded cove where I saw a heron feeding.

At 5.8 miles, the trail reaches Boat Mooring Area 3. Follow the lakeshore past a cul-de-sac and a canoe-storage rack. You'll find a LAKESIDE TRAIL sign by a picnic table on the right. Continue through the woods right next to the lake. At this point, the hike enters a secluded section of the park as it follows the boulder-strewn lakeshore.

At 7 miles, the trail reaches the northeast end of the lake at the dam. Although you can't walk across the dam, take a walk out on it for a wonderful view of Pinchot Lake. From the dam, descend an old gravel road into a parking area by Beaver Creek, the outflow from the lake. Walk out of the parking area and cross the bridge on a paved sidewalk. As soon as the pavement ends, you'll see a blue blaze on the guardrail. Step over it and walk down some steps. Walk through woods parallel to the road until the trail climbs and heads to the left away from the road. Soon it climbs a series of wooden steps before reaching a parking area by the dam. A sign indicates that the Lakeside Trail follows the fence southwest around the dam's spillway. This is the last of the trail signs.

As soon as the trail meets the level of the lake again, you'll find a beautiful spot at a cove for relaxing on the left. Just beyond that the trail crosses Rock Creek where the creek tumbles over small ledges. Beware: The creek would be impassable after heavy rain. The blue blazes end at the creek.

Cross the creek and climb generally uphill to the left. At 7.3 miles, the path meets the Equestrian Trail. Turn left and watch for woodpeckers in this area. The trail parallels the lakeshore, though above it a fair distance. Stay on this trail for what feels like a long 0.6 mile. At times the track gets very rocky and follows watercourses that climb away from the lake. At 8 miles, you'll reach a significant, though unmarked, trail junction just beyond a heavily washed-out section of the Equestrian Trail. The junction is easily identifiable by the footbridge immediately left of the Equestrian Trail.

Turn left and follow the path through the woods for the next 0.35 mile until you reach the paved park road. En route, you'll pass a trail crossing marked by a NO HORSES sign and then a grassy cut in the woods that leads to a park-maintenance area to the left. When you reach the paved road, turn left and walk into the parking lot.

Nearby Activities

Gifford Pinchot State Park offers all sorts of activities, including a swimming area, several boat launches, fishing, a disk-golf course, picnic pavilions, and a campground.

GPS INFORMATION AND DIRECTIONS
N40° 04.974' W76° 53.017'

From Harrisburg, follow I-83 South to Exit 35 (Lewisberry/PA 177). Follow PA 177 south 6.9 miles to Mount Airy Road. The park office for Gifford Pinchot State Park is at the corner on the left. Turn left and follow the road about a half-mile to the parking area, at Boat Mooring Area 2.

53 Pole Steeple and Mountain Creek

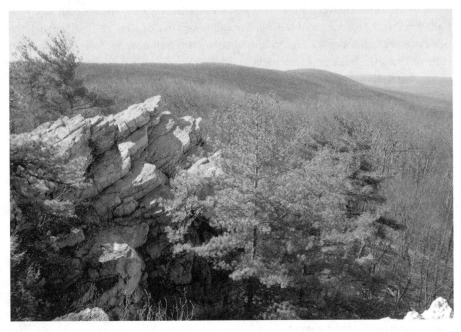

View from Pole Steeple

In Brief

After the short ascent of Pole Steeple, a quartzite outcrop along a mountain ridge, this hike picks up the Appalachian Trail (AT) and follows it west down to Railroad Bed Road. After joining the road, the hike follows Mountain Creek Trail along the creek, through wetlands, back to the parking area.

Description

From the parking area, walk across the road, the old South Mountain Railroad Grade dating back to the time of the forge and furnaces in the valley, to the trailhead marked by a sign and blue blazes just left of some private residences. The trail is wide with good footing as it climbs rather steeply at first through a forest of pine and fir trees, many of which show signs of woodpecker feeding. At about 0.5 mile, the trail forks and blue blazes go in both directions. If you take the right fork, the trail climbs more gently as it makes

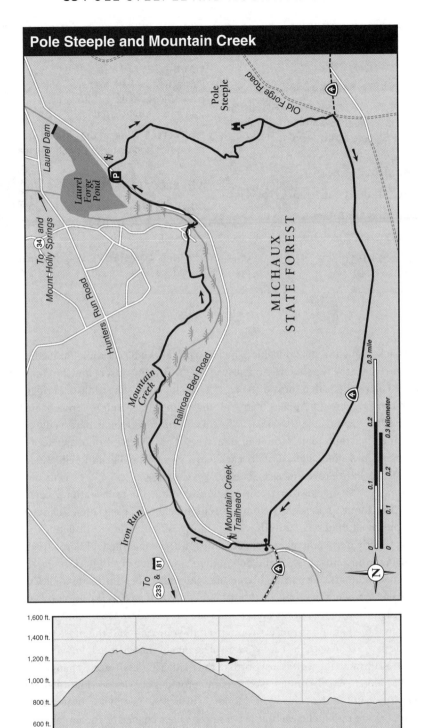

Pole Steeple and Mountain Creek

LENGTH 4.2 miles

CONFIGURATION Loop

DIFFICULTY Moderate

SCENERY Pine Grove Furnace State Park environs, a great view from the summit of Pole Steeple, halfway point of Appalachian Trail

EXPOSURE Mostly shaded

TRAIL TRAFFIC Moderately heavy

TRAIL SURFACE Dirt

HIKING TIME 2–3 hours

DRIVING DISTANCE About 9 miles from PA 233 and I-81

ACCESS Sunrise–sunset

MAPS USGS *Dickinson;* Pine Grove Furnace State Park map available at the park office or online at tinyurl.com /pinegrovefurnacespmap.

FACILITIES None at the parking area; restrooms and water are available nearby at Laurel Lake.

WHEELCHAIR TRAVERSABLE No

CONTACT Pine Grove Furnace State Park, 717-486-7174, tinyurl.com/pinegrove furnacesp

SPECIAL COMMENTS Use caution atop the cliffs at Pole Steeple.

switchbacks along the steep hillside. The left path takes a direct route up the hill. Both join again where the terrain levels out just above the fork and just below the cliffs of Pole Steeple. Follow the path a short distance to a trail junction at a saddle on a ridge with a sign pointing right to the Appalachian Trail and a bench (0.65 mile). Turn left and follow the blazes to Pole Steeple (0.8 mile). The hike to this overlook is deservedly popular. Surrounded by stout Table Mountain pine trees, Pole Steeple is a quartzite rock outcropping about 75 feet high. It offers excellent views of the Sunset Rocks Ridge to the north and the Pine Grove Furnace State Park, including Laurel Lake, directly below.

From Pole Steeple, return to the saddle and follow the trail south up a gentle rise to the AT at about 1 mile. At this point, the climbing for the day is done. The trail junction forms the hub of several trails radiating as spokes in different directions. The AT crosses directly perpendicular to the Pole Steeple Trail and the Old Forge Road cuts a diagonal in from across the AT and downhill to your left. Turn right onto the AT, here an old roadbed marked by white blazes, and descend a pleasant grade for 1.5 miles to the railroad grade in the valley. At about 1.5 miles, you'll pass a clearing surrounded by pines and in a few more minutes reach Railroad Bed Road by Mountain Creek.

From the AT, the most direct route back to your car—and the most common—is along the paved road with the cars. A more pleasant alternative is to follow the Mountain Creek Trail through the woods just north of the road. This less-traveled path follows and crosses Mountain Creek through wetlands and provides considerably more opportunity for viewing wildlife than the road. Mountain Creek is habitat for beaver and mink, though both are rather elusive. But you'll never have a chance of encountering either if you follow the road. The trail is well marked with red blazes the entire length, and with some care at the end, you should have no trouble following it.

To make this 1.5-mile excursion, turn right on Railroad Bed Road and after about 100 yards you'll see a trailhead on the left identified by a sign that says FOOT TRAFFIC ONLY. Turn left onto the trail and follow the red blazes generally along the course of the creek through the woods. About 0.75 mile from the trailhead, the trail crosses the creek at a good log crossing, obviously constructed since the floods. I've often seen white-tailed deer bedded down in the area north of the creek. At about 1.4 miles, the trail enters a small clearing at the edge of the creek, and then veers left away from the creek into a wetlands area. Finding the route gets a little tricky around here, as the blazes seem to disappear for a short distance. Look to your left, away from the creek, and you should see a small footbridge over a braided stream, which at the time of this writing was in disrepair due to the flood. Balance over the bridge into the wetlands area, and you should begin to see blazes again. After about 25 yards, you'll cross another stream braided over some timbers. Just beyond these timbers, the obvious trail continues straight; however, keep your eyes trained to your right for the red blazes and a less distinct path onto which you will turn right (about 20 feet beyond the timbers). Follow this to the cul-de-sac at the end of Ice House Road and a good bridge over Mountain Creek. The trail is much more well defined in the area of Ice House Road.

If you should miss the path, you will come quickly to a presentation area with benches and a fire ring beneath some cabins on a small hill. These are all part of a YMCA camp. Turn back and look for the junction. If you still have difficulty locating it, return to the presentation area and pass it through the woods, keeping it to your left, following the hillside with the cabins above. You will meet the trail within 50 yards or so near the bank of creek. Cross the good bridge over the creek, turn left on the road, and follow it for 0.25 mile back to your car.

Nearby Activities

Pine Grove Furnace State Park is a wonderful place with loads of activities. It has two lakes with swimming areas, picnic areas, biking and hiking trails, and the site of the old Pine Grove Furnace. It also has a wonderful campground. Your best bet is to stop by the park office at the intersection of PA 233 and Pine Grove Road for a park map and information on current events.

GPS INFORMATION AND DIRECTIONS
N40° 02.290' W77° 16.218'

Take Exit 37, PA 233, from I-81 and follow PA 233 south 8 miles to the park office at the intersection with Pine Grove Road. Turn left on Pine Grove Road and follow that east 1.5 miles to Railroad Bed Road, just beyond the Laurel Lake Day Use Area. Turn right. The parking area is on the right just above the outlet to the lake across from a couple of private cabins.

54 Rocky Knob

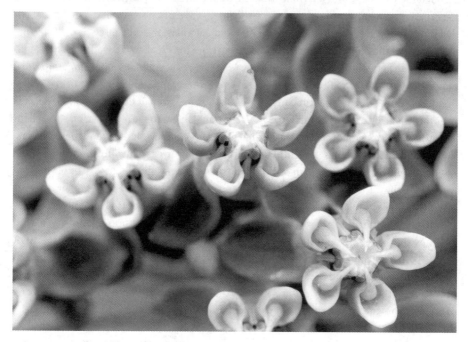

Common milkweed

In Brief

This hike follows the Rocky Knob Trail from Ridge Road south over Sier Hill to a saddle beneath Rocky Knob. From the saddle, the hike descends into a hollow and follows an old Civilian Conservation Corps (CCC) road back to the trailhead. An additional spur leads through the lower hollow from the junction with the CCC road out to a trailhead on Birch Run Road to the south.

Description

If you have any doubts about what mountain laurel looks like, this hike should alleviate those doubts forever. In late May and early June, the woods are filled with blossoms unlike any place I have seen before. During the summer, the forest is thick with the understory. Come autumn, the terrain begins to thin out a little bit and the trees put on a brilliant display of color.

This hike begins by following an old roadbed south from the parking area. The road was constructed by the CCC in 1937 in an attempt to make a connecting road between Ridge Road to the north and Birch Run Road to the south. The project was

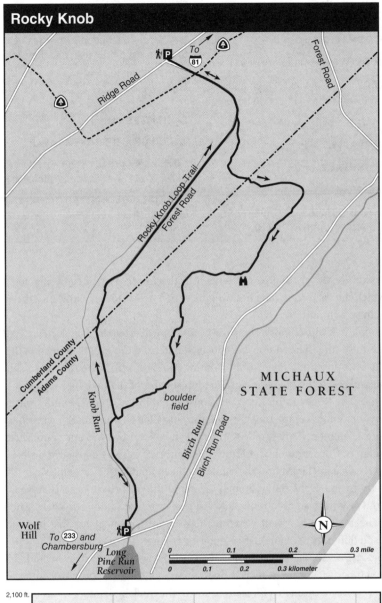

Rocky Knob

Ridge Road

To 81

Forest Road

Rocky Knob Loop Trail

Forest Road

Cumberland County
Adams County

Knob Run

boulder field

MICHAUX STATE FOREST

Birch Run

Birch Run Road

Wolf Hill

To 233 and Chambersburg

Long Pine Run Reservoir

N

| 0 | 0.1 | 0.2 | 0.3 mile |

| 0 | 0.1 | 0.2 | 0.3 kilometer |

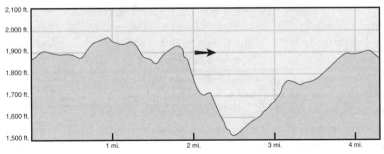

LENGTH 4.3 miles	**ACCESS** Sunrise–sunset
CONFIGURATION Loop	**MAPS** USGS *Caledonia Park;* Michaux State Forest public-use map; Keystone Trail Association *Appalachian Trail, PA Route 94 to US Route 30 (Sections 12 and 13)*
DIFFICULTY Easy–moderate	
SCENERY Mountain laurel highlands and beautiful view of Long Pine Run Reservoir	
EXPOSURE Mostly shade	**FACILITIES** None
TRAIL TRAFFIC Moderate	**WHEELCHAIR TRAVERSABLE** No
TRAIL SURFACE Dirt	**CONTACT** Michaux State Forest, 717-352-2211, tinyurl.com/michauxsf
HIKING TIME 2–2.5 hours	
DRIVING DISTANCE 18.5 miles from I-81 and PA 233 south of Carlisle	**SPECIAL COMMENTS** A popular hike in South Mountain that never gets too crowded.

unsuccessful, however, due to the terrain in the lower part of the unnamed hollow along which the road runs. The hollow gets very narrow down below and its flanks are covered in large boulders.

A couple of hundred yards along the road, you will cross the Appalachian Trail (AT). A sign for the orange-blazed Rocky Knob Trail is located there, explaining that the trail is for day-use purposes and hikers only. Continue straight across the AT and in about 0.25 mile you will reach the beginning of the loop section of the hike by a signpost marked NUMBER 1. The Rocky Knob Loop was constructed in 1977 by the Youth Conservation Corps. In addition to completing the trail, they installed 14 posts marking stations of natural interest. An interpretive guide to the trail and its stations was once published by the Department of Conservation and Natural Resources. I found a copy several years ago at the DCNR office in Harrisburg, though I have been unable to locate one since. The trail remains pretty much the same, though several of the posts have been removed. In particular, the original trail used to include a side spur to the summit of Rocky Knob. That spur has been closed in recent years, perhaps because of incidents that have occurred along it and difficulty of maintenance—it was extremely steep and rugged.

From the beginning of the loop, turn left leaving the CCC road behind. The hike walks much better clockwise than it does counterclockwise. The trail continues along mostly level terrain through a forest of oak with the thick understory of mountain laurel, sassafras, and blueberry. You'll pass several stations along the way. Station number 2 provides an orientation to forest strata, calling attention to the diverse understory. Station number 3 was marked to call attention to examples of tropisms, how trees and plants grow in response to the available light that makes its way through the forest canopy. Station number 4 is a fairly obvious one pointing out a colony and mound built by Allegheny mound-building ants, one of several such mounds alongside the trail.

As the trail continues, you will contour around the edge of Sier Hill. During the fall and winter you'll have nice views to the east across Birch Run Hollow. At 1.4 miles, you'll reach station number 9, an overlook that offers an excellent view to the southeast of Long Pine Run Reservoir and the South Mountain countryside. From there, the trail continues along a ridge until a set of double blazes marks the beginning of a descent to the saddle between Sier Hill and Rocky Knob. The descent is short, but rather steep and requires care. Upon reaching the saddle, the terrain levels out and at station number 10 you will be at a point just below the large quartzite boulder field that forms the north shoulder of Rocky Knob. The boulders are huge. This is a nice place to take a break in the shade.

Continue from the saddle down the trail toward the west. The arrangement of station posts gets a little confusing here as the next two posts you pass will be numbered 7 and 8. About 50 yards beyond them is the junction with the old summit spur. Please refrain from exploring as the terrain is closed and quite hazardous. At about 2.4 miles, you will reach the lower end of the CCC road at station 13. To complete the hike, turn right and follow the road up a steady but gentle hill for nearly 2 miles back to the trailhead.

A worthwhile side trip begins at station 13 and follows the recently constructed footpath down the hollow out to Birch Run Road at the Long Pine Run Reservoir. The walk through this lower part of the hollow is quite beautiful as it is filled with thick rhododendrons growing along the banks of the creek that provides cover for the local wildlife. I came across a bear here recently. We were both spooked by the encounter. It thundered off through the brush, while I stood astonished and caught my breath. The trail stays to the left (east) of the creek for most of the way before crossing it a couple of hundred yards shy of Birch Run Road. It is marked for its length with prolific orange blazes. Walking the lower section adds about a mile to the loop hike.

You might alternately begin the excursion from Birch Run Road rather than from Ridge Road. The trailhead is located about 50 feet past the guardrail to the west on Birch Run Road.

Nearby Activities

Pine Grove Furnace State Park, on PA 233 to the north, has two lakes with swimming areas, picnic area, biking and hiking trails, and the site of the old Pine Grove Furnace. It also has a wonderful campground. Your best bet is to stop by the park office at the intersection of PA 233 and Pine Grove Road for a park map and information on current events.

GPS INFORMATION AND DIRECTIONS
N39° 58.693' W77° 26.478'

From I-81, take Exit 37 (Newville/PA 233). Follow PA 233 south 14 miles to Shippensburg Road. Turn right on Shippensburg Road and follow it up the ridge 2.5 miles to Ridge Road on the left. Turn left and follow Ridge Road 2 miles to the parking area. The parking area is on the right and it has room for five or six cars. The trailhead is directly across the road, identified by a forest-usage sign. Just past the trailhead on Ridge Road is a wooden milepost marked Number 10.

55 Rocky Ridge County Park

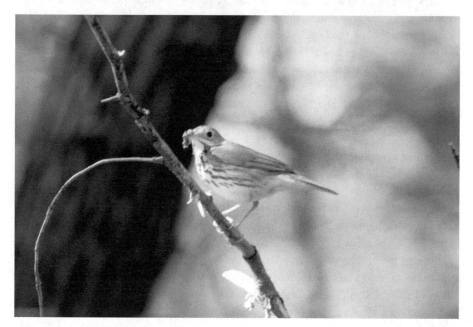

Ovenbird

In Brief

This hike follows several of the park trails along the south perimeter of the park before visiting the north overlook and returning to the car.

Description

Located on a ridgetop just a few miles northeast of York, the 750-acre Rocky Ridge County Park is a popular location for local bird-watchers. During the spring, it is visited by a variety of warblers, including black and white warblers, ovenbirds, chestnut-sided warblers, redstarts, blue warblers, yellow throats, and green warblers. In both the fall and spring, the two park overlooks provide excellent vantage points from which to view the seasonal hawk migrations. And the woods are home to a variety of woodland species, including scarlet tanager, thrushes, nuthatches, yellow-billed cuckoo, blue jays, downy woodpeckers, and flycatchers. It is a popular park that can be crowded on weekends, though you can always find some degree of solitude on the many trails that traverse its pretty oak forest.

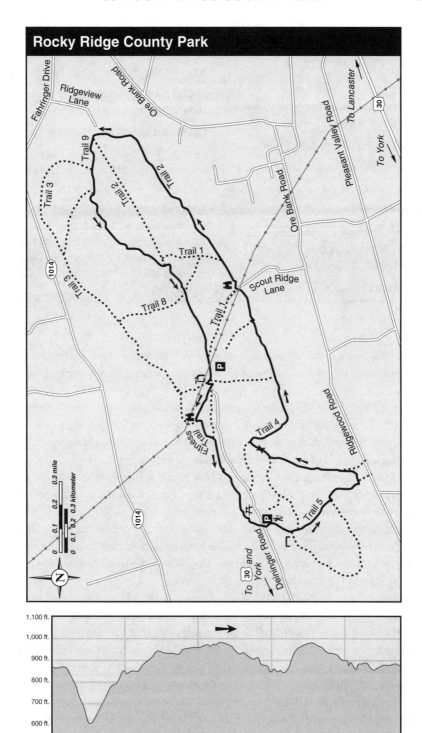

Rocky Ridge County Park

LENGTH 4.8 miles

CONFIGURATION Loop

DIFFICULTY Moderate

SCENERY Nice walk through the woods, 2 nice views at park overlooks

EXPOSURE More shade than sun

TRAIL TRAFFIC Moderate

TRAIL SURFACE Dirt and cinders, some paved sections

HIKING TIME About 2.5 hours

DRIVING DISTANCE About 3 miles from US 30 and PA 24 east of York

ACCESS 8 a.m.–sunset

MAPS USGS *York Haven;* a park map of the trails is available at parking areas and online at tinyurl.com/rockyridgeparkmap.

FACILITIES Toilets and water available at parking area

WHEELCHAIR TRAVERSABLE No

CONTACT York County Parks and Recreation, 717-840-7440, tinyurl.com /rockyridgepark

SPECIAL COMMENTS A good hike for warbler-watching in the spring. The park trails are all numbered and can be a little confusing. A park map available at the park and online can be helpful for orienting yourself.

This hike begins from the parking lot for the Wildlife Picnic Area, the first area on the right as you enter the park. Walk out of the back of the parking lot in a southerly direction by a NO PARKING sign between two spruce trees onto the obvious trail, a wide old logging path. Follow the trail to where it forks at a bench and keep left. Green-fiberglass signposts for Trail 5 mark both directions. In a short distance, another Trail 5 goes left, but you continue straight, and then another trail heads off to right. Again, continue straight and pass through a small clearing with many wildflowers growing in it.

At about 0.25 mile, you'll come to a half-log bench at a trail junction where you will veer left. You are now on Trail 6. Descend a rather steep, washed-out section of hillside, passing some water bars and another trail junction with signs for Trail 6. Just beyond that intersection, the main roadbed continues straight, but this route on Trail 6 goes left at an obvious turn onto more of a footpath. You are heading north at this point. Traverse into a hollow just above a creek and join a major path. Walk up the scenic hollow on a nice dirt trail passing some lovely rock outcrops.

At about 0.9 mile, Trail 6 turns left and crosses over a footbridge by an old pump house. Stay to the right here and climb for a short distance to a footbridge across a small creek. Just beyond, you'll reach Trail 4, a major path. Turn right (south) and cross another footbridge by a bench. Continue along Trail 4, which is smooth and level, staying right at all the trail junctions, until you come out to a power line and a junction with a major gravel path (1.8 miles). This is Trail 1, onto which you will turn right (east). An observation deck lies ahead and it provides an excellent view of the Conestoga Valley to the south. Follow Trail 1 for a couple of hundred yards into the woods to a dirt footpath that departs to the right (Trail 2). Keep right (still east) and follow the footpath as it bends around to the north until you reach a major trail junction (2.75 miles).

Trail 2 heads left here. You can follow that (and cut about 0.2 mile off the hike) or continue straight on Trail 9, which provides a nice trek through the woods. Following Trail 9, you will soon pass the junction with Trail 3, descending quite precipitously to the right. Continue straight, heading west and traversing the hill first descending and then ascending. Soon Trail 9 reaches the ridge again where it joins the wide gravel path of Trail 1, just 100 feet west of where that trail and Trail 2 come together. Turn right (still west) on Trail 1, and follow it to the large parking area (3.9 miles).

Walk through the lot angling toward its northwest corner, near some restrooms. Pick up the gravel path leading to the north observation deck, and walk out to the deck past some cherry trees. You'll have a view from the observation deck that will give you a good idea of how the park got its name. From the observation deck, follow the Fitness Trail straight into the woods. (Don't follow the path that heads downhill!) Hike along the Fitness Trail to a trail junction. Turn right and follow the path alongside the park road for a couple of tenths of a mile until you reach the pavilions at the Hidden Laurel Picnic Area (4.6 miles). Walk through the picnic area, across the parking lot, and then across the park road into the Wildlife Picnic Area parking lot to your car.

Nearby Activities

With its picnic pavilions, playgrounds, volleyball court, and trails, the park is the obvious location for additional activities. However, if you want a real treat, take a tour of the **Harley-Davidson** motorcycle factory just a few miles away in York. Information on tours is available at harley-davidson.com.

GPS INFORMATION AND DIRECTIONS
N40° 00.485' W76° 39.737'

From US 30 east of York, take the Mount Zion/PA 24 exit and follow PA 24 north 1.25 miles to Deininger Road. Turn right on Deininger Road and follow it into the park. Park in the Wildlife Picnic Area parking lot, the first picnic area on the right.

56 Samuel S. Lewis State Park

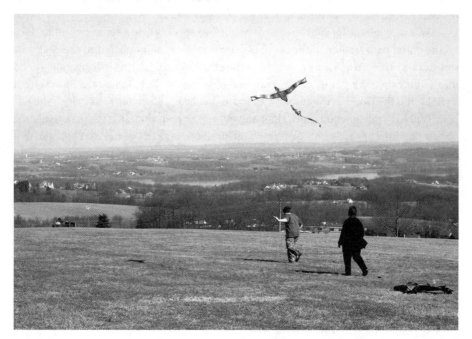

Kite-flying atop Mount Pisgah

In Brief

Following the established Hill Top Trail, this pleasant hike makes a loop around the perimeter of Samuel S. Lewis State Park just below the top of Mount Pisgah, finishing on the hilltop.

Description

Samuel S. Lewis State Park is located atop the 885-foot Mount Pisgah in east-central York County. Lewis, for whom the park is named, served as Secretary of the Pennsylvania Department of Forest and Waters from 1951 to 1954. He also served as Secretary of Highways under Gifford Pinchot during his term as governor.

The park was opened in 1954 and was initially cobbled together from three tracts of land: some farmland owned by Lewis, an arboretum owned by Walter Stine that is still part of the park, and an additional tract of farmland owned by a local family. The park is

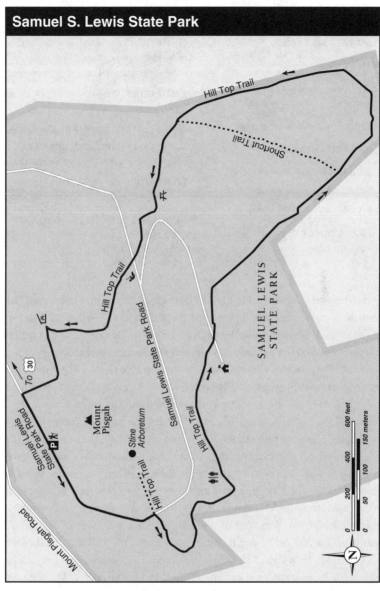

Samuel S. Lewis State Park

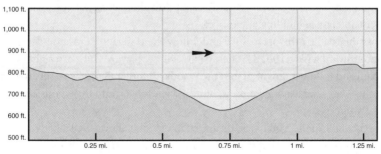

LENGTH 1.3 miles	**ACCESS** Sunrise–sunset
CONFIGURATION Loop	**MAPS** USGS *Red Lion;* a park map is available at the park and online at tinyurl.com /lewisspmap.
DIFFICULTY Easy	
SCENERY Nice views of York and Lancaster Counties	**FACILITIES** Restrooms, water, picnic facilities
EXPOSURE More sun than shade	**WHEELCHAIR TRAVERSABLE** No, but the park roads and summit of Mount Pisgah are accessible by wheelchair.
TRAIL TRAFFIC Heavy	
TRAIL SURFACE Dirt with stretches of paved trail	**CONTACT** Samuel S. Lewis State Park, 717-252-1134, tinyurl.com/samuelslewis
HIKING TIME 45 minutes–1 hour	**SPECIAL COMMENTS** The meadow in the center of the park is popular with kite-flying enthusiasts.
DRIVING DISTANCE 2.8 miles from US 30 at Wrightsville	

located on an upland layer of the Piedmont Physiographic Province in Pennsylvania, consisting mostly of rolling farmland, south of the Cumberland Valley and east of South Mountain. The park is part of the Pennsylvania Trail of Geology and a comprehensive guide to its geology and the surrounding countryside is available at the park.

This short hike provides a loop around the park and to the top of Mount Pisgah. The park tends to be rather busy, especially on weekends, but it is a lovely place for a picnic and a walk. This hike is a great outing with the kids, and the views toward the Susquehanna River and the east are expansive. On a clear day you can see as far as Governor Dick Hill in Lebanon County, 18 miles to the northeast, and the Safe Harbor Dam to the south.

Being higher than the surrounding terrain, the park always seems to have a nice breeze blowing through it, even in the summer. Be sure to bring a kite for flying from the top of Mount Pisgah. The hilltop's exposure, however, does subject it to some rather high winds at times. Much of the arboretum, in fact, has suffered from wind damage.

Begin this hike by walking out of the main parking area west and south along the park road. In about 200 yards, you'll come to a sign for the Hill Top Trail entering the woods on the right. Turn right and follow the orange blazes through a beautiful stand of old fir trees with an understory of mountain laurel and holly bushes. At the end of the fir trees, you'll pass some restrooms and then cut downhill across a large meadow toward the park maintenance building and office.

Cross the road by the park office and follow the trail along the shoulder of the park road south toward a playground. When you reach the playground, turn right (southeast) on the path and follow it downhill into the woods. Before it descends, a dirt road departs to the right. That road leads a couple of hundred yards back into the woods before ending at private property.

After about 0.7 mile, you'll pass the junction with the Short Cut Trail, departing to the left. If you don't feel like doing the lower part of the loop to see a beautiful stand of pine trees, turn left (north) here; you'll reach the Hill Top Trail in a couple of hundred yards, saving about 0.3 mile. Otherwise, continue downhill for a short distance farther. The trail bends left across the hillside and enters a meadow with a beautiful grove of mature pine trees. Walk across the field, turn left and follow the fence line and the pine grove uphill for 0.25 mile to the upper junction with the Short Cut Trail, entering from your left.

From the junction, angle left toward the rock outcrop and pass it to its right. At the end of the rocks, you'll find some picnic tables near the park road. Cross the road and make a beeline for the pavilion in the middle of the large meadow on the top of the hill. The park arboretum will be to your left as you make your way up the hill and is worth a walk over to visit. Several trees are marked with plaques identifying them. European beech, persimmon, English yew, among other species of trees can be found there.

The pavilion atop Mount Pisgah offers shade and picnic benches, and the meadow surrounding it offers the best views and best kite-flying in the park. You'll find an interpretive sign that identifies some of the points on the distant landscape at the pavilion. To return to your car, walk along the paved path from the pavilion back to the parking area.

Nearby Activities

Aside from the attractions of hiking and kite-flying, the park has many picnic tables and a ballfield. The hilltop is a wonderful place for viewing the stars, and local clubs often organize stargazing events in the park. Contact the park for information: 717-432-5011.

GPS INFORMATION AND DIRECTIONS
N39° 59.768' W76° 33.009'

From US 30 east of York, take the Wrightsville exit and head south on Cool Creek Road for 1.5 miles. Turn right on Mount Pisgah Road. The park entrance will be ahead on your left.

57 Strawberry Hill Nature Preserve

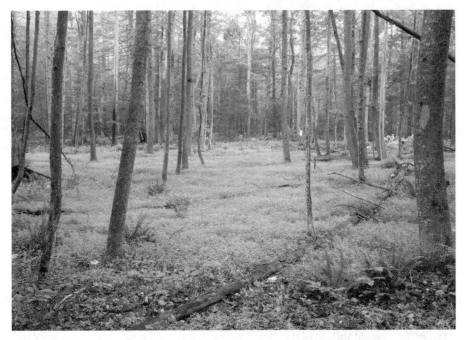

Ferns and poplars along Swamp Creek

In Brief

This hike follows the Nature Trail out of the parking area to the Swamp Creek Spur and the Swamp Creek Trail, east of the creek. Near the confluence of Swamp Creek's east and west forks, the hike picks up the 4-mile Foothills Trail loop, which circumnavigates private land before rejoining Swamp Creek Trail west of the creek.

Description

I learned about the Strawberry Hill Nature Center from Audubon Pennsylvania's *Susquehanna River Birding and Wildlife Trail Guide*. It is a little-known gem of an area well worth the trip. Located just 9 miles from Gettysburg in a valley in the southeast section of South Mountain, the center and preserve are oriented toward the interests of nature lovers. It has more than 12 miles of trails that wind through mature forest and wetlands. The nature

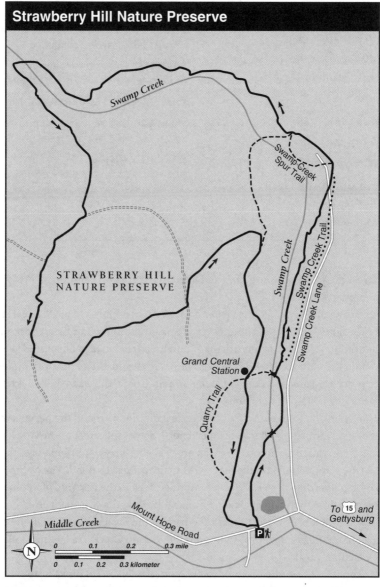

Strawberry Hill Nature Preserve

Swamp Creek

Swamp Creek Spur Trail

STRAWBERRY HILL
NATURE PRESERVE

Swamp Creek

Swamp Creek Trail

Swamp Creek Lane

Grand Central Station

Quarry Trail

Middle Creek

Mount Hope Road

To 15 and Gettysburg

N

0   0.1   0.2   0.3 mile
0   0.1   0.2   0.3 kilometer

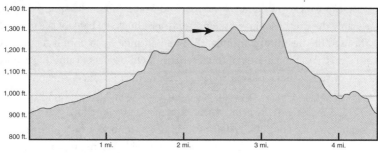

LENGTH 4.5 miles	**MAPS** USGS *Iron Springs;* a trail map is available at the trailhead and online at tinyurl.com/strawberryhillmap.
CONFIGURATION Loop	
DIFFICULTY Moderate	**FACILITIES** Portable toilets and pump water
SCENERY Beautiful woodlands	
EXPOSURE Shade	**WHEELCHAIR TRAVERSABLE** No
TRAIL TRAFFIC Light	**CONTACT** Strawberry Hill Nature Preserve, 717-642-5840, strawberryhill.org
TRAIL SURFACE Dirt	
HIKING TIME 2–3 hours	**SPECIAL COMMENTS** The nature preserve is a wonderful place for kids, and many shorter variations of this hike can be created as needed.
DRIVING DISTANCE About 13 miles from US 15 and US 30 east of Gettysburg	
ACCESS Sunrise–sunset	

center has an exhibit on the local flora and fauna, and provides educational programs for school groups and the public.

The tract of land on which the center is located was established in 1986 by Hans and Frances Froelicher, who sought to preserve its natural beauty and to support environmental education. The Froelichers originally purchased the small pond located just across the road from the nature center. In order to preserve the quality of the pond water, they gradually purchased much of the land along Swamp Creek, the watershed that feeds the pond, creating the 500-plus-acre preserve.

This hike links several of the trails to create a nice loop around the perimeter of the nature preserve. From the parking area, head north across the street toward the log cabin and hiking information station (trail maps are available here). Continue past the cabin and follow the Nature Trail into the pines next to the preserve's pond. The Nature Trail is marked by prolific white blazes. Cross a footbridge over to the east side of Swamp Creek in a forest of mature tulip poplars, and continue following the wide path aside the creek. You'll soon see pink blazes, which mark the path of the Swamp Creek Trail. Just before crossing a second footbridge, turn right onto the Swamp Creek Trail, which follows the old Fort Chamber Road.

After about 200 feet, the Swamp Creek Spur (also blazed in pink) heads to the left while the Swamp Creek Trail follows the roadbed to the right. The spur passes through what is arguably the prettiest part of the preserve as it hugs the bank of the creek. Follow the spur through the beautiful bottomlands for a half-mile or so until it reconnects with the Swamp Creek Trail in an area of thick ferns and tall poplars (1 mile). Turn left, and after 100 feet or so the trail and spur split again for a short distance. Stay on the trail this time, and in 100 yards or so the trail and spur join again by junction with the green-blazed Foothills Trail, departing to the right. A trail sign marks the junction.

Turn right onto the Foothills Trail (heading northeast now), which follows an old haul road initially and then departs from the roadbed to avoid private property. The trail gets

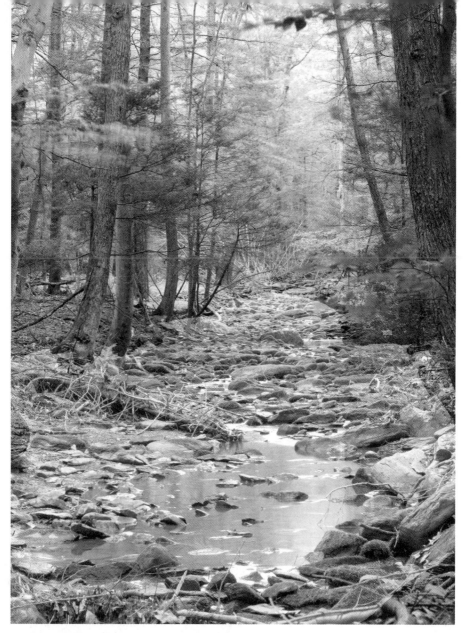

Swamp Creek flows through the preserve.

rather rugged for a short distance as it winds through some swampy and rocky woods, crossing several boards. The green blazes are abundant, however, so finding your way should be no problem. Soon the trail becomes more distinct, and it makes a sharp right turn uphill and then joins a road heading left and passing beneath some clear areas.

Follow the path as it wanders through the upper part of the hollow in a beautiful forest of huge tulip poplars, beech trees, and carcasses of old pine trees filled with holes that make wonderful nesting places for owls, woodpeckers, and squirrels. At about 2 miles, you'll reach a small clearing at a gated road. Turn left and cross the creek. Shortly thereafter, the trail makes a sharp left turn south into the woods at a turn marked by double green blazes. Follow the path left, traversing the top of the hollow. If you come to this area in July, be ready to spend some time sampling the wild raspberries.

After passing through the hollow, you'll reach a significant dirt road (2.5 miles) onto which you'll turn right (southwest). Follow that past an old cabin to an intersection where the main road goes to the right. Continue straight at the intersection, following the green blazes downhill on an old roadbed for a fair distance until you come to a junction with another dirt road, marked by green blazes (2.9 miles). Turn left and climb for a ways, passing some private property on the right before crossing over a ridgetop. The trail descends quite steeply from the ridge for a short distance before meeting up with another significant dirt road below. Turn left (east) on this road and follow it for 50 feet to a place where the green blazes head off to the right downhill along a smaller road. Turn right and follow the path around to the right, dropping into Swamp Creek. Soon you'll reach the Swamp Creek Trail again (3.7 miles), at which point you will turn right.

Continue walking along the trail above the creek until you reach a major junction of trails, called Grand Central Station. It is marked by a sign and has a nice bench where you can rest your weary feet. From Grand Central Station, continue straight following white blazes past the red-blazed Quarry Trail on the right. Shortly afterward, you'll reach the parking area and the log house.

Nearby Activities

You can take in the scenery at the pond, which has a platform for turtles to sun themselves, or visit the nature center. **Gettysburg National Military Park** (nps.gov/gett) is 9 miles to the northeast. Visiting there after a hike at Strawberry Hill makes for a reasonable and full day.

GPS INFORMATION AND DIRECTIONS
N39° 48.202' W77° 24.867'

From US 15 east of Gettysburg, follow US 30 west through the center of town. At the traffic circle, head south on Business 15 to PA 116 West (one block south of the circle). Turn right onto PA 116 and follow it south 7.2 miles to Bullfrog Road on the right. Turn right on Bullfrog Road and follow it to a stop sign (1 mile). After the stop sign, Bullfrog Road turns to Mount Hope Road. The parking area is about 2 miles along Mount Hope Road on the left. The trailhead is directly across the street next to a small pond and cabin.

58 Sunset Rocks

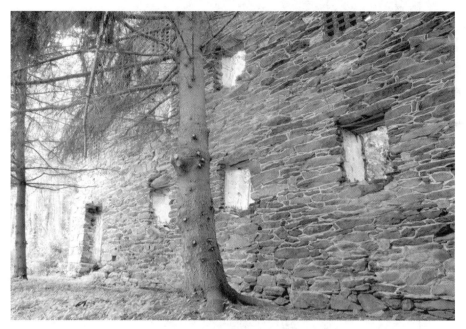

The ruins of Camp Michaux, just south of the Appalachian Trail

In Brief

This popular hike follows the Appalachian Trail (AT) from Pine Grove Furnace State Park for several miles to the Toms Run Shelters. Just beyond the shelters, it picks up the Sunset Rocks Trail and follows that over Sunset Rocks and Little Rocky Ridge back to the AT, about 1.5 miles from the parking area.

Description

In addition to passing through some extraordinarily beautiful forest and by the ruins of Camp Michaux, this hike offers some of the best views in South Mountain from the Little Rocky Ridge. You'll want to take extra care on the ridge, as traversing it requires using your hands to scramble over and among several large rock outcrops.

Begin this hike at the Furnace Stack parking area across from the general store at Pine Grove Furnace State Park. Following the AT past the front of the store and along Bendersville Road out to PA 233 following the white AT blazes. At the stop sign, turn left (west) and walk along the shoulder for 0.25 mile. Turn right (north) and cross the road at

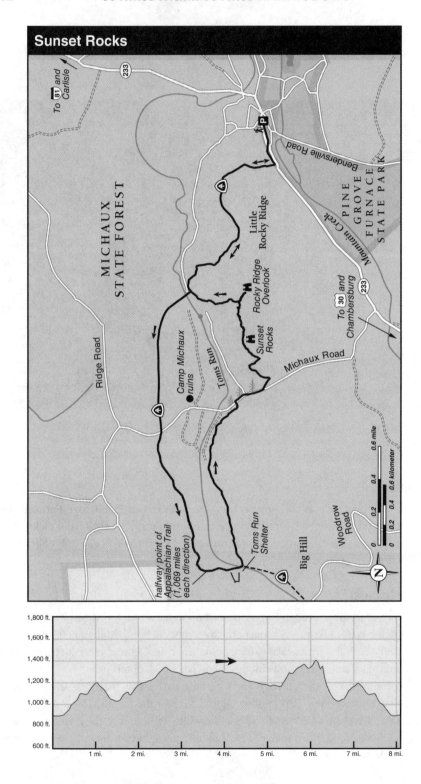

Sunset Rocks

To 81 and Carlisle

233

MICHAUX STATE FOREST

P

Bendersville Road

PINE GROVE FURNACE STATE PARK

Little Rocky Ridge

Mountain Creek

Rocky Ridge Overlook

To 30 and Chambersburg

233

Sunset Rocks

Camp Michaux ruins

Toms Run

Michaux Road

Ridge Road

halfway point of Appalachian Trail (1,069 miles each direction)

Toms Run Shelter

Big Hill

Woodrow Road

0.6 mile

0.2   0.4   0.6 kilometer

0   0.2   0.4

N

1,800 ft.
1,600 ft.
1,400 ft.
1,200 ft.
1,000 ft.
800 ft.
600 ft.

1 mi.   2 mi.   3 mi.   4 mi.   5 mi.   6 mi.   7 mi.   8 mi.

LENGTH 8.1 miles	**MAPS** USGS *Dickinson;* Michaux State Forest public-use map; Keystone Trail Association *Appalachian Trail, PA Route 94 to US Route 30 (Sections 12 and 13)*
CONFIGURATION Balloon	
DIFFICULTY Moderate hiking with some difficult scrambling on Little Rocky Ridge	
	FACILITIES Water and restrooms near trailhead in Pine Grove Furnace State Park
SCENERY Forest, Toms Run, excellent views of South Mountain area	
	WHEELCHAIR TRAVERSABLE No
EXPOSURE Mostly shade	
	CONTACT Michaux State Forest, 717-352-2211, tinyurl.com/michauxsf
TRAIL TRAFFIC Generally light	
TRAIL SURFACE Dirt	**SPECIAL COMMENTS** Little Rocky Ridge can be time-consuming to scramble over and is not a good place for young children. A good pair of boots is useful for this hike. Walk the loop section of this hike counterclockwise.
HIKING TIME 4–5 hours	
DRIVING DISTANCE 7.3 miles from I-81 and PA 233 south of Carlisle	
ACCESS Open	

the AT sign and follow the blazes along a dirt road, past private property, through a forest of pine trees and tall oak trees. The trail is lined with a thick understory of rose hips and honeysuckle.

Soon you'll cross a little creek and then wind your way through a lovely forest to the footbridge over Toms Run. The east end of the Sunset Rocks Trail departs to the left here, and you can follow that directly up to the ridge and the rocks, making an out-and-back trip of about 3 (very steep!) miles. To follow our hike, though, cross Toms Run and follow the AT along a hillside to a significant gravel road. You can continue along the AT crossing the road, which will bypass the ruins of Camp Michaux. To visit Camp Michaux turn left (west) on the road and follow that past the Halfway Spring (on the left).

Follow the road for a distance until a track leaves it to the right under some telephone lines (2.3 miles). In 100 yards or so, you will pass the ruins of Camp Michaux. Once a church camp shared by the United Presbyterian Church and the United Church of Christ, the ruins are unusual in that they resemble more of an old military outpost. Interestingly, it served as a Civilian Conservation Corps camp during the 1930s and then a prisoner of war camp during World War II.

After admiring the scenic ruins, walk out to Michaux Road and then to the right and along the road to where the AT crosses the road enters the woods on the left (2.65 miles). Upon entering the woods, you will pass through some of the most beautiful fern-filled forest you can imagine. Saunter your way through this small paradise. In another mile, you'll reach the current halfway point of the AT, a location that changes every few years as sections of the trail get rerouted and the trail gets longer or shorter. (Five years ago, for instance, it was located on the descent from Pole Steeple; see page 260.) A regal post and a sign identify its location. Just beyond, you'll reach the Toms Run Shelter (3.85 miles).

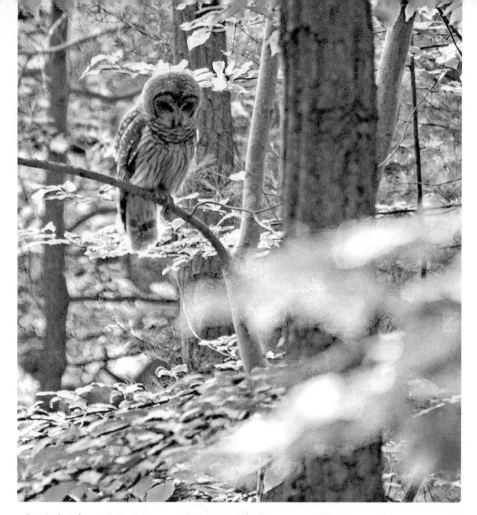

Barred owl

When I did this hike, the first thing that I noticed upon reaching the shelters was a healthy population of chipmunks. When I sat down for a break, I had the good fortune of seeing a beautiful barred owl land in a tree about 100 feet away from me. The sighting made sense, of course. With all the chipmunks in the area, the owl had plenty to feed on.

From the shelters, continue along the AT for 100 feet or so, crossing Toms Run. Just beyond the creek, you'll find the west terminus of the Sunset Rocks Trail on your left (blue blazes). Turn left and follow that path over some rocky terrain through an unusual hollow filled with saplings of what appear to be red birch trees. You'll pass two small clearings, the second of which you'll skirt to the right. I found both of the clearings to be populated by an inordinately large number of bees. I didn't get stung, but if you have allergies, you should bear this in mind.

Follow the trail through a swampy area, over some boardwalks, and past a large forest management area on the right. This is an excellent place to see pileated woodpeckers. Continue past the clearing until you come out to Michaux Road. Turn right (south) and follow the shoulder over the crest of a hill for 0.3 mile. The trail reenters woods on the left, just beyond the crest by a private drive numbered 111 (5.25 miles). You'll find double blazes on a tree to the right of the drive.

Follow the trail back into the woods, passing a nearby private residence on the left. Continue uphill into the woods until you reach the Little Rocky Ridge by a couple of boulders. This is a good rest spot and it offers a good view to the south.

Follow the blazes along the ridge uphill to the east. As you progress farther along the ridge, the going gets more rugged and you'll need to be prepared to do some scrambling and some route finding. It is an amazing ridge, however, with quartzite rock outcrops among hickory, oak, black gum, and pine trees. Mountain laurel grows from the crevices, and the views are incredible.

Working your way across the ridge is a time-consuming proposition, and at times the blazes can be a little mystifying. Just continue your way among the rocks, resisting the temptation to descend some inviting deer path too soon. Follow the ridge to a prominent saddle with blazes and a *very obvious* and well traveled descent path to the left (6 miles). From the saddle, a small side path takes you farther out on the Little Rocky Ridge to a wonderful, vertiginous overlook after about 200 yards. The walk to the overlook is worth every bit of effort and is a great place for a long rest. It has arguably the nicest view in South Mountain and definitely on the hike.

From the overlook, return to the saddle and follow the descent trail downhill to the north for 0.6 mile, at which point you will reach the eastern terminus of the trail at the Toms Run crossing on the AT. Turn right and follow the AT back to your car at Pine Grove Furnace.

Nearby Activities

Pine Grove Furnace State Park, on PA 233 to the north, has two lakes with swimming areas, picnic areas, biking and hiking trails, and the site of the old Pine Grove Furnace. It also has a wonderful campground. The **Appalachian Trail Museum** is right next to the parking area, and it has several very interesting exhibits on the AT, as well as a gift shop. Visit atmuseum.org for hours.

GPS INFORMATION AND DIRECTIONS
N40° 01.900' W77° 18.312'

From I-81, take Exit 37 (Newville/PA 233). Follow PA 233 South 7.8 miles to the intersection with Pine Grove Road at Pine Grove Furnace State Park. After PA 233 turns right, turn left toward the campground, furnace stack, and general store. Park in the Furnace Stack parking area, on the left across from the general store.

59 White Rocks and Center Point Knob

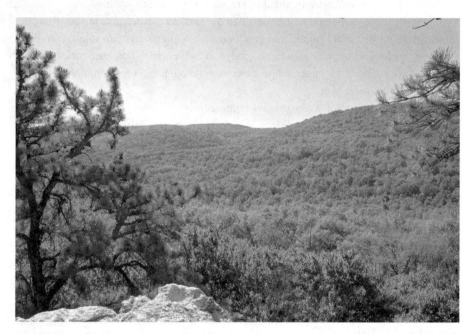

South Mountain from White Rocks

In Brief

This pleasant hike follows the White Rocks Trail from Kuhn Road up to and over White Rocks to the Appalachian Trail (AT) below Center Point Knob. A short walk along the AT takes you to the top of the Knob before retracing the route back to the car.

Description

This hike offers some lovely scenery, with large quartzite rock outcrops (popular with area rock climbers), a beautiful understory of mountain laurel, and great views. It is the only place that I have seen a gray fox, which makes it distinctive in my mind. It would be a nice hike to do with older kids, though some care needs to be taken passing the rock outcrops.

The hike begins at the prominent blue-blazed trail, about 100 feet uphill and along the shoulder of Kuhn Road from a yellow forest gate. A sign indicating that it is indeed the

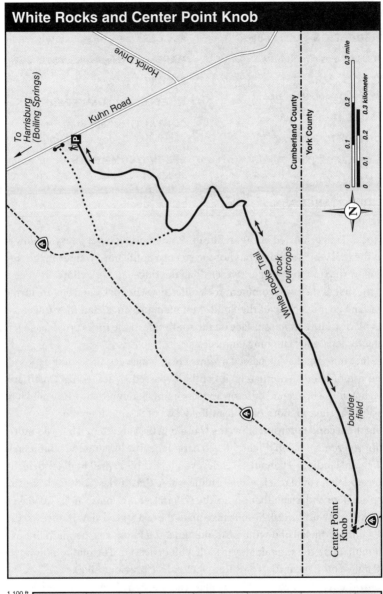

White Rocks and Center Point Knob

To Harrisburg (Boiling Springs)

Horick Drive

Kuhn Road

P

White Rocks Trail

rock outcrops

boulder field

Center Point Knob

Cumberland County
York County

N

0.3 mile
0.2
0.1
0

0.3 kilometer
0.2
0.1
0

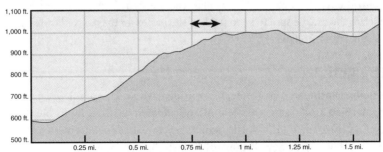

1,100 ft.
1,000 ft.
900 ft.
800 ft.
700 ft.
600 ft.
500 ft.

0.25 mi.   0.5 mi.   0.75 mi.   1 mi.   1.25 mi.   1.5 mi.

LENGTH 3.25 miles	from US 11 and PA 641 west of Harrisburg
CONFIGURATION Out-and-back	**ACCESS** Open; on state forest land
DIFFICULTY Easy–moderate	**MAPS** USGS *Mechanicsburg* and *Dillsburg*
SCENERY Quartzite outcrops and nice views of South Mountain area	**FACILITIES** None
EXPOSURE Mostly shade	**WHEELCHAIR TRAVERSABLE** No
TRAIL TRAFFIC Moderate	**CONTACT** Michaux State Forest, 717-352-2211, tinyurl.com/michauxsf
TRAIL SURFACE Dirt	**SPECIAL COMMENTS** Be cautious about loose rocks when passing over the outcrops, because rock climbers may be below you.
HIKING TIME 2 hours	
DRIVING DISTANCE About 22 miles	

White Rocks Trail is located at the trailhead. Route finding is very easy. Follow the blue blazes as the trail winds steadily, but not too steeply, uphill until you reach the ridge (0.75 mile). Follow the trail to the right (west) along the ridge, and in a short distance you will come to the first of the two prominent rock outcrops. The rock outcrops are formed from hard quartzite characteristic of the South Mountain province, and they tower as high as 40 feet in places. The precipitous face on the south side of the rocks provides several practice routes for local rock climbing enthusiasts.

The first outcrop may be passed over its crest, which requires some exposed scrambling and use of hands. Alternately, it can be bypassed by following a path around its north (right) side. The second outcrop appears immediately after the first, and it is passed quite easily over the top. Both offer beautiful views of South Mountain.

From the second outcrop, follow the trail along the ridge. You'll have no more scrambling until you return. If you do this hike in early June, the blossoming mountain laurel in this area is outstanding. At about 1.4 miles, you'll pass by a small boulder field, and then not far beyond that you'll reach a small saddle where the AT descends to the north. There is a campsite here and a sign that points the way to Center Point Knob, 1,060 feet, north along the AT. It is worth the 0.25-mile hike up to the top for the view it offers to the north, especially during the fall and winter. At one time, the knob was the midpoint of the AT, and a monument on the summit attests to that bit of history. The midpoint is now located about 18 miles south, near the Toms Run Shelter (see previous hike).

Follow the AT to the top, which is marked by a sign. After a nice rest, retrace your route back to the car. Be sure to keep track of the blazes on the descent from the ridge, as the path splits in several places.

Nearby Activities

Nearby **Boiling Springs** is a charming, historic town with restaurants and a beautiful park. The **Appalachian Trail Conference Mid-Atlantic Regional Office,** in the heart of town at 4 E. First St. (717-258-5771), is worth a stop. They have loads of information about the AT and the surrounding area, as well as maps, T-shirts, hats and the like.

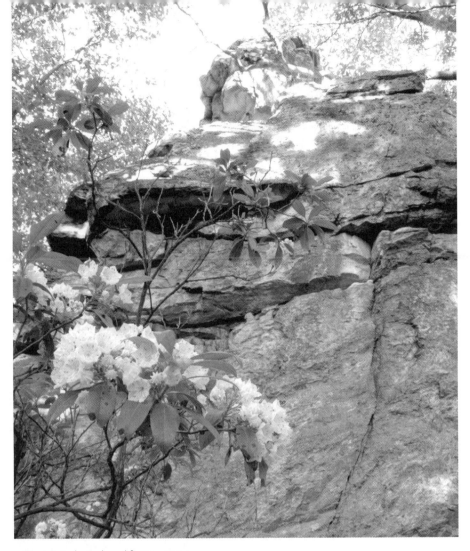

Mountain laurel and first outcrop

GPS INFORMATION AND DIRECTIONS

N40° 07.958' W77° 05.297'

From US 11 west of Harrisburg, take PA 641/Trindle Road west toward Mechanicsburg. Follow PA 641 for 7 miles to PA 174/Boiling Springs Road. Turn left and follow PA 174 for 12 miles to Boiling Springs. Keep your eyes open for the Allenberry Resort and Playhouse on the left just before Boiling Springs. After passing the Allenberry, look for Bucher Hill Road on the left. Turn left and follow that alongside the pond and town park. Turn left onto Mountain Road at the stop sign before crossing the pond. Cross over Yellow Breeches Creek and turn left onto Ledigh Drive. Follow Ledigh Drive 1.8 miles to Kuhn Road. Turn right. The parking area is about 0.7 mile along Kuhn Road on the right by a yellow gate. The main trailhead is about 100 feet farther up the road. It has a sign and a set of blue blazes.

60 William H. Kain County Park

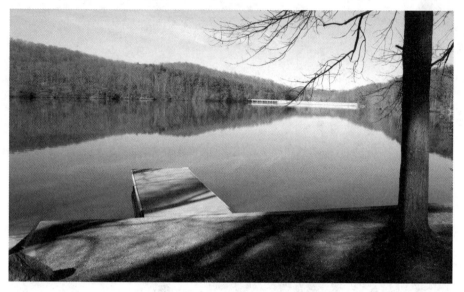

Looking across Lake Redman from the parking area

In Brief

This hike follows Trail 4 as it passes above Lake Williams to the Lake Redman Dam. At the top of the dam, it makes a side loop of about 1.9 miles following Trail 1 above Lake Redman. Returning to the dam, this hike drops to the parking area along South George Street, where it picks up Trail 2. It follows this trail the rest of the way around Lake Williams, completing a circuit of the lake.

Description

This is a very pleasant walk along wooded and grassy trails. The trail system can be a little confusing; there are primary trails (1, 2, 3, 4, etc.) and secondary trails to all of those classified by letters (1a, 1b, etc.). A park map, available online and at the parking area, can help to clarify the directions; however, all secondary trails along this hike which depart from a primary trail ultimately end up joining the primary trail again.

To begin, walk to the back of the parking loop at the Lake Williams Activity Area, where you will find Trail 4 (identified by a numbered green-fiberglass post). An old roadbed, it heads uphill away from the lake over a large log placed to keep motor vehicles off

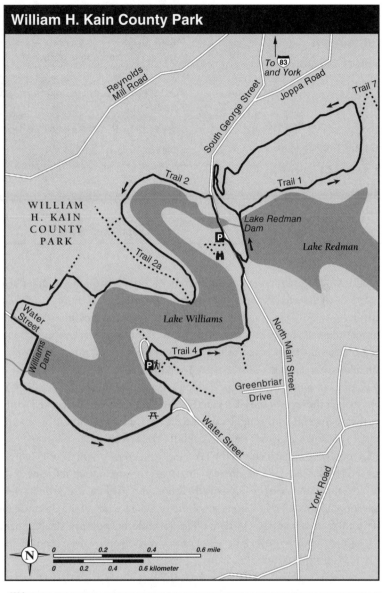

William H. Kain County Park

Reynolds Mill Road

To 83 and York

South George Street

Joppa Road

Trail 7

Trail 2

Trail 1

WILLIAM
H. KAIN
COUNTY
PARK

Trail 2a

Lake Redman Dam

Lake Redman

Water Street

Lake Williams

Trail 4

North Main Street

Williams Dam

Greenbriar Drive

Water Street

York Road

N

| 0 | 0.2 | 0.4 | 0.6 mile |

| 0 | 0.2 | 0.4 | 0.6 kilometer |

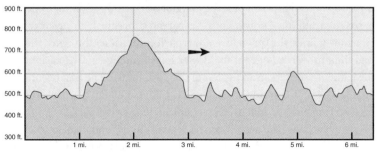

LENGTH 6.4 miles	**ACCESS** Sunrise–sunset
CONFIGURATION Figure-eight	**MAPS** USGS *York;* park map available at parking area and online at tinyurl.com /kainparkmap.
DIFFICULTY Moderate	
SCENERY Lake Williams and Lake Redman	**FACILITIES** Water and toilets at parking areas
EXPOSURE Mostly shaded	**WHEELCHAIR TRAVERSABLE** No
TRAIL TRAFFIC Moderate	**CONTACT** York County Parks and Recreation, 717-840-7440, tinyurl.com /wmkainpark
TRAIL SURFACE Dirt	
HIKING TIME 3–3.5 hours	
DRIVING DISTANCE About 3 miles from I-83 and PA 182 south of York	**SPECIAL COMMENTS** Trails in the park are used frequently by mountain bikers and can get busy on weekends.

of the trail. Don't confuse this with a second trail, a footpath without a number beginning about 50 feet or so to its left. That trail heads over toward the lakeshore.

Walk up the hill to a clearing with a little bench and a trail crossing. Turn left (northeast) onto an old carriage path and follow it into the woods and eventually above the shore of the lake. Like most of the trails in this part of the park, this one is popular with mountain bikers and it can get busy especially on the weekends. The path above the lake is pretty among tall pine trees and the walking is on a pleasant smooth grade. When the trail drops to near the level of the lake, you'll reach a junction of trails marked with several numbers that seem a bit confusing. Head straight on Trail 4 to continue around the lake. (*Note:* A spur of Trail 4 also goes right and uphill at this point.)

Walk around the eastern end of the lake until you come out to South George Street by a gate across from the Lake Redman Dam. Cross the street, turn left, and walk up to and across the top of the dam, heading north. From the end of the dam, you'll take a short secondary loop hike of 1.9 miles along the shore of Lake Redman for a distance and then back over a hill from the north. The dam offers a wonderful view of Lake Redman. From the north end of the dam, turn right (east) onto a nice open carriage road, Trail 1. The walking here is quite pleasant.

Soon the trail begins to climb away from the lake through a forest of spruce trees, and near the top of the hill you'll pass the junction with Trail 7. Continue climbing Trail 1 until you pass beneath some power lines that extend above the highway to your right. Just beyond the power lines, the trail makes a sharp left turn, passes through a short section of forest, and then proceeds beneath the power lines heading east. After about 0.25 mile, follow the path into the woods to the left of the power lines. The trail becomes more of a footpath as it descends around the edge of the hill. As you circle closer to the dam, the hillside gets steeper and the trail makes a couple of long switchbacks.

When you reach the dam again, walk back across its top and then down to the parking area by the outflow of Lake Redman. From the south edge of the parking area, you can walk up a path to a viewing platform overlooking Lake Williams. According to the information sign at the parking area, the park is rich in cultural history. Native Americans lived in the area and stone tools have been found nearby. The creek supported 16 mills in the late 1700s to early 1800s. The old gristmill was located across the creek from the parking area.

Much of the land around the shore of Lake Williams is characterized as a wetland. This means that for at least part of the year the land is saturated with water, it has typically dark soil, and it is populated by plants that enjoy a wet habitat. Just across the creek, you can see a stand of cattails and black willows, both wetland species. Ospreys and bald eagles both nest in the area, and the lake is home to wood and black ducks as well as scads of frogs and turtles who can be seen sunning themselves on logs in the spring.

From the parking lot, cross the creek and walk along the road for 50 yards in front of the yellow house. At the drive to the house, turn left through a gate and pick up Trail 2, another carriage road. You'll follow this trail most of the way around Lake Williams. About a mile from the parking area, you'll come to a bench on the shore of the lake at the point of a peninsula. Trail 2a enters here from atop the peninsula. Continue along the shore of the lake for another 0.3 mile, enjoying the excellent views, to a marshy area and a junction with a trail heading uphill to your right. Leave the shore of the lake and follow that trail for a short distance until it ends at a T-intersection. This is Trail 2. Turn left (west) and follow the trail downhill past some horse farms and out to Water Street.

When you reach Water Street, turn left (southeast) and you will see a sign welcoming you to William H. Kain County Park. Follow the road down to the dam at the outflow of Lake Williams, about 0.25 mile. Walking along the road is not unpleasant. Cross the dam and follow Water Street as it climbs up and around the lake. At 0.75 mile from the dam (6.14 miles total), you'll pass a picnic area on the left. Just beyond the picnic area, Trail 4 enters the woods to the left. Turn left (east), walk through the woods for a short distance to the day-use access road. Turn left on the road, and walk back to your car.

Nearby Activities

The York County Parks Department has built a 350-foot ADA-accessible walking deck at the **Lake Redman Activity Area,** near the Iron Stone Hill Road parking lot. For maps and information, check the website at tinyurl.com/williamkaincountypark.

Richard M. Nixon County Park is just across Water Street from the Lake Williams Activity Area. It has its own system of trails and an environmental-education center.

GPS INFORMATION AND DIRECTIONS
N39° 53.412' W76° 43.251'

From I-83, take Exit 4 (PA 182 West). Follow 182 to South George Street. Turn left. Follow South George Street south, past the Lake Redman Dam, into the town of Jacobus. Turn right on Water Street. The entrance to the Lake Williams Activity Area is about 1 mile on the right.

Appendix A:
SOME USEFUL MAPS AND GUIDES

Appalachian Trail in Pennsylvania, Sections 1 Through 6: Delaware Water Gap to Swatara Gap. Published by Keystone Trails Association, Cogan Station, PA.

Appalachian Trail in Pennsylvania, Sections 7 and 8: Swatara Gap to Susquehanna River. Published by Keystone Trails Association, Cogan Station, PA.

Appalachian Trail, Susquehanna River to PA Route 94 (Sections 9, 10, and 11). Published by the Potomac Appalachian Trail Club, Inc., Vienna, VA.

Appalachian Trail, PA Route 94 to US Route 30 (Sections 12 and 13). Published by the Potomac Appalachian Trail Club, Inc., Vienna, VA.

Guide to the Horse-Shoe Trail. Published by the Horse-Shoe Trail Conservancy, Inc. Southeastern, PA.

The Pennsylvania Atlas and Gazetteer. Published by DeLorme, Yarmouth, ME.

A Public Use Map for Michaux State Forest. Published by the Pennsylvania Department of Conservation and Natural Resources, Bureau of Forestry.

A Public Use Map for Tuscarora State Forest. Published by Pennsylvania Department of Conservation and Natural Resources, Bureau of Forestry.

Susquehanna River Birding and Wildlife Trail Guide. Published by Audubon Pennsylvania, Harrisburg.

Tuscarora Trail, Map J: Appalachian Trail, PA, to PA Route 641. Published by the Potomac Appalachian Trail Club, Inc., Vienna, VA.

Additionally, an excellent online resource for maps of Pennsylvania state game lands is the **Pennsylvania Game Commission Mapping Center:** tinyurl.com/pagamemappingcenter.

Appendix B:
LOCAL HIKING AND OUTDOOR-EQUIPMENT STORES

HARRISBURG

Bass Pro Shop
3501 Paxton St.
Harrisburg, PA 17111
717-565-5200

Blue Mountain Outfitters
103 S. State Road
Marysville, PA 17053
717-957-2413

Dick's Sporting Goods
5086 Jonestown Road
Harrisburg, PA 17112
717-652-3174

Gander Mountain
5005 Jonestown Road
Harrisburg, PA 17112
717-671-9700

LANCASTER

Eastern Mountain Sports
541 Park City Center
Lancaster, PA 17601
717-397-8120

YORK

Dick's Sporting Goods
PA 30 and Kenneth Road
York, PA 17404
717-848-1696

Dunham's Sporting Goods
411 Eisenhower Drive
Hanover, PA 17331
717-630-0074

Gander Mountain
1880 Loucks Road
York, PA 17404
717-767-2002

HAMBURG

Cabela's
100 Cabela Drive
Hamburg, PA 19526
610-929-7000

Appendix C:
HIKING CLUBS AND NATURE PRESERVATION/CONSERVATION ORGANIZATIONS

Central Pennsylvania Conservancy   centralpaconservancy.org

Cumberland Valley Appalachian Trail Club   cvatclub.org

Friends of Wildwood Nature Sanctuary
   wildwoodlake.org/support/membership-application.aspx

Keystone Trails Association   kta-hike.org

Lancaster County Conservancy   lancasterconservancy.org

Lancaster Hiking Club   lancasterhikingclub.angelfire.com

Mason-Dixon Trail System   mason-dixontrail.org

Ned Smith Center for Nature and Art   nedsmithcenter.org

Pennsylvania Department of Conservation and Natural Resources
   dcnr.state.pa.us

Potomac Appalachian Trail Club   patc.net

Susquehanna Appalachian Trail Club   satc-hike.org

York Hiking Club   yorkhikingclub.com

Index

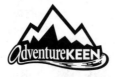

The Story of AdventureKEEN

We are an independent nature and outdoor activity publisher. Our founding dates back more than 40 years, guided then and now by our love of being in the woods and on the water, by our passion for reading and books, and by the sense of wonder and discovery made possible by spending time recreating outdoors in beautiful places.

It is our mission to share that wonder and fun with our readers, especially with those who haven't yet experienced all the physical and mental health benefits that nature and outdoor activity can bring.

In addition, we strive to teach about responsible recreation so that the natural resources and habitats we cherish and rely upon will be available for future generations.

We are a small team deeply rooted in the places where we live and work. We have been shaped by our communities of origin—primarily Birmingham, Alabama; Cincinnati, Ohio; and the northern suburbs of Minneapolis, Minnesota. Drawing on the decades of experience of our staff and our awareness of the industry, the marketplace, and the world at large, we have shaped a unique vision and mission for a company that serves our readers and authors.

We hope to meet you out on the trail someday.

#bewellbeoutdoors